BASIC AND ADVANCED
VITREOUS SURGERY

BASIC AND ADVANCED VITREOUS SURGERY

Edited by

George W. Blankenship
   The Bascom Palmer Eye Institute
   University of Miami School of Medicine
   Miami, Florida

Susanne Binder
   First University Eye Clinic
   Wien, Austria

Michel Gonvers
   Hôpital Ophtalmologique
   Lausanne, Switzerland

Mario Stirpe
   Fondazione Oftalmologica
   "G.B. Bietti", Roma, Italy

FIDIA
RESEARCH
SERIES
Volume 2

LIVIANA PRESS
Padova

Springer-Verlag Berlin Heidelberg GmbH

FIDIA RESEARCH SERIES

An open-end series of publications on international biomedical research, with special emphasis on the neurosciences, published by LIVIANA Press, Padova, Italy, in cooperation with FIDIA Research Labs, Abano Terme, Italy.

The series will be devoted to advances in basic and clinical research in the neurosciences and other fields.

The aim of the series is the rapid and worldwide dissemination of up-to-date, interdisciplinary data as presented at selected international scientific meetings and study groups.

Each volume is published under the editorial responsibility of scientists chosen by organizing committees of the meetings on the basis of their active involvement in the research of the field concerned.

© 1986 by Springer-Verlag Berlin Heidelberg
Originally published by Springer-Verlag Berlin Heidelberg New York Tokyo in 2002
Softcover reprint of the hardcover 1st edition 1986

ISBN 978-1-4757-3883-4   ISBN 978-1-4757-3881-0 (eBook)
DOI 10.1007/978-1-4757-3881-0

The concept of this book is based on the Vitreous Surgery Course which was held at the Urbaniana University, Rome, in September 1984. The course was organized in memory of G.B. Bietti.

After the course we were urged to present the contributions in a more durable form, and we are grateful to the partecipants that they accepted our invitation to prepare manuscripts of their lectures and to include current information. It is hoped that this volume may be of value to all who are interested in the study and practice of vitreo-retinal surgery.

The Editors

CONTENTS

VIII

III. COMPLICATIONS OF SILICONE OIL

XV. MEDICAL THERAPY

BASIC AND ADVANCED
VITREOUS SURGERY

Basic and advanced vitreous surgery
G.W. Blankenship, M. Stirpe, M. Gonvers, S. Binder (eds.)
Fidia Research Series, vol. II,
Liviana Press, Padova © 1986

DEVELOPMENT OF VITREOUS SURGERY
(G.B. Bietti memorial lecture)

Robert Machemer, M.D.

Professor and Chairman of the Department of Ophthalmology,
Duke University Medical Center,
Durham, North Caroline

Ladies and gentlemen, I feel very proud that you have invited me to talk to you about what has interested me during the last 15 years.

When I was in Miami, Florida, Prof. Bietti was one of the early visitors to our clinic. I was impressed that a man of his age would take part in what was at that time still an unknown, controversial, and non-evaluated technique. He showed further interest by sending his pupil, Mario Stirpe, to Miami to make sure that this technique, called vitreous surgery, would also be known in Italy.

I am happy that I can give this lecture in his memory and I thank you for inviting me.

I would like to give you a small personal account of vitreous surgery as it has developed over the years.

In 1968 and 1969 the first enthusiasm developed about open sky surgery in Miami. David Kasner had purposefully opened the eye to remove diseased vitreous. Vitreous loss and removal of the prolapsed vitreous has happened a lot of times to all of us who have done cataract surgery but we did not open the eye purposefully to eliminate

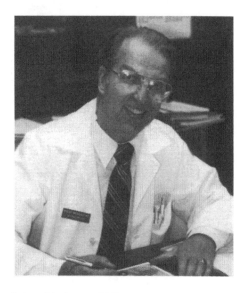

Robert Machemer, M.D.

diseased vitreous. His daring approach was the beginning of vitreous surgery. If it was not for David Kasner who developed open sky vitreous surgery technique, we would not be where we are today when we talk about closed vitrectomy.

I remember when he demonstrated how this open sky technique was to be done. He used scissors and sponges and after taking out the cornea and lens he would grasp the vitreous and cut it away.

At that time available instruments were coarse, made for anterior surgery but not for use inside the eye. As you can easily imagine, this stimulated us to design an instrument that would not touch the cornea nor the iris and that would especially allow good observation of the operation field as well.

We went into our laboratory garage and in this laboratory we demonstrated with a drill inserted into an egg that removal of egg white was possible when the drill was surrounded by a tube (Fig. 1a, b).

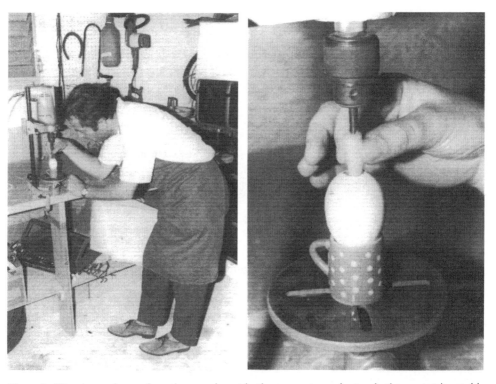

Figure 1. The above photos show the experiment in the garage to evaluate whether or not it would be possible to remove the egg white by a rotating drill inserted into a tube.

Now how do you miniaturize this instrument? We went to a toy shop and bought a long so called airplane drill that is used for model planes. The drill bit was put into a hypodermic needle and driven by a small electrical motor. All of this was placed into a syringe with a battery connection and a little switch (Fig. 2). This was the first vitrectomy instrument designed for open sky vitrectomy to be used after removing the cornea. Case number "0" showed that we could successfully remove vitreous with this small instrument.

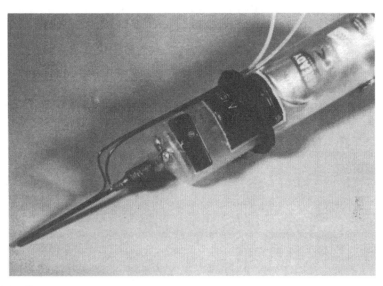

Figure 2. The first pars plana vitrectomy instrument with infusion and suction used successfully on a human eye on April 20, 1970.

But why should we have to cut the cornea? Why was it necessary to remove the lens to get to the vitreous? The ideal would be to avoid destruction of the anterior segment.

I thought it might be a good idea to enter the eye in an area where there was no retina, no ciliary body, namely the pars plana. This indeed became the approach to what we call today closed vitrectomy.

The idea was to use instruments as small as possibile with combined functions. The first instrument was called the vitreous infusion cutter and had several functions: it could cut the vitreous, it could remove the vitreous, and now that we had a closed system we had to replace the fluid by infusion to avoid collapse of the eye. Finally we added intra-ocular illumination; with this instrument we performed the first closed vitrectomy in April 1970.

This man had been blind in one eye for 5 years; he had a vision of finger counting at 2 feet, a slight cataract, and his vitreous was opaque. We were very lucky to select a patient with a condition that we know today to be the easiest to treat, just a hemorrhage. We were also lucky that we did not have any complications. One can imagine the enthusiasm that we had when the first operation was a full success and the patient could see 20/50.

Very exciting developments occurred in a rapid sequence. A multitude of problems had to be solved. The solution to these problems would not have been possible if Jean-Marie Parel had not become a member of the Bascom Palmer Eye Institute and helped in the design of new instruments.

What were the problems that we had to solve? With Parel's knowledge an electrically driven combination instrument was designed. Other vitrectomy instruments were quickly discarded such as one that had diathermy capability built in, a plastic instrument made of nylon. We did not know that nylon swells. As we used the instrument, the rotary parts would not function after a while. Finally we ended up with what we called the Visc X, the tenth design of the vitrectomy instrument.

What principles guided us in this development? We wanted an instrument that one could build easily, could take apart, and that allowed easy replacement of its parts. Vitrectomy, despite all accessories that we have today, and despite all the sophistication that we think necessary, is still very simple in its principles. One should be able to operate the instrument with very little means if necessary. A simple infusion bottle provides fluid by gravity, and simple syringe can aspirate the fluid from the eye. Sophisticated accessories are helpful additions but are not a necessity.

Very rapidly a multitude of vitreous cutters developed; however two basic principles are still today functional: the rotating and the reciprocal instrument. We decided on the rotating principle. The tip of the vitreous cutter is composed of an outer tube and an inner tube. The inner tube rotates. Both tubes have an opening so when the openings coincide fluid is aspirated and will pass through the inner tube out of the eye. Vitreous will incarcerate in the opening with suction applied and with rotation of the inner tube its blade passes through the opening, cuts the vitreous off and removes it from the eye. Fluid is simultaneously infused between the two tubes and enters the eye near the end of the tip so that the volume of the eye can be maintained.

The other very popular instrument, the OCUTOME, is fascinating for its very simple design and its small size. It uses a reciprocating hollow piston that cuts the vitreous.

Once we had a cutting device that was working well, many other problems had to be solved. Put yourself back into those years when no specialized instrumentation was available and everything had to be developed. At the time we used the OPMI II of Zeiss because it had co-axial illumination to bring light into the eye. The pupil had to be well dilated in order to get this light into the eye. All anterior segment surgeons liked side illumination but we needed light as coaxial as possible. The problem remained that we still could not see well; many pupils did not dilate enough. There was too much light dispersion, too much reflection from the various surfaces. We therefore thought of using a slit lamp attached to the operating microscope. The narrow beam was used to shine a light into the eye at a very narrow angle and indeed this was an improvement. A movable slit lamp was designed so that we could vary the angle of the incident light.

We came up with another idea. Why make such a desperate attempt to put the light into the eye from outside? Why not try to peek into a room through a key hole with the light switched on in the room rather than trying to illuminate the room through the key hole? This was how the fiber optic light was born. The fiber optic light was so superior in its quality to the slit lamp approach that we immediately discarded the slit lamp.

Just think of what an advantage we now had: not only could we illuminate the part that we wanted to work on with very high intensity but we also avoided the multitude of reflections on the corneal surface, the posterior surface of the cornea, the anterior surface and posterior surface of the lens and the scattering of light that occurs in hazy media. The improvement in illumination and visibility was dramatic. By placing a light pipe around our instrument tip the problem of visibility inside the eye was solved.

TRAINING OF VITREOUS SURGERY

Although vitreous surgery is simple in principle, it is a difficult technique that necessitates longer and more intense training than ab externo surgery. For this reason I would like to spend the remaining time on how to prepare oneself for vitreous surgery by using an animal model.

The eye is a very small organ and considerable training is needed to learn the fine manipulations inside the eye. To resolve this problem animal surgery offered the best opportunity for experience.

A rabbit is anesthesized with sodium pentobarbital and retrobulbar and topical anesthesia to the eye. The animal should be positioned just like one would do with a patient. One should not move the head of the animal during surgery just as one would not adjust the patient's head. One has to learn to do everything from one position only, just as in the operating room.

It is very helpful to remove the third lid and do a canthotomy to have easier access to the lateral part of the eye. Traction sutures are placed under the four recti muscles.

The rabbit has a slightly different anatomy from the human eye: the lens is much larger and there is no pars plana. When you enter the eye you either have to pass into the eye anteriorly through the iris base or posteriorly through the retina. In the first case the lens has to be removed, in the second only a small part of the vitreous can be removed.

How do you remove the lens? One can use the vitrectomy instrument or a phacoemulsifying instrument. The lens of the rabbit is very difficult to remove even with the best of instrumentation because it is like rubber. Only animals of less than 1.5 kg weight have a soft lens which can be removed with the vitreous cutter. Heavier animals need a phacoemulsifyer.

The posterior approach is very good to teach one to remove the vitreous without touching and destroying the lens. The entry site is about 6 mm posteriorly from the limbus. Vitreous in the rabbit is adherent to the retina and therefore one pulls easily on retina. Since vitreous surgery is more difficult in the rabbit eye than in the human one performing successful vitreous surgery on the rabbit will be very helpful for the human experience.

At the perforation site preplaced sutures help keep the wound tight. Once the instrument is inserted into the vitreous cavity one can learn to hold the instrument properly, learn to rotate the tip, learn to tilt the instrument, and move it in and out.

Basic and advanced vitreous surgery
G.W. Blankenship, M. Stirpe, M. Gonvers, S. Binder (eds.)
Fidia Research Series, vol. II,
Liviana Press, Padova © 1986

TRAINING FOR VITREOUS SURGERY: ANIMAL SURGERY

Robert Machemer

Duke University, Dept of Ophthalmology Durham, North Carolina
(Reported by Severino Fruscella)

Vitreous surgery calls for the surgeon's skilled and thorough practice with surgical situations and sophisticated technical instruments along with good clinical judgement. In order to avoid any risk to the patients, it is therefore advisable for the surgeon, at the beginning, to train for this delicate operation on animals. Although monkey eyes are more similar to human ones from the anatomic point of view, it seems better for economical and practical reasons to practice vitrectomy on the eyes of rabbits.

The latter have many anatomical differences from the human eye; in fact, they are smaller, the ora serrata is 3 mm behind the limbus, and the lens is larger in relation to the whole size of the eye. Due to the position and size of the lens, instrument insertion cannot take place at the ora serrata, but rather through the retina behind the lens. In order to prevent retinal injuries when instruments are introduced, the area of insertion should be treated with cryotherapy one week before the vitrectomy.

The operation must be performed under general anesthesia with an operating microscope and the same instruments that are used for human vitrectomy. Because of the structure of the rabbit's orbit, the chosen quadrant of access for instruments is the inferonasal area.

The second instrument is to be inserted in a similar plane 90 to 180 degrees from the infranasal access. A peritomy of the limbus is undertaken and four traction sutures are placed under the four recti muscles. A suture is preplaced at the sclerotomy site in order to allow quick sealing of the scleral opening after the completion of vitrectomy and after the instruments have been taken out. A scleral cut is performed equatorially, in the inferonasal quadrant in that area which was pretreated with cryotherapy. A pointed knife is used for the cutting. The circumference of the knife will vary according to the size of the instrument to be introduced.

Illumination is provided by the paraxial light of the microscope; focusing is eased by the contact lens which is manipulated by the assistant.

The transparent mid-vitreous posterior to the lens has to be removed first; then vitrectomy near the retinal plane can be performed. This practice can be made easier by applying the technique of Dr. S. Charles, that is, the injection into the vitreous cavity of 10% fluorescein through the infusion instrument. Fluorescein uniformly stains the vitreous with a thick yellow-green color. In this way areas where the vitreous is removed become clear, while the other parts keep fluorescein coloration. Practice is needed in handling the instruments in order to develop such skills as rotation, in and out movement, tilting of the instrument pivoted at the sclerotomy and shifting of the eye by using the instrument as a lever.

The assistant must acquire the skills necessary for manual aspiration with a large syringe, and he learns how to distinguish if the vitreous or infusion fluid is encountered, according to the suction resistence.

When the surgeon has enough practice on normal eyes with or without fluorescein, he must begin surgery on pathologic eyes. A wounded eye is simulated in the rabbit by performing a perforating injury one week before the scheduled surgery. After anesthesia of the animal, the injury is made with a blunt pointed knife deeply inserted into the globe 6 mm posterior to the limbus and perforating through the eye into the posterior wall one disc diameter below the optic disc. Inside the vitreous cavity, the surgeon will then encounter along with the vitreous, blood, fibrin and proliferative tissue which have to be removed during surgery.

The pathologic vitreous is more easily operated upon by performing a two instrument technique. A 22 gauge hypodermic needle with a 100 degree bent tip attached to a syringe is generally used. The needle lifts and gets fibrin and condensed vitreous, otherwise inaccessible to the vitrectomy instrument, closer to the vitreous cutter; retinal injuries are better prevented as the vitrectomy instrument is allowed to work far from the retinal surface.

We can confirm that the rabbit's eye offers the best opportunity for training of vitrectomy techniques. The surgeon, along with improving the technique, can test the instrument sharpness and other relevant features before using them on human eyes.

Basic and advanced vitreous surgery
G.W. Blankenship, M. Stirpe, M. Gonvers, S. Binder (eds.)
Fidia Research Series, vol. II,
Liviana Press, Padova © 1986

INSTRUMENTATION FOR VITREORETINAL SURGERY

P.K. Leaver

Moorfields Eye Hospital, City Road, London EC1V 2PD

Since the introduction by Machemer and his colleagues of pars plana vitrectomy, the range of microsurgical instruments for closed intraocular microsurgery has proliferated. Moreover the original instrumentation has been developed and modified constantly.

The Vitreous Infusion Suction Cutter, Rotoextractor, Vitrophage, Vitreous Stripper and other early vitrectomy instruments were all multifunction, single probe designs incorporating cutting, suction, infusion and illumination in the one module. In the early 1970's O'Malley introduced the concept of common-gauge, single function instrumentation whereby each function is undertaken by a single small instrument introduced separately into the eye. This change in approach had two fundamental advantages: firstly by decreasing the size of the instruments and ports, surgical complications such as retinal dialysis and late complications associated with vitreous incarceration and fibrovascular ingrowth were reduced, and secondly the common-gauge instrumentation introduced greater flexibility. Fiberlight pics, vitreous scissors, intraocular foreign body forceps and other accessories were developed while Charles advanced the system further with his flute-needle and endophotocoagulation probe.

The access to the retinal surface and excellence of visualization provided by closed microsurgical techniques have enabled us to treat conditions which were hitherto nearly or completely inoperable. Thus the removal of vitreous opacity in diabetic eye disease progressed to dissection and removal of surface membranes and retinal reattachment, while in massive periretinal proliferation the methods of Cibis and early workers have given way to microsurgical epiretinal membrane dissection and fluid/gas or fluid/silicone-oil exchange.

Vitreoretinal instrumentation can be broadly divided into 4 aspects:

1. *Visualization*
   Microscopy
   Illumination
   Contact Lenses

2. *Cutting/Aspiration Instruments for:*
   Vitreous gel
   Preretinal membranes
   Anterior segment revision/lensectomy

3. *Infusion/Exchange with:*
   Physiological fluids
   Gases
   Silicone-oil

4. *Endocoagulation/Adhesion with:*
   Bipolar endodiathermy
   Endophotocoagulation
       — xenon
       — laser
   Endocryopexy

VISUALIZATION

At Moorfields we are currently using the Zeiss Op Mi VI microscope with X-Y coupling, Clinitex light-pipe with Keeler cold-light source and the Machemer infusion contact lens. Optimal positioning of the patient's head is achieved and maintained throughout surgery using a Lamtec head-support with adjustable wrist rests. The pupil is kept widely dilated by injecting 0.3 mls of Mydricaine subconjunctivally at the commencement of surgery.

CUTTING/ASPIRATION

Excision and aspiration of the vitreous gel are achieved with the Ocutome Mark II. Preretinal membranes are peeled and dissected with a bent 20 gauge needle and vitreous scissors manufactured in London by Osborn and Simmons. Removal of the lens is sometimes aided by using the Fragmatome.

INFUSION/EXCHANGE

A standard 2.5 mm infusion cannula connected to a bag of Hartmann's solution by a standard infusion set with a 3-way tap is used, but cannulae of 4 and 6 mm lengths are available for cases with choroidal thickening.

Air and Sulphexafluoride/air mixture are injected with a 50 ml syringe connected to the infusion cannula via the 3-way tap. Mixtures of Sulfurhexafluoride with air greater than 1 part SF6 to 4 parts air (20% mixture) are never used.

Silicone-oil of 1000 centistokes viscosity is injected in similar fashion, but a compressed air-powered 20 ml syringe operated by a foot-pedal is used. If silicone-oil of viscosities greater than 1000 centistokes is used an 18 or 19 gauge infusion cannula is available.

ENDOCOAGULATION/ADHESION

Bipolar endodiathermy of forward new blood vessels is achieved using the Mentor wet field coagulator and Charles clips attached to the vitrectomy instruments. Single probe bipolar instrumentation is also available.

The Clinitex Xenon Arc endophotocoagulator with Charles endoprobe is used for endophotocoagulation, but an endo laser facility is at present being installed. Cryopexy is always applied externally through full-thickness sclera and neither endocryopexy nor cyanoacrylates are used at Moorfieds for achieving chorio-retinal adhesion.

In summary, the wide and expanding range of instrumentation now available for vitreoretinal microsurgery has enabled us to approach increasingly difficult surgical problems with a greater degree of success.

Basic and advanced vitreous surgery
G.W. Blankenship, M. Stirpe, M. Gonvers, S. Binder (eds.)
Fidia Research Series, vol. II,
Liviana Press, Padova © 1986

HOW AUTOMATIC INFUSION AND SUCTION HAVE CHANGED DURING THE LAST FIVE YEARS

Ing. Manfredi Orciuolo

Fondazione Oftalmologica 'G.B. Bietti', Piazza Sassari, 5, Roma

Ocular hydrodynamics during vitrectomies because of its particular conditions are completely different from the physiological. The main differences are due to the fact that there is a forced infusion, so the inflow is exclusively conditioned by the source of pressure, by the dimension of the inflow tube, by intraocular pressure and by positive or negative resistance to the outflow. Therefore, outflow depends on the levels of suction applied by the I/A machines, on the average section of the outlet tubes, on the leakage of the sclerotomies and on intraocular pressure.

Ocular pressure depends on inflow/outflow and it is conditioned by scleral rigidity which is completely different from the physiological one. It is important to stress that this ocular rigidity does not only depend on the rigidity of the bulb, but mainly on the amount of air present in the inlet-outlet tubes. The presence of air within the tubes connected to the eye during surgery, hardly decreases the rigidity to 1/10 of its average values. (In fact, since the eye is no longer filled with incompressible fluid:

$$PV = KnRT$$

is valid for the gases contained within the tubes).

We accomplished some tests with a Schiotz tonometer and have observed that the values of ocular rigidity were lower than average, in fact, the plunger of a tonometer indents normal eyes more because it compresses the air present in the bulb and stops only because of corneal rigidity. We should take into account the fact that the irrigation is refluxed, and small variations of volume do not produce big variations of eye pressure.

Indeed, ocular pressure in the case of refluxed infusion fluid is the capacity to provide the eye with sufficient fluid at different flows without varying its pressure.

Let us now examine which pressure is advisable to maintain during vitrectomy surgery. Let us start from the only available data: the normal pressure of an eye, which is the pressure considered the lower limit capable of maintaining the choroidal flow. The eye during surgery is evidently different from the physiological one, and therefore it is advisable to maintain a pressure of at least 5-6 mm Hg more, which avoids further complications during surgical manoeuvres. Furthermore, there is a maximum limit of pressure suggested by glaucoma pathologies; when the cornea is kept at a pressure higher than 30 mm Hg edema will develop in a short time. We have observed with a pressure of 35 mm Hg the cornea to develop edema in less than 30 min, and with a pressure of 45 mm Hg in 20 min.

The ideal intraocular pressure is about 25 mm Hg.

Let us examine the situation in which an eye is fed by a bottle with physiological solution through a sclerotomy. In order to maintain the ideal pressure of 25 mm Hg, the bottle should be positioned 25×13 mm over the level of the patient's head.

The bottle positioned at a height of 30 cm over the level of the patient's head may clearly seem too low, but till now nothing can prove that this may be wrong.

Let us start taking into account the maximum flow of a bottle with infusion of about 44 cc/min. Normal leakage due to sclerotomies is about 1/10 to 3/10 of this value; however if higher leakage occurs, it is advisable not to continue until sclerotomy leakage is reduced. We can say that the sclerotomy leakage of the infusion, at so little flow, is simply proportional to the flow, and the pressure will be lower by 3-7 mm Hg. When suction starts, the situation will surely worsen even when utilizing aspiration by a syringe, we will have an outflow of 50% to 200% more than the maximum value obtainable by the infusion line.

The surgeon should never exceed a 50% suction flow, or the ocular pressure may drop to 10 mm Hg or even lower, thus provoking a collapse of the bulb.

It is impossible to position the bottle at a higher height because it would increase the pressure up to 50 mm Hg, and this pressure is clearly dangerous to the cornea.

This problem can only be resolved by lifting and lowering the bottle during aspiration.

We have already described the parameters which are to be controlled and combined to obtain an automatic regulation, and came to the conclusion that the only possible way to control the whole system was to use a computer (Fig. 1).

Let us now show the system after five years of continuous changes.

First of all the two pumps of infusion and suction have been differentiated. The infusion pump has 10 rollers with a capacity which is lower than that of the suction pump. The infusion pump has to provide a constant flow according to the amount of outflow. It can also manage to cope with leakages amounting to 30 mm Hg, which seems very simple if we consider that the pressure during the tests exceeded 500 mm Hg (Fig. 2).

The suction pump has 3 rollers, because we are not interested in a constant flow here, but more in increasing pressure-velocity and the level of suction (-500 mm Hg) (Fig. 3).

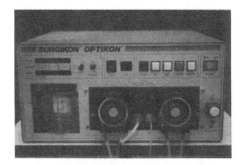

Figure 1. Automated infusion/aspiration unit.

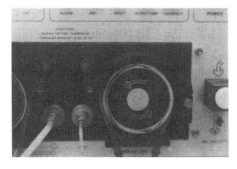

Figure 2. Peristaltic suction-pump.

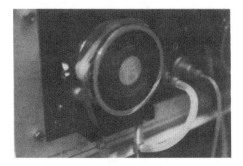

Figure 3. Infusion peristaltic pump.

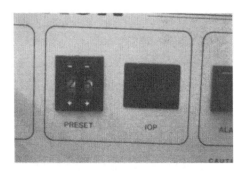

Figure 4. IOP display and preset.

The most important piece of the unit is represented by the infusion control. A transducer measures the pressure of the liquid of infusion near the eye. It is only from the transducer that we obtain the most important data about the right function of the pump. We can also control the level of suction and thence perform a correct aspiration.

THE VARIOUS PROCEDURES

We set a pressure of 25 mm Hg (Fig. 4). The infusion pump delivers liquid till the transducer sets the exact pressure. It is obvious that during surgery the flow is set by the computer in accordance with the change of leakage in the line. This would be like reading the intraocular pressure and then depending on it to lower or to raise the bottle. However, this is performed by a computer, and every measurement lasts less than 1/20 of a sec. A constant leakage can be counterbalanced by increasing the pressure of infusion, and waiting until the pressure reaches normal levels. This is a pressure to flow control. This means that every time the preset pressure varies, there is a change of velocity of the pump, excluding of course when there is no leakage and the pump remains still.

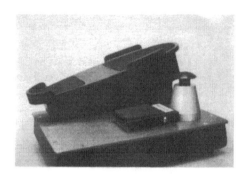

Figure 5. Linear control foot switch.

Once the flow and vacuum (linear control) have been set for the desired aspiration, suction will function automatically, and will also control the infusion to balance leakage (Fig. 5).

In unusual cases, when vacuum and flow exceed the standard working conditions of infusion, suction does not allow further negative variations in the intraocular pressure.

Thus, the control we described is capable of elaborating the various data it receives from the operator, testing the conditions of the eye during surgery and deciding what to do.

We will now illustrate some typical situations in vitrectomy and how we can cope with them utilizing the Surgikon.

Insertion of the scleral infusion trocar and checking its correct position

This is considered the most important and critical moment of the surgical procedure. An obstruction by the vitreous near the sclerotomy prevents a correct infusion of liquid (Fig. 6, 7).

The Surgikon does not recognize the standard pattern of the eye, because the volume of infusion is too low, and informs the surgeon that it is necessary to check the situation.

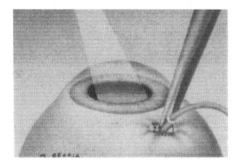

Figure 6. Cannula insertion in the eye.

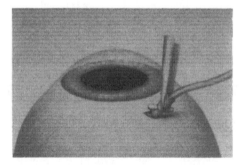

Figure 7. Ophthalmoscopic check of the cannula's correct position.

Pressure control during subretinal fluid drainage

There is another critical moment in the pressure balance of the eye, when there is external subretinal liquid release (Fig. 8). During the initial phase of surgery, the pressure, because of compression, may increase artificially up to 80 mm Hg, or even more. Then during the liquid release the pressure rapidly drops; however, it can remain too high and consequently cause incarceration. A correct procedure would be to maintain a normal pressure (25 mm Hg) during the initial phases even when there are abrupt variations of volume (muscle tractions), keeping a balanced pressure during scleral buckling, maintaining a pressure lower than 10 mm Hg during the liquid release, and increase it again when the situation has become less critical. The Surgikon is programmed to accomplish such difficult operations. It is equipped with a device that varies the pressure either positively or negatively by rotating the pump in both directions.

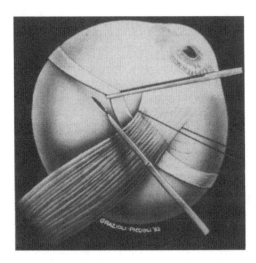

Figure 8. Subretinal drainage incision.

Aspirate viscous vitreous and checking its state of hydratation

There are different things that we have to take into account when cutting and aspirating the vitreous:
- Its transparency
- How much of it has to be cut
- Which is the right suction rate
- Its state of hydratation
- When it is still there and it cannot be visualized

We can do this by selecting an appropriate suction pressure (vacuum), in the case of the vitreous - 300 mm Hg.

Suction is set by pressing the foot switch (linear control) at not more than 50 mm Hg; if the vitreous does not flow, the unit gives a sound alert meaning that the vitreous is engaged in the vitreoctome tip. It is sufficient to press the foot switch till the signal disappears, to be sure that the vitreous is aspirated in the correct way (Fig. 9).

It is better to start at a lower pressure if the vitreous is hydratated and can be removed at a low pressure. If the pressure is at 25 mm Hg or lower, it means that we aspirate only water. Naturally, these suction controls are continuously adjusted by infusion. Even with uncontrolled suction due to a mistake, the ocular pressure will be maintained at acceptable values by the unit.

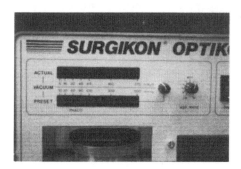

Figure 9. Vacuum control on the front panel.

CHANGING THE INSTRUMENTS THROUGH THE PORT AND AVOIDING THE RISK OF HYPOTONICITY

Frequently during the procedure the surgeon needs to change the instrument because of different situations.

A very critical and difficult moment is when an instrument has to be replaced by another one. In fact, the sclerotomy remains open and when working with the bottle, the pressure decreases too much unless we have already increased it, but this increase in pressure can easily cause vitreal incarceration.

All these problems can be avoided by using the automatic infusion. An increase in the flow does not correspond to an increase in pressure, therefore, incarceration will not represent a problem.

POSSIBILITY OF KEEPING LARGE INCISIONS OPEN WHEN EXTRACTING FOREIGN BODIES

A particular case is the extraction of a foreign body when the incision is not very large; however, it is possible to do it without having the risk of an ocular collapse.

AUTOMATIC CLEANING OF THE VITREOUS CHAMBER UNDER CONSTANT PRESSURE

There are some particular advantages that can be used for hemorrhages occurring during surgery:
    a) We can increase the pressure in order to obtain complete hemostasis
    b) We can completely control the eye during the cleaning phase.

Let us take into account the situation in which there is a drop in the pressure of some vessels at 25 mm Hg. Pressure is to be increased to 35 mm Hg to stop the hemorrhage (Fig. 10). We should now clean the vitreous chamber in order to have a clearer view

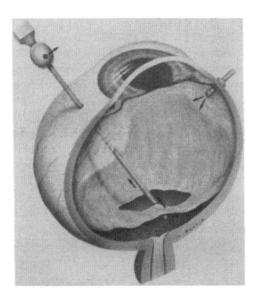

Figure 10. Vacuum cleaning technique.

of it. However, if we utilize the bottle every time, we would surely decrease the pressure and produce another hemorrhage, setting an endless circle.

For this reason, some authors suggest not to touch the eye for some minutes. However, if this solves the problem of a hemorrhage, it allows the formation of coagulates which are very difficult to remove.

We will also be able to remove the blood located on the retina with a constant pressure and perfectly controlled suction (P constant).

SOME CONSIDERATIONS ON THE USE
OF COMPLEX INSTRUMENTS

One of the disadvantages represented by this kind of complex instrument is that sometimes the surgeon is afraid of not being able to handle a particular situation and of not being capable of doing something in case of breakdown or of wrong utilization of the instrument. However, the automatic infusion device is not as complicated as it may seem.

According to our opinion these worries are well grounded, but the utilization of these instruments has allowed us to resolve some very complicated cases.

However, if the surgical procedure will not take more than an hour, it is pratically absurd to utilize such a complex instrument. But when dealing with very serious cases it is necessary to be well organized.

Indeed this kind of surgical procedure requires a good team of physicians, where at least one person should know the instrument well and another one should be a skilled assistant of the surgeon.

LIQUID-GAS EXCHANGE

We will now describe the Liquid-Gas exchange, that we have been using for 4 years. The peristaltic infusion pump can either work with water or with air. A two-way tap connecting on one side the physiological solution, and on the other one or more Millipore filters (Fig. 11) is placed at the input. When one wants to inject air, turn the tap and air will enter into the irrigation line. The aspiration can be performed by the unit at very low levels (10-15 mm Hg) or using a flute cannula (Fig. 12). The automatic control of the IOP remains and you can, therefore, exchange liquid-air at constant pressure.

The vacuum level can be further controlled to avoid loss of the eye pressure. The unit indicates when the liquid is finished and you are aspirating air; infact, as air reaches the tip of the aspiration cannula, the unit will feel the weight of the column of liquid in the aspiration line and the pump will stop rotating.

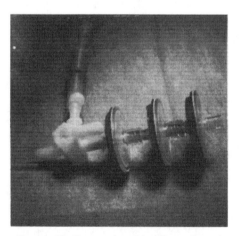

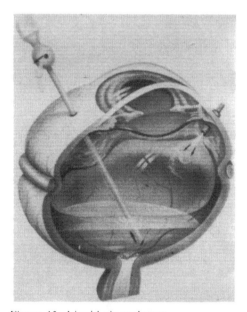

Figure 11. Stopcock with filters for air-infusion.

Figure 12. Liquid-air exchange.

Basic and advanced vitreous surgery
G.W. Blankenship, M. Stirpe, M. Gonvers, S. Binder (eds.)
Fidia Research Series, vol. II,
Liviana Press, Padova © 1986

"LE SYSTEM": A UNIFIED MICROSURGICAL CENTER

Jean-Marie Parel, Ing. ETS-G

The Bascom Palmer Eye Institute, Department of Ophthalmology,
University of Miami School of Medicine, Miami, Florida, USA

Fifteen years ago, vitrectomy instrumentation was quite simple. Gravity infusion and manual aspiration did not require complicated apparatus. The first vitrectomy machine's (the VISC) cutting function was controlled by a single foot-switch (1). The microscope foot-pedal controls activated the fine focus and, in some instances, a motorized zoom magnification changing device. Although motorized automated vitreous scissors already existed, they were rarely used during vitreous surgery (2). Basically, the surgeon had two simple pedals at his disposal: one for the microscope and one for operating the vitreous cutter, hence one for each foot.

This simplicity did not last very long. By 1972, the microscope included X-Y translation stage controls, room and coaxial light controls, rapid column retraction controls, the motorized 60 degree photo slit-lamp controls as well as controls for 35 mm and movie cameras. Each of these features required additional surgeon operated foot-switches which were added to the microscope foot-pedal (3).

With time, other surgical modalities were added to the armamentarium of the vitrectomist: high frequency diathermy was incorporated into the vitrectomy instrument to treat bleeders. This modality was quickly replaced by the bipolar "wet-field" type cautery. Later, medium frequency bipolar coaxial instruments designed for treating the surface of the retina were introduced (4). Each requires a different foot pedal. In the middle 1970's, other methods were introduced. First came the endocryogenic probes and the Xenon endophotocoagulating probes. The latter was replaced by yet another intraoperative photocoagulating modality: the endolaser probe (5). All of these foot-switch controlled modalities are still in use today.

The aspiration of diseased vitreous with a syringe manually operated by the surgical assistant was replaced by various automated aspirating devices. These devices were later improved by the addition of pressure-feedback systems, leading to a variable flow control named "linear suction" control by Charles (6).

The peeling of retinal membranes and the manipulation of delicate intraocular tissues led to the development of specialized automated microsurgical instruments exemplified by the MPC, the automated Sutherland scissors and other single action cutting, gripping and fixation devices. The instantaneous control of the patient's IOP during surgery required another type of automated apparatus: the Blankenship EPA, a fully motorized and remote controlled, infusion pole (7). Fluid-gas exchange was also automated by the introduction of motorized gas injectors. Constant pressure air pumps are now being widely used. The resurrection of silicone oil as a tamponade and, in some cases, as a vitreous substitute, led to the development of other kinds of automated devices: the silicone oil injectors (8). Each of the above mentioned instruments requires its own power supply and a separate foot-pedal for its control.

The above list is certainly incomplete. With each passing day, another foot-switch controlled automated device is introduced, adding to the burden of the vitreo-retinal surgical staff. The surgeons and their operating room staffs are faced with a problem: each time another instrument is introduced, it requires additional table-top space for its power module. Thus, the operating suite quickly becomes further crowded under the compounded mass of machines and cables.

In order to resolve this problem, in 1977 at the Bascom Palmer Eye Institute, we attempted a vertical integration of some of the above mentioned modalities. The existing power consoles used for the operation of a vitrectomy instrument, motorized scissors, ultrasonic phacofragmentation, automated aspiration and a fiber optic cold light source were stacked on top of each other. The assembly was bolted to a 4-wheeled cart. A special multi-function foot-switch was designed to control each of the above functions separately. This solution quickly became obsolete, as the vertical integration of existing consoles could not accommodate additional modalities, nor could it accept newer instrumentation.

In 1981, we introduced a new concept: the selectable modular approach. We named it "Le System". In this concept, each surgical modality is confined to a miniaturized module having similar dimensions. It allows the user to stack them in a variety of configurations to suit his or her particular surgical speciality. In addition, all modules make use of a common remote-controlled interconnecting system. Thus, any of the modules or any combination of modules can be controlled by a single device. Such a device can be a handheld keyboard, a digital computer, a radio-frequency controlled system or a simple foot-switch.

As each module has its own built-in power source, it can also be used as a stand alone device. This concept has the additional advantage of being obsolescence proof: when new modalities are introduced, they can be integrated into the modular array in a few minutes. The plug-in principle is easy to understand and can be performed by the OR staff. Also, with this concept, any defective module can be quickly replaced by a newer model.

In our first experimental prototype (9), the modules are supported by a movable cart (Figure 1). This cart hosts the motorized infusion pole, a vacuum pump, the nitrous oxide gas bottles, provides storage space for the various surgical probes and supplies, as well as storage for the multi-function foot pedal. In addition, it provides the nursing

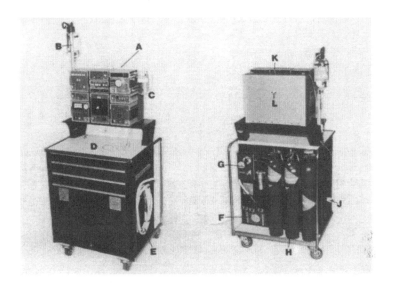

Figure 1. Front and Rear Views of "Le System" and it's Supporting Cart. "Le System" consists of the modular array, the module selector and the unitized foot-switch. The cart and the other devices described are only ancilliary equipment. A: Modular array; B: EPA motorized infusion pole; C: Collection cannister and fluid lines; D: Storage mobile cart; E: Foot-pedal cable in storage position; F: Foot-pedal; G: Nitrous Oxide high pressure manometer and bottle selector; H: Nitrous Oxide bottles; J: Power cable in retracted position; K: Connection to external OR vacuum supply; L: External/internal vacuum switching valve.

staff with an illuminated semi-sterile instrument table top. A single retractable power cord supplies the whole modular array, eliminating the usual octopus-like cable confusion found in the operating room.

The modular array has 8 modalities, 7 of which are foot-operated by the surgeon (Figure 2). In addition to miniaturization, each modality was optimized to conform with the surgical state of the art of the Bascom Palmer Eye Institute clinical faculty. For flexibility, most modules have been fitted with various adjustments to suit the vitreo-retinal surgeons as well as those surgeons favoring the anterior segment specialties.

The *Fiber optic cold light source module* (Figure 2A) has two front-loaded halogen lamps and can be fit with 5 different filters for intraoperative fluoroscopy, blue-light hazard protection, photography and other specialized functions, such as the detection of HpD in tissues. To allow for the multiplicity of existing fiberoptic cords and probes used in the same surgical case, the source will accept as many as 3 probes simultaneously.

The automated *Infusion/Aspiration module* (Figure 2H) has a variable flow rate controlled by the surgeon's foot as well as a means of monitoring the patient's IOP during the case. The vacuum upper limit can be pre-set at the start of the case to between 10 and 600 mm Hg. The pressure indicator is self-illuminated and digital for ease of reading. A provision for instant irrigation cut-off, required for ECCEs and

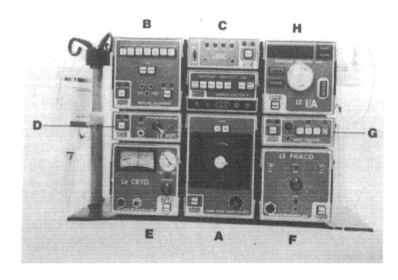

Figure 2. "Le System": A Selectable Modular Array. All miniature modules have similar dimensions and, based on the building block principle, can be interconnected as desired. The centrally located module selector permits a single foot-pedal to control any of the modalities selected. In addition to the linear aspiration modality, a maximum of two other modalities can be selected for simultaneous use (see text for symbol explanation).

phacoemulsification surgery, is integrated into the module and is also foot-switch controlled. The surgical fluid lines and the collection bottle are fully flash autoclavable for fast reuse.

The *Vitrectomy module* (Figure 2G) powers the various cutters designed at Bascom Palmer, including the VISC, the STAT, the TAC and the VITAC series of instruments. In addition, it also powers the PhacoExcavator.

The *Phacoemulsification module* (Figure 2F) generates the power needed for anterior segment or pars plana ultrasonic phacoemulsification of the nucleus. It has an automated frequency tuning circuit and works on the jack-hammer principle for deeper and faster tissue penetration. It accommodates both the probes described by Shock and Girard as well as those I have designed.

Both the Vitrectomy and the Phacoemulsification modules were designed to work in conjunction with the above described infusion/aspiration module as well as with commercially available automated irrigation/aspiration consoles.

The *Cryogenic module* (Figure 2E) operates on the principle described by Amoils. It has a tip temperature adjustment and a single pulse timing device for controlled cryo application. The application duration can be adjusted from 1 to 10 seconds. The surgeon can override the timed application simply by increasing the pressure on the foot-switch control. The probe tip will defrost immediately upon foot-switch release. Safety features include a probe heater fault-detector.

The *Diathermy module* (Figure 2B) operates exclusively in the bipolar mode for safety reasons (4). It generates a 1.25MHz sine wave, which can vary in intensity from

0.5 to 32 Watts. The module is a foot-switch operated timing device for controlled applications. This device allows a single pulse of energy to be delivered to the tissue. Energy can be adjusted from 0.125 to 8 Joules per pulse. The module will accept any kind of bipolar endodiathermy and exodiathermy probes.

The *MPC module* (Figure 2D) will power all solenoid operated surgical devices, including the MPC, a guillotine type cutter and the automated Sutherland scissors. The cutting rate is adjustable from 1 to 9 cuts per second. For gripping or holding instruments such as automated forceps, the unit is operated in an on/off mode. The module features foot-switch operated control allowing the surgeon to hold the instrument's blades or jaws closed during wound insertion or retraction.

The IOC module (Figure 2C) is reserved for specialized automated instrumentation, such as motorized trephines, automated anterior capsule cutters, silicone oil injectors, motorized micro staplers designed to hold the retina, such as the Norton Ligator, etc. This module automatically detects which type of instrument has been connected, and automatically provides the necessary energy and required foot-switch control functions.

All 3 of the above modules are battery powered, have automated charging circuits, short-circuit protection, and battery low level detection for safety.

The control of any of the above 7 modalities is performed by a single unitized foot-pedal (Figure 3). The foot-pedal is electrically connected to the module selector, which in turn directs the appropriate signals to the various modules via a series of interconnecting cables (Figure 3L). For simplicity of use, the module selector was designed to be operated by the scrub technician or assistant nurse. This person can easily select a particular modality by merely pushing the desired button with a disposable sterile "Q" tip or other sterile item. The normally red illuminated push button will turn green when selected, giving a visual feedback to the OR staff. The module selector also provides energy for the simultaneous recharge of four of the above described modules (Figure 3K).

The pedal was designed to be operated with one foot only. It has 6 different switches. The right treadle bar (Figure 3A) is the variflow, sometimes also called "linear" aspiration control: the greater the foot pressure applied, the greater the suction applied to the instrument. This same device will operate either the vitrectomy or the ultrasonic fragmenting instrument. The choice is made simply by pushing the appropriate button on the right side of the module selector (Figure 3G). In certain surgical situations, it is of benefit to the surgeon to use the surgical instrument as a simple aspiration cannula. A switch is thus provided to cut power to the surgical tool (Figure 3E). Another switch was provided for rapid change of the tool's cutting rate (Figure 3F) as is necessary when operating in close proximity to the retina, to the posterior capsule or other delicate tissues. The left treadle bar (Figure 3B) controls all other surgical modalities, such as cryo, diathermy, scissors, trephines, injectors, etc. The choice is made simply by pressing the corresponding button on the left side of the module selector (Figure 3H). The left treadle bar provides for two functions which are selected by the surgeon's foot pressure. This feature serves, for example, to override the cryo and diathermy timers, to choose between the automated scissors cutting action and blade closure. It also allows for fast flow reversal during fluid/silicone exchange, etc.

The unitized pedal has two additional controls; one operates the infusion ON/OFF pinch-valve (Figure 3D) and with the other, the surgeon controls the height of the EPA motorized infusion pole (Figure 3C).

26

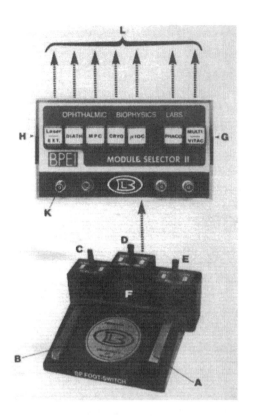

Figure 3. Unitized Foot-Pedal and Module Selector. The foot-pedal is operated with one foot only, but allows for the control of more than 6 functions without requiring changes to the module selector. With the 7 stage module selector, the combination of controls available to the surgeon are greatly enhanced (see text for symbol explanation).

Certain surgical modalities have large space and power requirements and are difficult to integrate into a unitized system. The Argon endolaser is a typical example. In our "Le System" prototype, one of the module selector functions, labeled EXT/LASER, was dedicated to such extraordinary modalities. When adequately connected to the module selector, any kind of laser, including Argon, Krypton, CO_2 and Nd:YAGs, can be controlled by the unitized foot-pedal.

We never made a second prototype of "Le System". Not only did it cost a fortune, it also took months (nine to be exact) to build and countless sleepless nights. Today, technology has further advanced and it should be possible to reduce the size of our apparatus to the extent of making it a truly portable system. I noted with pride that many of the leading ophthalmic instrumentation firms have finally adopted our approach; a unified modular control center equipped with a single unitized foot pedal.

ACKNOWLEDGMENTS

Izuru Nose, B.S., William Lee, David Denham, M.S., Woody Moore and Willi Aumayr provided many of the technical refinements, fabricated Le System's prototype and many of the described microsurgical instruments. Barbara French, B.A., prepared the illustrations and Marilyn Maxwell, M.B.A., wrote this paper in English. I am grateful to Professor E.W.D. Norton, M.D. for his continued support and to the members of the clinical staff of the Bascom Palmer Eye Institute for sharing their ideas and surgical experiences with me.

REFERENCES

1. Machemer R, Buttner H, Norton EWD and Parel J-M (1971): Vitrectomy: a pars plana approach. Trans. Am Acad Ophthalmol Otolaryngol 75:813-820.
2. Parel J-M, Crock GW, O'Brien B, Henderson PN, Galbraight JEK and Pericic L. (1970): Prototypal Electromicrosurgical Instruments. Med J Austr 1-709.
3. Parel J-M, Machemer R and Aumayr W (1974): A new concept for Vitreous Surgery, 5: An Automated Microscope. Am J Ophthalmol 77-161.
4. Parel J-M, Machemer R, O'Grady G, Crock GW and Nose I (1983): Intraocular diathermy Coagulation. Von Graefes Arch. 221:31-34.
5. Fleishman JA, Swartz M and Dixon JA (1982): Argon Laser Endophotocoagulation. An Intraoperative Trans-Pars Plana Technique. Arch Ophthalmol 99:1610-1612.
6. Charles S and Wang K: Linear Suction Control System. Ocutome/Fragmatome Newsletter. Vol. 4, 3.
7. Blankenship G, Lee W and Parel J-M (1984): An electronic Infusion Pole Adjuster. Ophthalmic Surgery, 15 (4): 317-318.
8. Zivojnovic R, Mertens DAE and Peperkamp F (1982): Das Flussige silikon in der Amotiochirurgie. (II) Bereicht ueber 280 Fallenweitere Entwiklung der Technik. Klin Mbl Augenheilk. 181:444-452.
9. Parel J-M, Blumenkranz M, O'Grady G, Blankenship G, Nose I, Denham D, Lee W and Norton EWD (1982): Advances in Vitreoretinal Microsurgical Instrumentation. Ophthalmology, 89(9S): 186.

Basic and advanced vitreous surgery
G.W. Blankenship, M. Stirpe, M. Gonvers, S. Binder (eds.)
Fidia Research Series, vol. II,
Liviana Press, Padova © 1986

THE PHACOEXCAVATOR: A NEW APPROACH TO LENTECTOMY

Jean-Marie Parel, Ing.ETS-G

The Bascom Palmer Eye Institute, Department of Ophthalmology,
University of Miami School of Medicine, Miami, Florida, USA

Before discussing a new instrument and technique designed for the removal of a cataract during vitrectomy, I would like to present a short review of the most commonly accepted methods.

KELMAN

The removal of hard cataracts through a single, small incision while maintaining intraocular pressure at normal levels was resolved by Kelman in 1969 (1). Kelman used the magnetostrictive ultrasonic technology invented for dentistry by Cavitron chief engineer Anton Banko. The 18 gauge intraocular active portion of his instrument is made of titanium and vibrates 25,000 times per second. With magnetostrictive technology, the ultrasonic motions are multi-dimensional and not solely limited to back and forth motions along the axis of the tip. The vectorial combination of these vibrations can emulsify up to degree 3$^+$ nuclear sclerotic cataracts. His instrument was specifically designed to fit the anterior segment limbal entry and cannot easily be used via the pars plana because of restrictions in tip length. In addition, Kelman's instrument requires a continuous flow of infusion surrounding the 18 gauge tip to remove the heat generated by the ultrasonic vibrations. Should the flow of infusion fluid be interrupted during ultrasonic emulsification, the temperature of the aqueous can be raised well above 44°C in less than one minute. In addition to the reported endothelial cell damage caused by ultrasonic energy and the use of large volume of fluids (2), I attribute this heat generation as another cause of endothelial cell loss. To prevent conduction of heat to the edges of the wound and to the surrounding intraocular tissues, Kelman employs a 2.0 mm diameter silicone sleeve to provide for large infusion flow. Due to its inherent softness, this 14 gauge sleeve easily collapses and cannot be used without difficulty through the pars plana.

GIRARD AND SHOCK

Two other ultrasonic devices originally designed for dentistry were adapted in the middle 1970's for cataract surgery; the Girard Fragmatome (3) and the Shock Fragmenter (4).

Both have long intraocular 20 gauge needle tips for aspiration of emulsified nucleous tissue but lack infusion capability. Thus, a separate infusion port is necessary to maintain the IOP at a normal level. Instead of using the magnetostrictive technology employed by Kelman, both the Girard and Shock units make use of piezoelectric technology for the generation of ultrasonic motion. Piezoelectric technology has the distinct theoretical advantage of limiting the tip motion to a back and forth movement, thereby considerably reducing heat generation. In addition, both the Girard and Shock systems have lower ultrasonic output power than the Kelman unit. Thus, infusion cooling of the intraocular tip is unnecessary, except possibly at very high power levels, at which point one can observe tissue shrinkage at the pars plana entrance site. The upper power limit for the Girard Fragmatome is a degree 2 cataract and for the Shock unit a degree 3 cataract.

Besides being very expensive, all above ultrasonic instruments have a common mechanical limitation: a reduction in the diameter of their tips translates to an ultrasonic power loss, thus smaller tips can no longer emulsify hard nuclei. For example, when equipped with a 20 gauge tip, the most powerful unit presently available (Kelman's) can no longer emulsify cataracts harder than degree 2 instead of a degree 3 cataract.

MACHEMER

Vitrectomy instruments like the VISC are more than adequate to remove soft lenses via the pars plana (5). Dr. Robert Machemer pioneered this mechanical technique early in the 1970's. Special VISC tips were developed for lentectomy through the pars plana. These tips were relatively large (2.3 mm in diameter) and would not work well with cataracts harder than degree 1$^+$. The obvious advantages of this solution are low cost and the ease with which the surgeon can switch from lentectomy to vitrectomy.

PHACO-ERSATZ

My interest in lentectomy techniques stemmed from a very different approach to cataract surgery. In 1980, I started an experimental project known as "Phaco-Ersatz": the lens contents are removed through a very small hole made in the periphery of the capsule. The emptied capsule is then refilled with a substitute gel-like material I dubbed "Ersatz". With this technique I hope to preserve accommodation after cataract surgery (6). In 1981, my collegues and I stumbled onto a major problem: for ideal results the capsular bag had to be emptied while maintaining the capsular walls at respectful distances. That meant we had to infuse while aspirating the fragmented lens tissues. For this procedure to succeed, the outer diameter of the instrument has to be as small as possible, probably below 1.0 mm to minimize damage to the elastic capsule. Our attempts at reducing the size of the 2 mm diameter Kelman instrument were unsuccessful. We then attempted to adapt infusion devices to both the Shock and the Girard instruments and to further reduce the diameter of their tips. With all 3 instruments, the attempted miniaturization reduced the ultrasonic power beyond clinical usefulness. We then searched for alternative technology.

WILSON

Late in 1981, Dr. Donald Wilson, Chairman of the Midwest Eye Center, located in Indianapolis, suggested the use of a rotating fork encased in a small stainless steel tube as a means of excavating the nucleus. He had made a prototype of this new device by modifying his oldest VISC-X cutting tip. The inner rotating portion of the tip had been fitted with two small needles. A VISC-X coaxial fiber optic light pipe served as a protecting sleeve. The surgeon could shield the rotating needles while entering the eye by moving the light pipe tube forward. The blades' rotational speed was approximately 120 cycles per minute.

Wilson's instrument was 2.3 mm in outer diameter, thus a perfect fit for the standard VISC-X pars plana cannula. It provided a forceful irrigation flow capable of flushing the fragmented nucleous pieces while maintaining an adequate IOP. This instrument had proven experimentally quite capable of excavating holes in a lens nucleous. After excavation, it was possible to remove the lens remnants using the VISC-X vitrectomy instrument. Wilson named his invention the "PhacoExcavator".

Besides its unwieldy size, this instrument had the tendency to induce rotation of the nucleous, a fact described earlier by Kelman (1). Wilson's PhacoExcavator device had the definite advantage of simplicity.

PHACOEXCAVATOR

With the hope of resolving our Phaco-Ersatz dilemma, infusion and aspiration channels were added. We then miniaturized Wilson's original PhacoExcavator instrument by reducing the outer diameter to 1.65 mm (Figure 1). This made it compatible with the available full-function unimanual and 2-port vitrectomy probes advocated by Machemer (7). To increase its cutting efficiency, the excavating tip was fit with 3 sharp blades each 30 gauge in size. In order to satisfy the surgeons using Steve Charles' 3-port technique, the infusion channel was designed as a removable sleeve. Two types of sleeves were made, a 1.65 mm diameter metallic type (Figure 2A) for pars plana entry and a 2.0 mm diameter soft silicone type for surgeons favoring the anterior limbal entry (Figure 2B).

Thus, the PhacoExcavator can also be used as a 19 gauge instrument. In this case, a separate infusion cannula is needed to maintain the IOP at normal level. A spring loaded mechanism was added to automatically shield the blades for both the protection of delicate tissues at the surgical entrance site and the sharpness of the blades. To avoid spinning the nucleous, the rotation speed of this second generation instrument was set to 9,000 cycles per minute (8). In a 3rd generation, we made the PhacoExcavator fully autoclavable for fast reuse, further increased its speed to 12,000 cycles per minute, and designed it to fit commonly available aspiration sources. To avoid power system

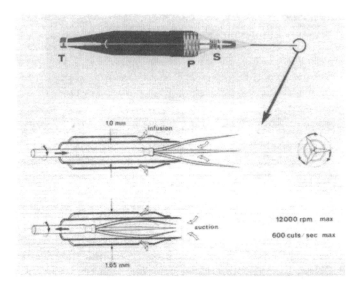

Figure 1. 3rd and 4th Generation PhacoExcavator Handprobe. Both instruments have identical outside appearances. In the 4th generation, the infusion sleeve has a diameter of 1.0 mm instead of 1.65 mm and an internal diameter of 0.65 mm instead of 1.0 mm. S: Spring return mechanism of the blade shield; P: Retractable finger platform to unshield the blades; T: Infusion, aspiration and electrical supply lines termination.

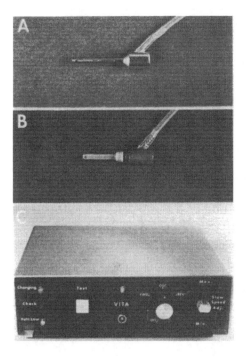

Figure 2. Photograph of the Infusion Sleeves and Power Unit. A: Pars plana 1.65 mm stainless steel infusion sleeve (3rd generation only); B: Limbal 2.0 mm silicone infusion sleeve (Kelman type); C.: Experimental power module designed to achive speeds of over 18,000 cycles per minute.

redundancy, the PhacoExcavator was designed so that its electrical power could be provided by commercially available VISC-X and VITAC multi-purpose power modules (Figure 2C).

The third generation PhacoExcavator prototype was then tested surgically. In Indianapolis, Dr. Wilson performed an experimental double blind clinical trial in 30 rabbits (Figure 3). Cornea endothelium cell count and histopathology tests were conducted in these animal eyes. This trial proved the PhacoExcavator safe for human use. Since then, Dr. Wilson has utilized the PhacoExcavator in all his pars plana vitrectomy cases requiring lentectomy. Wilson's surgical technique is very different from that pioneered many years ago by Dr. Charles Kelman. Instead of prolapsing the nucleous in the anterior chamber and then proceeding with its ultrasonic emulsification, in Wilson's technique, the excavation of the nucleous is performed in situ or "in the bag" (Figure 3B and 3C). The anterior and posterior capsule surfaces are maintained intact while the nucleous is excavated by the instrument. Hence the anterior chamber, and in particular the cor-

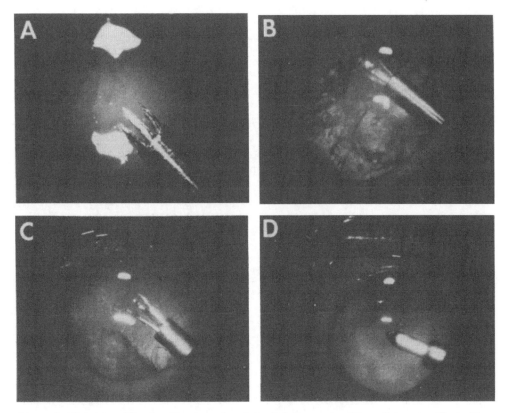

Figure 3. High Magnification Photographs of the 3rd Generation PhacoExcavator Tip in Use. A: Blades' integrity and rotation speed inspection before entering the eye; B: Start of the excavation process in a rabbit nucleous; C: Cortex remnant (lower left) at the end of the excavation process; D: Posterior capsule and cortex removed with VITAC III (TAC handpiece) fitted with the 1.65 mm diameter infusione sleeve. The anterior capsule is intact.

neal endothelium and iris structures, are protected during the excavating process. The posterior capsule and the remnant cortex are then removed with a commonly available 1/A handpiece or, as Dr. Wilson suggests, with a vitrectomy instrument (Figure 3D). The surgeon can then elect to remove the anterior capsule at the end of the lentectomy or after completing his vitrectomy.

In my opinon, the above technique is the logical solution to fluid-silicone vitreous substitution. An intact anterior capsule could provide the ideal barrier to the silicone bubble. Together with the remnant pars plana vitreous base, the anterior capsule could be a protecting agent against silicone infiltration in the anterior chamber. An intact anterior capsule might prevent silicone induced band keratitis and glaucoma.

In order for us to gain further clinical knowledge, two additional models of the PhacoExcavator 3rd generation were constructed and sent for clinical testing by Dr. Machemer, Chairman of the Duke University Eye Center and by Dr. O'Grady of the Veterans Administation Hospital Miami Center. Both surgeons reported that the PhacoExcavator performed as succesfully as the ultrasonic or mechanical instrument counterparts they were using prior to these tests.

CONCLUSION

The above information shows that we provided the vitreous surgeon with another modality for pars plana lentectomy, but this instrument was still too large. We had not solved the Phaco-Ersatz dilemma. In addition, further "in vitro" tests performed on cadaver eyes in our laboratory under very high magnification demonstrated that the 3rd generation prototypes could still induce the spinning of fragments of a partially excavated nucleous. Thus, additional modifications were made. The outer diameter of the instrument was further reduced to 1.0 mm (19ga) and the three 30 gauge moving elements were replaced with 33 gauge stainless steel triangular shaped blades. In addition, the blade rotation speed was increased to 18,000 cycles per minute. With this 4th generation PhacoExcavator prototype, we are able to excavate and remove a lens nucleous through a 1 mm hole performed near the equator of a rabbit lens in less than 5 minutes.

ACKNOWLEDGMENTS

David Denham, M.S., and William Lee provided many of the technical refinements and fabricated the Phaco-Excavator prototype handpieces. Izuru Nose, B.S., designed and fabricated the electronical control systems. Barbara French, B.A., prepared the illustrations. Marilyn Maxwell, M.B.A., wrote this paper in English. I am grateful to Dr.E.W.D. Norton for his continued support.

REFERENCES

1. Kelman CD (1975): Phacoemulsification and aspiration: the Kelman Technique of cataract removal. Birmingham, AL, Aesculapius.

2. Olson LE, Marshall J, Rice, NSC and Andrew, R (1978): Effects of ultrasound on the corneal endothelium: I. The acute lesion. Brit J Ophthalmol 62:134-244.

3. Girard LJ and Hawkins RS (1974): Cataract Extraction by Ultrasonic Aspiration. Vitrectomy by Ultrasonic Aspiration. Trans Am Acad Ophthalmol Otolaryngol 78:1.

4. Shock JP (1976): Phacofragmentation and Aspiration. Ann Ophthalmol 8:591.

5. Machemer R and Aaberg TM (1979): Vitrectomy. 2nd edition, New York, Grune and Stratton.

6. Parel J-M, Treffers F, Gelender H and Norton EWD (1981): Phaco-Ersatz: A New Approach to Cataract Surgery. Ophthalmology, 88 (9s): 95.

7. Machemer R (1984): 2-Port Technique. Presented at the Duke Advanced Vitreous Surgery Course, III. Durham, NC. April.

8. Wilson DL, Parel J-M and Egnatz T (1982): Phacoexcavator. Ophthalmology, 89: 187.

Basic and advanced vitreous surgery
G.W. Blankenship, M. Stirpe, M. Gonvers, S. Binder (eds.)
Fidia Research Series, vol. II,
Liviana Press, Padova © 1986

PNEUMATIC FORCEPS FOR THE REMOVAL
OF EPIRETINAL MEMBRANES

M. Stirpe M.D. and Ing. M. Orciuolo

Fondazione Oftalmologica 'G.B. Bietti', Piazza Sassari, 5, Roma

During the removal of epiretinal membranes, it is frequently easier, after elevating the edge of the membrane with a hooked needle, to use forceps for the complete removal of the membrane. The ordinary forceps used in this operation are not very effective because the membranes break easily and because they easily slip from the grasp of ordinary forceps. Moreover, for a safe removal, and in order to avoid lesions in the retina, it is necessary to alternately grasp and release the membrane and to apply the forceps constantly very near the point at which the membrane is attached to the retina. When the membrane is partially detached, the free portion frequently moves so as to cover the point at which the membrane should be correctly grasped for its safe removal.

For this reason, and in order to remove the detached portion of the membrane, pneumatic forceps have been devised (Fig. 1). The membrane is caught by aspiration

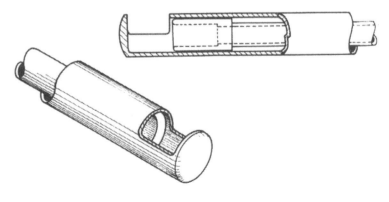

Figure 1

and grasped between two smoothed jaws. The piston inside the actuator, unlike that of other actuators, can move forward or backward with the same force, which is also high, due to the fact that the pressure of the inlet gas is at 9 Bar.

Such high force, applied to the inner movable jaw of the forceps, has the advantage of strongly grasping the membranes without any manual effort of the operator. Manual forceps have, in fact, the disadvantage of requiring strong manual pressure of the surgeon; but many times the membrane nevertheless slips out.

The advantages of pneumatic forceps for the removal of epiretinal membranes are:

1) the possibility of grasping the membrane at the point of adhesion to the retina;

2) the possibility for the surgeon to grasp and release the membrane without difficulty, because the forceps are run by foot control;

3) the possibility of keeping the field constantly free from the portion of the elevated membrane, which is aspirated into the cannula of the instrument;

4) the possibility of exerting a very solid hold on the membrane.

Basic and advanced vitreous surgery
G.W. Blankenship, M. Stirpe, M. Gonvers, S. Binder (eds.)
Fidia Research Series, vol. II,
Liviana Press, Padova © 1986

MECHANICAL SYSTEMS FOR IRRIGATION AND SUCTION OF HIGH VISCOSITY SILICONE OIL

Ing. Manfredi Orciuolo

Fondazione Oftalmologica 'G.B. Bietti', Piazza Sassari, 5, Roma

Among the various methods of tamponade, silicone oil is the most valid. The surgeon can utilize it when dealing with a particularly complex retinal situation that requires a prolonged tamponade in the vitreous chamber. In the past one of the most serious problems was the manipulation of the silicone oil; however, this does not create a problem anymore.

Silicone oil (dimethylpolysiloxane) is a very viscose liquid and the one we use has a value of 3000 centistokes.

First of all let us try to explain the concept of viscosity of a liquid. Viscosity is the property of a liquid that creates resistance to the flowing of two different layers of such liquid. Such resistance can be described:

$$R = \mu \times \frac{\Delta V}{\Delta Y}$$

Where μ is the dynamic viscosity, $\Delta V/\Delta Y$ is the quantity of volume "V" displaced for the space "Y". The unit of measurement of the dynamic viscosity is the Poise. However, the kinematic viscosity is much more frequently utilized because it can better define these properties.

The kinematic viscosity is the quotient between dynamic viscosity and density (mass of the unit of volume). The unit of measurement of viscosity is the Stock, which is divided in centistocks.

Let us now examine the problems connected with the use of silicone, and describe the different surgical techniques for its infusion.

SILICONE OIL INFUSION IN A NON VITRECTOMIZED CLOSED EYE
AS A METHOD TO DETACH EPIRETINAL MEMBRANES

The technique consists of the insertion of an 18 gauge or less needle via pars-plana. A port is opened in the epiretinal membrane under direct ophthalmoscope observation, through which silicone oil is injected. The injection of silicone oil underneath the membranes detach them further.

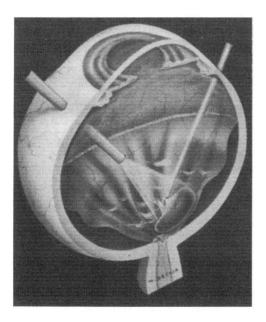

Figure 1. Infusion of silicone oil under the membranes.

LIQUID-AIR-SILICONE EXCHANGE

In some cases after vitrectomy it is necessary to proceed with a liquid-air-silicone exchange.

We start from a 3-port surgery: Irrigation (hr 4 or 7), instrument and optical fibers at hr 2 and 10. The instrument is an 18-gauge cannula with a suction control (flute cannula).

Forced irrigation (SURGIKON) is then turned from physiological solution to sterile air. The evacuation procedure is controlled through the microscope with a special air-lens. The bulb is emptied with positive pressure with no aspiration till the papilla-macular region is perfectly dry.

The instrument has to be withdrawn, the nasal incision is closed, and a provisional suture is tied on the temporal side. Air infusion is stopped, and a 14-gauge needle is inserted controlling it through the pupil. This procedure does not require a microscope.

Silicone oil is injected, and the scleral incision allows outflow of a sufficient quantity of air. At this point the eye has to be turned to have the needle on the top for a complete fill. During this procedure the ocular pressure has to be continuously con-

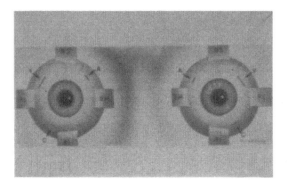

Figure 2. Position of incision on both eyes.

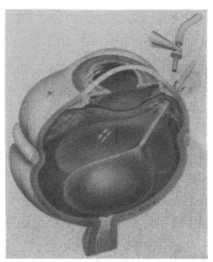

Figure 3. Silicone-air exchange.

trolled with a Schiotz or Perkins tonometer. When silicone oil appears around the needle, the exchange may be considered accomplished. However, some air may remain at the highest level; in this case it is advisable to open the temporal suture and let the air flow out. The same procedure may be used if one of the two paths is partially obstructed with vitreous. The final suture is now prepared and can be tied, with the eye at the correct pressure, after a little adjustment of the volume of the oil.

DIRECT LIQUID-OIL EXCHANGE

For this kind of exchange we need a particular two-port needle that can aspirate at the end and inject silicone oil laterally in the desired direction. Moreover, the needle is equipped with a hole that closes and opens. We start with a 3-port surgery.

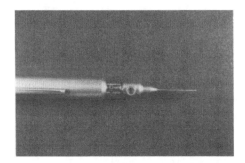

Figure 4. Cannula for direct exchange of liquid-oil.

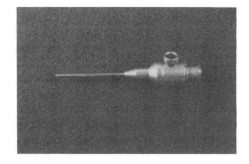

Figure 5. Assembled syringe with direct exchange liquid-oil cannula.

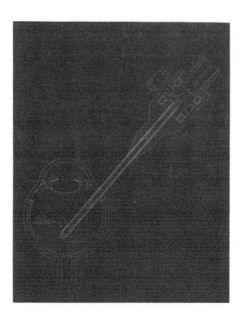

Figure 6. Use of the cannula for direct exchange of liquid-oil.

The special needle and the optical fiber have to be inserted in the vitreous cavity. The infusion hole is positioned by rotating the body of the needle to ease the retinal distension.

At this point the liquid irrigation is stopped and silicone oil is injected. The exchange is now only volumetric, because the solution and silicone are exchanged at equal volumes. The vitreous cavity liquid flows out of the hole, and when this does not happen, irrigation has to be immediately stopped. It should be controlled through a microscope so that the retina does not close the port of suction, causing an increase of pressure and a dangerous incarceration.

THE PNEUMATIC SYRINGE FOR INJECTION OF SILICONE OIL

The instrument has the following characteristics:
— Possibility of the use of very thin needles
— Easy to handle, just like a vitrectome
— Very light
— Possibility of different flow rates
— It can be sterilized
— Interchangeability of tips

The project specifications that we included in the instrument after the first experiences are the following:
— Volumetric capacity 6-14 cc.
— Max. irrigation pressure 10 kg/cm^2
— Source of gas pressure commonly used in a surgical theatre CO_2 or N_2O
— Standard connection (luer lock) either for needles or fittings.

The irrigation syringe is composed of a stainless steel cylinder of appropriate

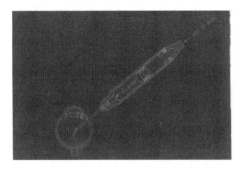

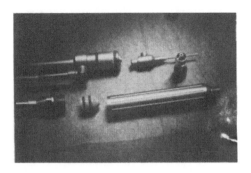

Figure 7. Section view silicone oil injection with pneumatic syringe.

Figure 8. Disassembled pneumatic silicone oil injection syringe.

thickness which contains a teflon piston sliding inside and designed to separate the fluid from the gas. The base is closed by a locknut and connected to the source of pressure by a small tube.

The front side of the syringe has a luer-lock fitting to accept the various needles required during surgery. Before connecting the cannula, the syringe must be loaded with silicone oil. The oil is first placed into a conventional syringe without any needle, and then the conventional syringe is connected to the front luer-lock fitting.

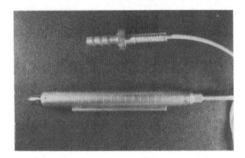

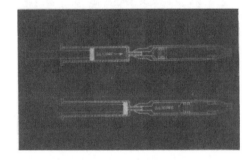

Figure 9. Silicone oil level indicator.

Figure 10. Silicone oil filling procedures.

By pushing the piston of the plastic syringe, the oil is easily injected into the pneumatic syringe until completely filled. At this time the operator can attach the cannula of choice. As explained previously, the source of power which activates the piston of the syringe is the compressed gas used in cryo units. To bring pressure down to lower levels, a pressure reducer is placed between the cryo unit and the syringe. A second model of this syringe can be connected to the special vitrectomy unit made by Optikon, which is already provided with the appropriate value of pressure for such application.

The use of the syringe is very simple:
1. Place the piston into the sterile body of the syringe.
2. Connect the syringe to the source of pressure (either the cryo or the VITREON unit).
3. Activate the piston and fill the syringe as explained previously.
4. Connect the required cannula and activate the syringe to remove the air from the cannula.

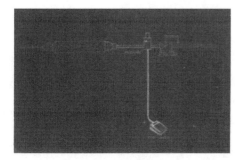

Figure 11. Silicone oil infusion system illustrated diagrammatically.

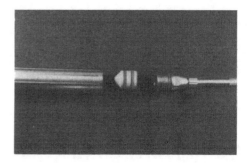

Figure 12. Piston insertion to the syringe's posterior.

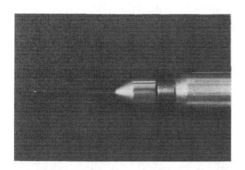

Figure 13. Silicone oil syringe tip.

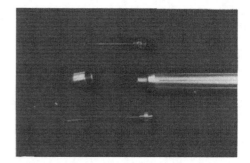

Figure 14. Disassembled syringe tip.

SAFETY PROCEDURES DURING IRRIGATION

It is important to notice that the irrigation of oil is performed at high pressure. In fact, if irrigation is performed into a closed volume, its pressure could reach the supply pressure (10 bar).

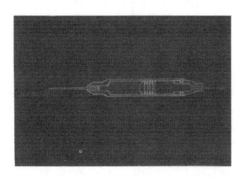

Figure 15. Silicone oil infusion.

In surgery, therefore, the irrigation of oil must be constantly performed under control of the eye pressure. The flow of irrigation can be adjusted in 3 different ways:
1. By changing the pressure of the gas which supplies the piston.
2. By varying the application time
3. By varying the size of the cannula
    During surgery points 2 and 3 are frequently applied.

Before surgery the operator can select the proper cannula to obtain the required flow. During surgery the operator can press the foot-switch on and off to obtain a perfect control of irrigation even when using large needles.

SILICONE OIL REMOVAL

The oil can be easily removed by performing a sclerotomy on the upper part of the operating field. Since oil is lighter than water, it will easily flow out, specially if an appropriate injection of BSS is performed via pars plana.

This manoeuvre can be dangerous to the structures of the eye (i.e., lens opacities), taking into account that these eyes have been already operated many times. A more advanced method consists in the direct aspiration of the oil under microscopic observation. A proper fiber optic illumination will allow the operator to see those membranes, which, compressed by oil, were sometimes invisible.

Opening two or three ports can avoid the loss of liquids as the exchange with the cannula remains strictly volumetric and the stability of the bubble at the tip of the cannula allows the operator to remove the oil completely.

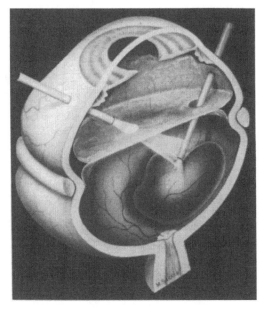

Figure 16. Silicone oil removal under the membranes.

Basic and advanced vitreous surgery
G.W. Blankenship, M. Stirpe, M. Gonvers, S. Binder (eds.)
Fidia Research Series, vol. II,
Liviana Press, Padova © 1986

PRE-VITRECTOMY ASSESSMENT BY ULTRASOUND

Pier Enrico Gallenga and Antonio Rossi*

Istituto di Oftalmologia, Università G. D'Annunzio, Chieti.
*Clinica Oculistica, Università di Ferrara

The first extensive monograph on vitreous body B-scan echography was presented by G. Bellone at the 1968 International Symposium on Ultrasound in Ophthalmology, organized in Turin by Professor Riccardo Gallenga.

Ten years before, A. Oksala had published in the American Journal of Ophthalmology his "Investigations on the structure of the vitreous body by ultrasound", using a Krautkrämer Impuls-Schallgerät Usip 9 with 4 MHz transducer.

At the time, we were in a position to make the diagnosis but had no possibility of surgical confirmation except in cases submitted to enucleation.

The true advance in quality was represented by contact B-scan with the instruments created by Bronson and Coleman which permit accurate topographic diagnosis, and by Ossoinig's standardized A-scan which is particularly suitable for differential diagnosis of tissues.

As a matter of fact, echographic diagnosis and vitrectomy have advanced together in a relationship of mutual dependence in so far as surgical verification during the latter lends support to the data presumed on the basis of the former, while the former in its turn allows progressively more precise indication, choice of approach, and prognostic orientation.

The purpose of presurgical echographic assessment is to detect, localize, differentiate, and determine the size and type of every interface that produces reflections observable in the vitreous chamber.

Oksala (1966) correlated the importance of vitreous opacities to the functional impairment:

— high echoes in the whole vitreous chamber: visual acuity 1/20 or less;
— low echoes in a quarter of the vitreous chamber: v.a. 1/10 to 5/10;
— minimal echoes or acoustic silence: v.a. ≥ 5/10.

DETACHMENT OF RETINA

Small tractional detachments are easily detected by B-scan while extensive ones which occupy one or several quadrants are best differentiated by A-scan.

Used concurrently, A-scan and B-scan have an over 80% probability of assuring correct diagnosis (Ossoinig, 1983). Differential diagnosis from membranes is based on differences in reflection as compared to scleral echo (selective echography, Oksala, 1962); see Ossoinig's classical table (1977) (Table 1), for which a standardized A-scan instrument is necessary (at present: Kretzechnik 7200 MA and Sonokretz Cilco-Sonometrics).

Table 1. *Quantitative echography II*

RETINA 100%		MEMBRANE >95%
6-15	BORDERLINE	20-36
>90%	16	<10%
~60%	17	~40%
~40%	18	~60%
<10%	19	>90%

△ DB = DIFFERENCE in decibels between maximal echoes from LESION and SCLERA of same eye

Ossoinig, 1977

When finding the T-shaped B-scan image described by Machemer as the pathognomic sign of MPP, the M-mode study of aftermovements of the intravitreal structure examined may be added: as shown by Cennamo (1983), vitreous membranes oscillate more than the retina which is all the more rigid the more it is involved in PVR.

POSTERIOR HYPHEMAS

These pools of fluid blood and serum are usually found in the retro-hyaloid space of the lower sector.

The posterior hyaloid lacquered blood/liquid interface is highly reflective and has often been confused with an inferior retinal detachment; it is however possible to arrive at a differential diagnosis "showing the strongly reflecting surface of the fluid blood (which resembles detached retina) in a strictly horizontal orientation (displayed with a sound beam aligned strictly perpendicular in space), and a typical shift of this strongly reflective surface toward the lowest fundus portion following a change in gaze direction or head tilt" (Ossoinig, 1983).

Using B-scan, it is sometimes possible to visualize the passage of the interface over the optic disk and thus to exclude retinal detachment.

Ossoinig (1983) also listed in this table, which he presented at the 24th International Congress of Ophthalmology in S. Francisco, the diagnostic possibilities of echography (standardized A-scan and B-scan) for the presurgical study of patients who might be submitted to vitrectomy (Table 2), as well as information essential for the planning of surgical strategy (Rossi and Gallenga, 1980).

Table 2. *Some of the conditions of the vitreous, retina, and choroid that can be determined with standardized echography prior to vitrectomy (Ossoinig, 1983)*

A. Vitreous
  1) Clear
  2) Opaque
    a) Morphology
      Homogeneous

	Mild	>0.1	
Density	Moderate	<0.1	Corresponding vision or
	Dense	<0.05	visibility of fundus
	Very dense	LP only	

      Dust-like (dispersed)
      Pseudomembraneous (eg, layered blood, veils)
      Membraneous (fibrovascular membranes; also bands, strands)

    b) Density   Thickness   Mobility

Tiny	Thin	Freely mobile
Moderate	Thick	Mobile
Dense	Compact	Reduced mobility (inserting into disc, retina, vitreous base)
Very dense	Fluffy	Immobile (stiff)

    c) Type
      Typical for hemorrhage (fresh vs. old)
      Pockets of fluid blood
      Typical for inflammatory changes (eg, peripheral uveitis vs. endophthalmitis, abscess, etc.)
      Cyclitic membranes
      Asteroid hyalosis
      Cholesterol crystals
      Synchysis scintillans
      Non-specific
    d) Distribution, location (eg, preretinal vs. midvitreal, posterior vs. peripheral, etc.)
  3) Detached
      Partially
      Subtotally (funnel-shaped posterior vitreous surface)
      Totally (retracted vitreous)
B. Subvitreal Space
  1) Clear
  2) Opaque
      Dust-like opacities (regarding implications for vision or visibility of fundus, see above)

	Mild
Density:	Moderate (sandstorm possible)
	Dense (sandstorm likely)
	Very dense (sandstorm likely)

Continued next page

Table 2. *Some of the conditions of the vitreous, retina, and choroid that can be determined with standardized echography prior to vitrectomy (Ossoinig, 1983)*

      Posterior hyphemas
    Height—measured in mm
    Quality—Thin (easy to remove)
              Thick (sticky)
              Corpuscular (sandstorm likely)

C. Retina-Choroid

  1) Within Normal Limits

  2) Thickening of Retinochoroid Layer
      Diffuse regular (eg, in hypotony)
      Nodular (eg, in endophthalmitis)
      With inserting membrane or band traction

  3) Retinal Folds

  4) Retinal Detachment
      Type
        Idiopathic
        Hemorrhagic
        Traction (tent-like, etc.)
      Height—measured in mm
      Localization
      Extent
        Small
        Large
        Subtotal
        Total (funnel shaped)
          Open funnel
          Narrowly open funnel
          Triangular detachment
          Closed funnel (T-shaped detachment)
      Quality
        Smooth surface
        Folded
        Thickened
        Thinned
      Mobility
        Mobile
        Poorly mobile
        Fixed (MPP)
      Occasional findings
        Large holes
        Ora disinsertion
        Rolled edges

  5) Retinoschisis

  6) Choroidal Detachment
      Type
        Serous
        Hemorrhagic
      Height—Measured in mm
      Location—peripheral, meridians involved, etc.
      Extent—Small peripheral vs. large, "kissing," etc.

Continued next page

Table 2. *Some of the conditions of the vitreous, retina, and choroid that can be determined with standardized echography prior to vitrectomy (Ossoinig, 1983)*

D. Subretinal and Subchoroidal Space
  1) Clear
  2) Opaque
      Hemorrhagic (fluid blood) (regarding implications for vision or visibility of fundus, see above)

      Density
        Mild
        Moderate
        Dense
        Very dense

      Hemorrhagic (coagulated blood)
      Cholesterol crystals
      Posterior hyphemas (rare)
      Subretinal membranes

Among this information, there is also data concerning the morphology of the anterior chamber which may be impossible to explore, e.g. in the presence of large leukomas or anterior chamber hyphema (these may mask abnormal situations: cfr. the case reported by R. Gallenga in the 13th Cavara Lecture, 1969) which may mask open traumatic cataracts or the presence of foreign bodies. However, most of the data deal with the morphology of the posterior segment.

The dicotomy between the "grass effect" in the vitreous body's A-scan examination, seen as "starring sky" in M-mode, and the inaccessibility to the ophthalmoscope due to vitreous colliquation is an unfavorable prognostic sign (Gallenga, 1973) and can be an indication for vitreous substitution (Rossi and Gallenga, 1981).

The vitreous, retrovitreal space, retina, subretinal and subchoroidal spaces can be investigated and a variety of pathological situations can be detected with different degrees of approximation. Until alternative non-invasive techniques of equally low cost and high specific *sensitivity* (correctly diagnosed cases as a percentage of those histologically and surgically proven pathologies in which a definite echographic diagnosis has been arrived at), *accuracy* (correctly diagnosed cases as a percentage of all histologically and surgically verified cases), and *reliability* (comparison of all positive echographic diagnoses with histological and surgical results) compared to new techniques - PETT, NMR, last generation CT - become available, echography will play a central role in pre-operative assessment as well as in post-operative follow-up and monitoring of the eye, also on account of the ease with which it can be repeated without undue discomfort to the patient, and finally in view of its highly positive cost/benefit ratio.

REFERENCES

1. Bellone G (1968): Studio ultrasonotomografico del corpo vitreo. In Gallenga R: Atti Simposio internazionale sulla diagnostica ultrasonica in Oftalmologia, Torino, p. 153-310, Italseber.
2. Bronson NR, Turner FT (1973): A simple B-scan ultrasonoscope. Arch Ophthal 90:237.
3. Cennamo G (1983): Diagnostica endobulbare. X Corso di tecnica e diagnostica ultrasonica in oftalmologia, Chieti.

4. Coleman DJ, Lizzi FL, Jack RL (1977): Ultrasonography of the Eye and Orbit. Lea Febiger, Philadelphia.
5. Gallenga PE (1973): Echographic classification of diseases of vitreous body. In Massin M, Poujol J: Diagnostica Ultrasonica in Oftalmologia, p. 183-188, Paris.
6. Gallenga R (1970): L'ultrasonografia diagnostica in Oculistica. Lectura ad V. Cavara Memorandum. Archivio e Rass It Oftal 1:9.
7. Gallenga R, Bellone G, Gallenga PE, Pasquarelli A (1971): Ultrasonografia clinica dell'occhio e dell'orbita, SOI.
8. Jack RL, Hutton WL, Machemer R (1974): Ultrasonography and Vitrectomy. Am J Ophthal 78:265.
9. Oksala A (1958): Investigations on the structure of the vitreous body. Amer J Ophthal 46:361.
10. Oksala A (1962): About selective echography in some eye diseases. Acta Ophthal Kbh 40:466.
11. Oksala A (1966): Development and significance of ultrasonic diagnosis in eye diseases. Ultrasonic in Ophthalmology, Munster 1:21.
12. Ossoinig KC (1983): Advances in diagnostic ultrasound. In P Hend: Acta XXIV Int Congr Ophthal, Lippincot.
13. Rossi A, Gallenga PE (1980): Ruolo dell'ecografia nella strategia della chirurgia vitreo retinica. Int Conf on Retinal Detachment, Roma.
14. Rossi A, Gallenga PE (1981): Importance of ultrasound in cataract surgery and visual rehabilitation. In François J, Maumenee AE, Esente I: Cataract Surgery and Visual rehabilitation. Milano, Ghedini, p. 53-59.

Basic and advanced vitreous surgery
G.W. Blankenship, M. Stirpe, M. Gonvers, S. Binder (eds.)
Fidia Research Series, vol. II,
Liviana Press, Padova © 1986

PREPARATION OF THE PATIENT FOR VITRECTOMY SURGERY

Harry W. Flynn, Jr., M.D.

The Bascom Palmer Eye Institute, Department of Ophthalmology,
University of Miami School of Medicine, Miami, Florida

Following the preoperative evaluation, preparation is started for vitreous surgery. This preparation includes a discussion regarding the benefits and risks of vitreous surgery (informed consent), selection of anesthesia, and medical consultation in many cases. This review will discuss the special preparations required for vitreous surgery.

INFORMED CONSENT

Since vitreous surgery has significant risks and is performed only on eyes with advanced disease, informed consent is an important part of patient preparation (1, 2). A brief discussion regarding the potential benefits of vitreous surgery, as well as possible complications, is included in this consent. The expected length of operating time, the length of hospital stay, and any special requirements (e.g. face-down positioning with intraocular gas) should also be discussed with the patient prior to vitreous surgery. The operative permit serves as documentation of the patient's informed consent for vitreous surgery.

SELECTION OF ANESTHESIA

Local or general anesthesia may be used for vitreous surgery. After evaluation of the ability of the patient to cooperate and review of the extent of the surgical problem by the vitreous surgeon, the patient may be allowed to participate in the decision for the type of anesthesia (3).

Local anesthesia with intravenous administration of sedatives can be used in the majority of patients undergoing vitreous surgery. Local with sedation anesthesia usually allows a shorter recovery period and is less likely to cause metabolic imbalance, which is particularly important in diabetic patients. General anesthesia is required for children and for patients unable to cooperate for the necessary time to complete vitreous surgery.

THE ROLE OF THE ANESTHESIOLOGIST

Because the length of operating time in vitreous surgery may be uncertain, the anesthesiologist should be involved in the administration of anesthesia for all patients having vitreous surgery. Whereas patients undergoing standard cataract extraction may have only local anesthesia, patients having vitreous surgery should be monitored by an anesthesiologist or by an experienced nurse anesthetist under supervision. The anesthesiologist will select the appropriate preoperative medications and will maintain an adequately sedated yet cooperative patient during local with sedation anesthesia.

THE ROLE OF THE INTERNIST

Consultation with an internist may be necessary for patients with advanced systemic illness. Minimal laboratory studies include complete blood count, urinalysis, electrocardiogram (in patients over 40), and chest x-ray. Based on the preoperative physical examination and laboratory studies, the internist will advise the vitreous surgeon regarding the patient's ability to tolerate the surgical procedure. Diabetic patients are often admitted to the hospital two days prior to vitreous surgery in order to evaluate and control the blood glucose levels under the supervision of the internist.

LOCAL ANESTHESIA WITH INTRAVENOUS SEDATION

Local with sedation anesthesia permits vitreous surgery on patients who would be at high risk for general anesthesia. The choice of anesthetic for regional block is variable, but most surgeons prefer to use a combination of short and long acting anesthetic agents, with hyaluronidase added. Lidocaine (Xylocaine 4%) and Bupivacaine (Marcaine 0.75%) is a commonly used combination of short and long acting anesthetic agents. The exact mixture of these agents may vary between 1:1 to 1:3, depending on physician preference. Lidocaine is rapid in onset of action but may last only one hour or less. Bupivacaine has a slower onset effect but may last several hours. Bupivacaine has been reported to cause sudden respiratory arrest and rarely endotracheal intubation may be necessary in patients receiving retrobulbar injection of this medication (4).

A facial nerve block may be achieved by a variety of standard techniques (5). In the Van-Lint technique, injection of subcutaneous anesthetic is given along the lateral margin of the orbital wall with the injections superiorly and temporally. In the O'Brien technique, injection is given anterior to the external auditory canal.

Retrobulbar administration of anesthetics requires the use of a one and one-half inch (38 mm) needle, which is usually a blunt tapered-tip needle or a disposable ''flat grind'' 23 gauge needle. The needle is introduced through the skin of the lower lid at the inferior lateral third of the orbital rim. The needle is directed posteriorly and towards the apex of the orbit. The syringe is tested by withdrawal of the plunger to rule out the possibility of venous penetration of the needle tip. Four to five milliliters of anesthetic is usually necessary for prolonged anesthesia and akinesia required in vitreous surgery.

GENERAL ANESTHESIA

General anesthesia is used in younger patients, in patients with an open ocular wound, and in patients unable to cooperate for the length of time required for vitreous surgery. The drawbacks of general anesthesia include a longer postoperative recovery period and the inability of the patient to cooperate by head positioning during vitreous surgery.

PREOPERATIVE MEDICATIONS

Preoperative medications are given to the patient to relieve anxiety and induce sedation. For general anesthesia, the preoperative medications are also necessary to achieve appropriate drying of secretions. Preoperative medications are selected by the anesthesiologist based on the general health and age of the patient. These medications are used to achieve a cooperative but calm patient ready for the administration of local anesthetic injections or for the induction of general anesthesia. The preoperative medications are intended to begin the sedation, but should not cause the patients to become disoriented or drowsy to the point that they cannot cooperate with the administration of local anesthetic injections.

Both active external ocular infections and systemic bacterial infections represent contraindications to vitreous surgery. External ocular infections should be treated with appropriate medications and become quiescent before undertaking vitreous surgery. Likewise, active systemic infections, such as an infection of extremities in diabetic patients, is usually a contraindication for vitrectomy. Vitreous surgery can be rescheduled after the infection has resolved.

Prophylactic preoperative antibiotics are not used by most vitreous surgeons. Since trimming lid lashes may reduce postoperative lid matter accumulation, many surgeons prefer to trim lashes before vitreous surgery.

THE HOLDING ROOM

The holding room, which is a part of the operating room, is an area for the final prepartion for vitreous surgery. An intravenous line is started, blood pressure readings are obtained, and electrocardiogram monitor leads are placed appropriately. In the holding room, the adequacy of pre-medications should be assessed and additional intravenous sedatives may be administered. Following evaluation of the patient by the anesthesiologist or the nurse anesthetist in the holding room, regional anesthetic injections are given. Adverse reactions to previous anesthetic agents or local injections can be observed prior to moving the patient into an individual operating room.

SPECIAL SITUATIONS

Patients with open ocular wounds undergoing vitreoretinal surgery usually require general anesthesia. Certain muscle relaxants used to facilitate intubation (e.g. succinylcholine) may cause a transient rise in intraocular pressure, presumably due to a contraction of the extraocular muscles. The anesthesiologist should be informed of the status of the eye and the need to avoid succinylcholine in patients with an open ocular wound.

Patients with a giant retinal tear may be required to change position during the operative procedure and local with sedation anesthesia may be preferable. With this patient cooperation and ability to change position on the operative table, the surgeon can perform an intraoperative fluid-gas exchange, with the patient in the face-down position. When a specialized rotating table is required in these cases, the anesthesiologist should be familiar with maneuvers using this operating table (6).

OPERATING ROOM PREPARATIONS

The patient's head is positioned in order to reduce instrument obstruction from facial prominences. This can be achieved by rotating the face slightly toward the opposite eye. The operative field is prepared in the standard fashion prior to application of self-adhering drapes. Topical anesthetics are also administered in the fellow eye in the event that inadvertent skin soap enters the fellow eye during preparation of the field for vitreous surgery.

A solid ring support is placed around the head of the patient to serve as a wrist rest during vitreous surgery (7). This ring also serves as a water trough, collecting excess irrigating fluid during surgery and acts as a site for temporary placement of instruments.

PUPILLARY DILATION

Maximum pupillary dilation is necessary for vitreous surgery. This dilation can be achieved by the use of Phenylephrine 10% drops and Cyclogyl 1% drops every 15 minutes four times prior to vitreous surgery. If the pupil is not adequately dilated, additional topical medications may be applied in the holding room prior to surgery.

OPERATIVE PREPARATIONS

The operating microscope is focused on the eye and the lateral movements of the microscope are tested. The viewing axis of the operating microscope is oriented vertically in order to permit a maximum view of the posterior segment. A wire speculum is most commonly used during vitreous surgery.

Vitrectomy instrumentation should always be checked for adequate function before vitreous surgery begins. The scrub nurse can observe the vitrectomy instrument for grossly correct performance but the surgeon must actually inspect the intrument under the operating microscope before entering the tip of the instrument into the eye (8).

The operating field should be set up in a manner familiar to the surgeon and the scrub nurse. A Mayo Stand over the patient's chest is a convenient way of displaying hand instruments. The assistant may sit on the same side of the patient as the eye undergoing surgery. The consoles and power pack for the vitrectomy instruments can be brought in from the opposite side.

REFERENCES

1. Bettman JW (1982): The issue of informed consent. Surv Ophthalmol 27:133-135.
2. Wells WT (1984): The surgeon's duty to warn of risks. Lancet, 8388:974.
3. Michels RG (1984): Vitreous surgery. In: Ophthalmic Surgery. Rice TA, Michels RG, Stark WI (eds). CV Mosby, St Louis, 1984, p. 222.
4. Beltranena HP, Verga M, Garcia J, Blankenship G (1982): Complications of retrobulbar marcaine injection. J Clin Neuro-Ophthalmol. 2:159-161.
5. Bron AJ, McKenzie PI (1984): Ocular anesthesia. In: Ophthalmic Surgery. Rice TA, Michels RG, Stark WI (eds). CV Mosby, St Louis, p. 11.
6. Machemer R, Allen AW (1976): Retinal tears 180° and greater: Management with vitrectomy and intraocular gas. Arch Ophthalmol 94:1340-1346.
7. Machemer R, Aaberg TM (1979): Vitrectomy. Grune and Stratton, New York, 1979, pp. 33-35.
8. Charles S (1981): Vitreous Microsurgery. Williams and Wilkins, Baltimore, pp. 21-31.

Basic and advanced vitreous surgery
G.W. Blankenship, M. Stirpe, M. Gonvers, S. Binder (eds.)
Fidia Research Series, vol. II,
Liviana Press, Padova © 1986

VITRECTOMY TECHNIQUES
FOR THE ANTERIOR SEGMENT SURGEON

Walter J. Stark, M. Bowes Hamill, Ronald G. Michels,
Arlo C. Terry, John D. Gottsch, Peter A. Rapoza

The Wilmer Ophthalmological Institute
Johns Hopkins Hospital, Baltimore, Maryland, 21205, U.S.A.

Since the introduction and development of the operating microscope by Harms in 1953 (1) and Barraquer in 1956 (2) an array of surgical tools, equipment, and technology has been added to the ophthalmic armamentarium. Examples include the microinstrumentation developed for cataract surgery (particularly for extracapsular extraction and intraocular lens techniques) and, importantly, microinstrumentation for surgical manipulation and management of the vitreous.

Vitrectomy instrumentation, however, is not applicable solely to the posterior segment. It can provide the anterior segment surgeon with a variety of new capabilities, namely, 1) "a closed-eye" system which maintains the normal configuration of the globe and allows the surgeon to control intraocular pressure and thereby decrease intraoperative bleeding. 2) It affords precise control for "bite by bite" excision of tissue. 3) It provides the capability for removal of lens material and other tissues from the anterior segment. 4) It provides unique capabilities for intraocular manipulation such as intraocular bipolar cautery. These techniques are the preferred management methods for some anterior segment conditions, and as alternates to currently used methods in other situations (Table 1).

INSTRUMENTATION

There are three major components of vitrectomy systems currently in use. These components are the cutter, the aspiration system, and the infusion system. Two major subgroups of cutters are available, rotary and oscillating or guillotine cutters. We prefer the oscillating or guillotine type cutters because they are not as prone to cause traction, a potential problem with the rotary systems.

Table 1

---

1. *Vitreous in the anterior chamber*
   a. vitreous loss in cataract surgery
   b. endothelial vitreous "touch"
   c. aphakic pupillary block
   d. vitreous incarceration in wound with persistent CME (Irvine-Gass)
   e. vitreous "wick"
   f. vitreous and glaucoma filtering procedures

2. *Inadequate pupillary opening*
   a. capsulo-lenticular membrane
   b. opacified posterior capsule
   c. other pupillary membranes

3. *Lens surgery*
   a. complicated cataract
   b. PHPV
   c. IOL-membrane formation
   d. retained lens fragments
   e. subluxed lens
   f. posterior IOL displacement

4. *Epithelial downgrowth*
   a. sheet-like
   b. cystic

5. *Hyphema*
   a. total hyphema

6. *The glaucomas*
   a. phacolytic
   b. aphakic pupillary block
   c. hemolytic

7. *Vitrectomy in keratoplasty*

Adapted from Taylor, Michels, and Stark. Methods in Anterior Segment Surgery. Ophthal Surg Vol 10, No. 10, Oct. 1979 p. 262.

In regard to the aspiration system, we have found it important to vary the suction according to the tissue cutting requirements. For example membranous tissue requires little suction, while thicker tissues require higher suction. Therefore, it is important to have a system with variable aspiration.

The infusion system may be introduced through a separate incision or through the same incision as the cutter via an infusion sleeve. The infusion system maintains the shape of the globe during excision and aspiration, and helps to control intraocular bleeding with incision of vascular tissues. When bleeding occurs, increasing the infusion elevates the intraocular pressure and maintains hemostasis.

TECHNIQUE

As in all surgical procedures, the specific technique depends upon the desired objective and the individual situation facing the surgeon. In general, the site of instrument entry for anterior segment techniques depends on the needs and preferences of the surgeon. We have generally found the limbal approach to be preferable when the procedure involves tissues and structures located anterior to the pupillary-lenticular plane. Conversely, the pars plana approach seems to work best for extensive vitrectomies, posterior tissue excision, or when fiberoptic illumination is required. In all cases, however, the technique is tailored to the specific situation.

VITREOUS IN THE ANTERIOR CHAMBER

The most common use for vitrectomy instrumentation in anterior segment surgery involves the removal of vitreous from the anterior chamber, usually during cataract extraction. With vitreous loss during intracapsular cataract extraction, the vitrectomy cutter is a valuable alternative to the "blot and cut" vitrectomy method. In the case of vitreous prolapsing through the wound, vitreous may first be excised by the "blot and cut" method utilizing ophthalmic sponges and scissors, taking care to avoid vitreous traction.The vitrectomy instrument can then be placed in the pupillary space for the removal of the remaining vitreous.

Following removal of vitreous from the anterior chamber, the vitrectomy instrument can be removed, and air placed in the anterior chamber to move the iris leaflets and vitreous face posteriorly. The anterior chamber may be checked for residual vitreous by identifying pupillary irregularities which may be caused by adherent vitreous strands. Any remaining vitreous may be removed by sweeping the surface of the iris or by reinserting the vitrectomy instrument. Following removal of residual vitreous, the wound edges should be blotted again and the wound closed.

During extracapsular surgery, vitreous most commonly presents following rupture of the posterior capsule. It may be removed from the wound using the sponge and scissors technique and the wound may then be closed and an anterior vitrectomy performed. (Cortical lens fragments are also easily removed with the vitreous cutter). Finally, an air bubble is placed in the anterior chamber, the wound is checked for adherent vitreous, and the wound is closed.

Endothelial vitreous touch with secondary corneal edema is readily eliminated using vitrectomy instrumentation. The authors limit surgical intervention to eyes with minimal corneal edema centrally and pre-existing endothelial disease such as Fuch's dystrophy. Corneal edema should be clearly demonstrable prior to surgical intervention, as not all vitreous touch results in edema. A pars plana or limbal approach may be utilized, and an anterior vitrectomy is performed to clear all vitreous from the anterior segment. An air bubble is placed in the anterior chamber in order to check for vitreous remnants and the wound is closed.

Tissue cutting and removal is greatly simplified by the use of vitrectomy techniques. Most tissues are soft and easily excised and aspirated. With dense tissue, however, it is helpful to first cut the tissue into segments with a knife or intraocular scissors and then excise and aspirate the remaining strips of tissue. Alternately, a two instrument technique may be employed, where in the tissue is supported from beneath with the cutter and is directed towards the cutter with a second instrument located anterior to the tissue. This technique works well with non-pliable tissues in locations which are accessible under direct visualization.

Specific instrument settings are given as guidelines, but each case should be evaluated individually. In general, when extracting vitreous, a fast cutting speed between 350-400 cycles per minute is recommended. This reduces the amount of vitreous traction because only a small portion of the vitreous tissue is drawn into the cutting port at any given time. In removing lens material, a slow rate of about 50 cycles per minute is efficacious as it allows time during the cycle for lens to be aspirated deep into the cutting port before the cutter acts. For cutting membranes, a moderately slow speed between 50 and 100 is used. Generally, stiffer tissues require slower cutting speeds, while tissues such as vitreous that may produce retinal traction should be cut at high speeds (3).

The port (or opening in the vitrectomy instrument) should initially be adjusted to one-half maximal aperture and re-adjusted as necessary. For vitreous cutting, a small opening is preferred (approximately 1/4 to 1/2 full opening), so that when used in combination with a fast cutting speed and low suction, small bites are taken. For membranes, the cutter should be adjusted so as to allow the tissue to fill the port and minimize concurrent fluid aspiration. By doing this, cutting efficiency is maximixed while the amount of circulating fluid passing in and out of the eye is kept to a minimum. The opening must be monitored and adjusted as different densities and types of tissues are encountered.

Hemostasis during vitrectomy procedures is achievable by two methods. The first is by elevation of intraocular pressure by raising the irrigating bottle (Table 2). High intraocular pressures for a sustained length of time should be avoided, however, as vascular catastrophies may result. If bleeding is not controllable by manipulation of intraocular pressure, bipolar cautery can be utilized. One lead of the bipolar circuit is attached to each of the two vitrectomy instruments in the eye and current is passed from instrument tip to instrument tip. This technique is especially helpful in situations such as cauterization of the hyaloid remnant in surgery for persistent hyperplastic primary vitreous. With bleeding in the filtering angle, one can cauterize across the eye by placing one instrument in the angle and the second instrument in a corresponding position on the external eye wall passing a current through the tissues.

Vitreous "wick" is a condition in which vitreous has prolapsed through either a surgical incision or a suture tract and presents outside the eye wall. This condition may be associated with irritation or secondary infection along the fistulous tract, or epithelial downgrowth through the opening. The treatment involves removing the vitreous and closing the fistula. External vitreous is excised with sponge and scissors following which a limited pars plana anterior vitrectomy is performed. Following

Table 2. *Increase in intraocular pressure*

IOP (mm Hg)	bottle height above eye	
	cm	in
1	1.36	1/2
15	20.4	8
20	27.2	10
30	40.8	16
40	54.4	21
50	68.0	24
60	81.6	30

Stern, W.H., Diddie, K.R., Smith, R.E. Vitrectomy techniques for the anterior segment surgeon, a practical approach. Grune and Stratton. NY, 1983, pp. 24.

vitrectomy and instillation of air into the anterior chamber, the tract should be opened slightly and the edges debrided prior to closing. This technique has been successfully employed by the authors in a number of cases.

Vitreous prolapse through a glaucoma filter may result in non-function of an anatomically good filtration fistula. An anterior vitrectomy can be performed either at the time of original filtration surgery, or as a separate procedure. It has been our experience that a separate pars plana vitrectomy with removal of anterior vitreous (especially superiorly) prior to the performance of the filtration surgery has been very successful. Another possible approach is the removal of vitreous with the vitrectomy cutter through the filtration fistula or through a separate limbal incision. Using the filtering tract as an entrance wound has some hazards, however, as the cutting tip is not always visable and vitreous posterior to the iris is difficult to remove.

PUPILLARY MEMBRANES

In an eye with an opaque pupillary membrane, a goal is to create an opening that is optically and cosmetically acceptable. A 4 to 5 mm opening improves visual function and allows adequate visualization of the fundus. Larger openings may cause the patient discomfort secondary to photophobia. The pupillary opening may be placed eccentrically in order to avoid corneal opacities or resection of dense fibrotic or vascular areas within the membrane.

The irrigation and cutting instruments are introduced into the anterior chamber through separate limbal incisions and the membrane is excised. Sufficient protruding vitreous should be removed to prevent postoperative vitreous prolapse. Following removal of the pupillary membrane, anterior vitreous displacement may be prevented by introducing air into the anterior chamber. The air pushes the iris and remnants of the pupillary membrane and vitreous face posteriorly. Following wound closure the air is replaced with saline. Vitreous prolapse may be detected by direct visualization or by peaking of the pupil.

Aphakic pupillary block occurs due to obstruction of the pupillary space and iridotomies by the vitreous face with subsequent posterior dissection of the aqueous humor. Vitreous continues to move anteriorly with ongoing production of aqueous, resulting in shallowing of the anterior chamber and eventual obliteration of the filtering angle. The initial therapy for this condition is medical and involves the use of nydriatics and hyperosmotic agents to attempt to relieve the pupillary block. Unfortunately, medical therapy is frequently ineffective, especially in cases where irido-vitreal adhesions have formed. Argon laser peripherial iridotomy may relieve this condition, but in the event that this is unsuccessful, vitrectomy is effective. The surgical goal is to excise the anterior vitreous and create a communication with posteriorly localized aqueous. Removal of vitreous also prevents subsequent attacks of pupillary block and glaucoma. A knife incision of the anterior vitreous face, via a limbal entrance, is sometimes effective,but often a pars plana vitrectomy is required. A central vitrectomy is performed, and a posterior vitreous detachment is frequently present. The posterior vitreous face can often be excised in the mid vitreous as it moves forward. Removal of the central vitreous core is curative. Following vitrectomy, air may be injected through a small limbal incision in order to separate the iris from the cornea and reform the anterior chamber.

Vitreous incarceration in the wound with persistent CME (the "Irvine-Gass" syndrome), is felt to result from vitreous traction. The role of vitrectomy in this condition is as yet unproven, but in the authors' experience, approximately 70% of patients regain vision following vitrectomy. Several factors need to be assessed in planning the surgery. The surgeon should ascertain whether or not vitreous is actually incarcerated in the wound, and CME should be demonstrable by fluorescein angiography. The authors prefer to perform surgery on patients whose vision is decreased to 20/80 or worse, and whose visual acuity has been decreased for nine months or longer. Improved visual acuity following a systemic steroid trial suggests a good prognosis for improved vision following vitrectomy (4).

The surgical approach is usually via the pars plana, although a limbal approach may be employed. All vitreous adherent to the iris and wound, as well as all cloudy or turbid vitreous, is removed. In considering the surgical procedure, careful attention should be paid to the location of vitrectomy instruments. The surgeon should attempt to introduce the instruments 90° from the adherent vitreous so that all vitreous strands present can be adequately engaged in the cutting port. When removing the vitreous, iris movement, such as jerking of the iris during cutting, indicates vitreous adhesions. Cessation of iris movement upon cutting is a good indication that adherent vitreous has been removed. Following anterior vitrectomy the surgeon should do a sweep of the anterior iris surface in order to free any iridocorneal vitreous connections that may remain. In our experience, patients operated for Irvine-Gass syndrome generally show a decrease in CME over 12 to 24 months following surgery.

LENS SURGERY

Vitrectomy techniques can be a valuable adjunct in cataract surgery, not only in the management of complications, but also as a technique to remove the lens primarily. Generally, vitrectomy techniques are reserved for subluxated or disrupted lenses, or for soft cataracts. The pars plana approach helps to avoid posterior dislocation of the lens. Cortical material and soft nuclear material are readily aspirated through the vitrectomy instrument. When dense nuclear material is encountered, the nucleus must be removed via a separate limbal incision.

Complicated cataracts generally involve extensive synechia and membrane formation, and removal of vitreous is frequently necessary. In eyes with microcornea, a pars plana approach may significantly decrease the risk of intraocular complications as well as avoid intraoperative damage to the corneal endothelium. The pars plana approach may also be used in cases of compromised endothelium resulting from Fuch's dystrophy or previous corneal injury. In performing lensectomy through the pars plana in an eye with endothelial compromise, the posterior capsule and lens should be removed first and the anterior capsule last, utilizing minimal irrigation in order to avoid further damage to the cornea. Vitrectomy is performed as required.

Persistent hyperplastic primary vitreous is a condition characterized by cataract and retrolenticular membrane. Surgery is usually not indicated in mild cases or is limited to an optical iridectomy in eyes with clear areas of lens and retrolenticular space. With significant involvement of the lens and optical axis, however, lensectomy and removal of the retrolenticular membrane is generally required. Because of the narrow pars plana in these eyes, and the possible pre-existing peripheral retinal detachment, the preferred approach is limbal. The goal is aspiration and removal of the lens and excision of the retrolenticular membrane which releases traction on the ciliary proceses. In these cases bipolar cautery is frequently helpful in order to close bleeding vessels of the ciliary processes, and to seal the central hyloid artery.

Retained lens fragments may be removed directly by utilizing vitrectomy techniques. Although most retained cortical fragments reabsorb spontaneously, in some cases it may be preferable to remove them surgically. When using a limbal approach, removing vitreous near the vitreous base or attempting a "core", vitrectomy should be avoided. In the event that firm nuclear fragments are encountered, these can be removed through a separate limbal wound.

A limbal approach may be technically difficult for excision of very dense membranes such as those occurring secondary to organization of retained lens or traumatic cataract. In such cases, it is generally necessary to cut the membrane with a knife or with scissors in order to create an edge which vitrectomy instruments can engage. The membrane may be cut either in strips or in a stellate fashion, and the resulting pupillary membrane excised with the vitreous cutter.

The pars plana approach is used when anterior vitrectomy must be performed. The surgeon should attempt to remove the vitreous and the central posterior vitreous surface in the mid vitreal cavity, and if a posterior vitreous detachment is present, the central posterior vitreous surface should be incised. As in the limbal approach, it is necessary to avoid vitreous prolapse from the entry wounds, and in the event that vitreous does prolapse through the incision, it can be picked up with a sponge and cut flush with the surface of the globe, following which the remaining vitreous is repositioned within the globe prior to suturing.

The "chopping block" technique is generally reserved for very dense pupillary membranes. In this technique, the irrigating instrument is introduced through a limbal wound, and the vitrectomy instrument is introduced through a pars plana incision. The pupillary membrane can then be directed into the cutting port of the vitrectomy instrument by the infusion instrument.

Removal of pupillary membranes by vitrectomy instrumentation has been found to be superior to other methods such as simple incision. By removing the tissue rather than simply incising it, the surgeon prevents the regrowth or reattachment of the membrane, and obviates the need for further surgery.

The most common pupillary membrane encountered is the opacified posterior capsule. Capsular opacification occurs frequently following extracapsular cataract extraction, and even if the posterior capsule is cleaned or "polished" at the time of surgery, it frequently becomes opaque because of proliferation of lens epithelium. In dealing with the opacified posterior capsule, vitrectomy techniques may be used as an alternative to discission with the Neodynium: YAG laser. This may be necessary in cases where retained lens material has resulted in a membrane too dense for laser discission. Other pupillary membranes such as those secondary to chronic uveitis or to resolution of hyphemas can also be excised in a similar fashion.

Subluxed lenses are occasionally encountered. If the lens is intact causing no inflammation, the management is generally conservative. If inflammation or glaucoma ensues, then removal of the lens is required. If the lens is in the anterior chamber, it may be removed with a cryoprobe. However, if the lens is disrupted and soft, removal with vitrectomy instruments through the pars plana is the preferred method of extraction.

EPITHELIAL INGROWTH

Epithelial ingrowth is a serious complication of intraocular surgery or trauma. Ingrowth generally occurs in one of two forms, sheet-like or cystic. Sheet-like epithelial ingrowth involves a thin layer of epithelial cells growing over the endothelium, iris, and/or ciliary body. The surgical treatment of these cases involves removing all of the accessible epithelium and killing all of the remaining epithelial cells with cryosurgery. Using a pars plana approach, the vitrectomy instrument is introduced into the anterior segment and the involved iris and the vitreous is excised down to the iris root. The fistula is closed and following air injection into the anterior chamber (which acts as a thermal insulator) the cryoprobe is placed over the areas of the downgrowth, and two cycles of freezing and thawing are employed to kill the epithelial cells.

In the cases of cystic epithelial involvement, the indications for surgery are a decrease in visual acuity secondary to blockage of the optical axis, or secondary complications arising from the cyst. It should be noted, however, that even the most careful surgical excision of these cysts may be followed by the development of a secondary sheet-like membrane with its attendant complications. The surgical technique in volves complete removal of the cyst without rupture. However, if the cyst is adherent to the iris or to the endothelium, such complete removal may be impossible.

In such cases, a needle is first introduced into the cyst to attempt decompression and the collapsed cyst is excised, following which secondary cryotherapy is applied.

HYPHEMA

Surgical treatment of hyphema is reserved for those eyes suffering from total or "eight ball" hyphemas with increased intraocular pressure and corneal blood staining. Ideally, surgery should be performed prior to the onset of corneal blood staining. The surgical technique is one of lavaging blood from the anterior chamber. This can be achieved by creating separate irrigation and aspiration entrances on either side of the anterior chamber and gently rinsing the anterior chamber. The vitrectomy cutter can then be used to excise any free clot that remains. Caution should be advised, however, as visualization is frequently difficult. Clot that remains adherent to the iris and does not easily rinse loose should be left in place because severe bleeding may result from its removal.

THE GLAUCOMAS

The glaucomas most amenable to treatment with vitrectomy techniques include aphakic pupillary block glaucoma and hemolytic or "ghost cell" glaucoma. In ghost cell glaucoma, the trabecular meshwork is blocked by the cellular remnants of lysed red blood cells migrating anteriorly from a vitreous hemorrhage. In these cases, if the pressure is not controllable with medical therapy, a limited anterior vitrectomy may be performed in an attempt to remove the offending cell membranes, and thus alleviate the glaucomatous condition.

Phakolytic glaucoma is a condition in which slow leakage of lens protein from a mature cataract may cause inflammation and secondary intraocular pressure rise. The treatment of choice for this disorder is removal of the lens either by intracapsular or extracapsular technique or by lens removal with vitrectomy instrumentation.

VITRECTOMY IN KERATOPLASTY

During keratoplasty in the aphakic eye, it is frequently necessary to remove anterior vitreous which is present in the anterior chamber. This can be performed most easily via the open sky technique following removal of the host corneal button. Irrigation is unnecessary in this technique as the vitreous meniscus provides an indication of the amount of vitreous remaining. It is generally recommended that the vitrectomy be extended well posterior to the iris diaphragm, almost to the equator, to prevent subsequent anterior movement of the vitreous in the postoperative period.

SUMMARY

Vitrectomy techniques and instrumentation have been used successfully to treat a number of conditions in the anterior segment. These include: 1) vitreous in the anterior chamber, 2) inadequate pupillary openings, 3) lens surgery, 4) epithelial downgrowth, 5) hyphemas, and 6) certain glaucomas. These methods offer several advantages to the anterior segment surgeon. The advantages are primarily those of a well-controlled tissue excision system, maintenance of the normal shape of the globe, and ability to control intraocular pressure.

ACKNOWLEDGMENTS

This work was supported in part by the Women's Committee of the International Medical Eye Bank of Maryland.

REFERENCES

1. Harms H, Ber (1953): Dtsch Ophthal Ges, 58, 119.
2. Barraquer JI, Amer J (1956): Ophthal, 42, 916.
3. Stern WH, Diddie KR, Smith, RE (1983): Vitrectomy techniques for the anterior segment surgeon, a practical approach. Grune and Stratton, NY, pp. 24.
4. Orth DH, Henry MD (1978): Current concepts of cataract surgery, selected proceedings of the fifth cataract surgery, retinal congress, Emery J, (ED) St Louis, CV Mosby, p 375.

Basic and advanced vitreous surgery
G.W. Blankenship, M. Stirpe, M. Gonvers, S. Binder (eds.)
Fidia Research Series, vol. II,
Liviana Press, Padova © 1986

THE CORNEA AND VITREOUS SURGERY

Severino Fruscella, Piero Ducoli and Giustino Boccassini[*]

Fondazione Oftalmologica 'G.B. Bietti', Piazza Sassari, 5, Roma
[*]Divisione Oculistica, C.T.O., Via S. Nemesio, Roma

The most common problems involving the cornea in vitreous surgery during the operation and the post-operative period will not be taken into account, but instead we will be dealing with particular and less frequent pathological conditions concerning the cornea during vitrectomy. Sometimes, these pathological situations may go beyond the specific field of the posterior segment, and therefore require the collaboration of a corneal surgeon. In other cases, the resolution of the pathology of the posterior segment may facilitate a probable surgery of the anterior segment.

The following pathological situations will be taken into consideration:
1) Cicatricial retrolental fibroplasia: the cornea is removed because of vitreous surgery requirements.
2) Corneal leukoma in an eye that is to be vitrectomized: a corneal transplant is performed using the temporary Landers keratoprosthesis.
3) Corneal bullous keratopathy as a consequence of vitrectomy or caused by silicone oil: a corneal transplant is performed in order to avoid corneal opacity that may occur after vitreous surgery.
4) Vitreous in the anterior chamber: a vitrectomy is performed in order to prevent the formation or extension of corneal opacities.

DISCUSSION

Cicatricial retrolental fibroplasia

Cicatricial retrolental fibroplasia represents a very particular condition in which, according to our experience, the cornea must be removed because of vitreous surgery requirements. In these cases, surgery is performed in two stages: in the first stage, open sky vitrectomy is performed after having removed the cornea and the lens. In the second stage, some months later, a closed vitrectomy through the pars plana is undertaken.

As a result of the particular anatomical conditions of the retina in this pathologic situation (Fig. 1), it will be noted that the insertion of the instruments through the pars plana may produce serious lesions of the peripheral retina, whereas the insertion of the instruments through the ciliary body may be harmful for this structure. It is for this reason that, during the first stage, we prefer to perform open sky surgery through the corneal aperture. After having removed the cornea and the lens, it will be easier to release the peripheral retina.

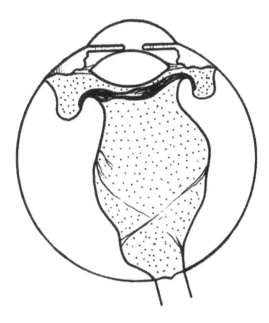

Figure 1. For the particular anatomical condition assumed by the retina in cicatricial retrolental fibroplasia, one may note that the insertion of the instruments through the pars-plana may produce serious lesions of the peripheral retina.

The operating steps are as follows: a corneal button of 8 mm diameter is removed and preserved in M.K. medium at +4 degrees centigrade during the entire procedure; the lens is removed, and the retrolental membrane is detached in order to release and remove the epiretinal proliferations on the anterior surface which cause the retina to shrink. In this way the retina acquires a certain mobility again. The previously detached corneal button is then sutured with a continuous suture and some air is let into the anterior chamber. We do not evacuate the subretinal liquid.

It is obvious that in the open sky technique the lens must necessarily be removed. On the other hand, for this kind of pathology, also during a closed vitrectomy, lensectomy must always be performed, otherwise it would be impossible to remove the retrolental membrane and the anterior epiretinal proliferations without the risk of a cataract. The air in the anterior chamber causes a backward retinal displacement, due to the fact that the retina has been released from the membranes which cause it to shrink on the anterior surface. During this step, retinal reattachment is not achieved, but only a backward displacement of the retina. However, this gives us the possibility, some months later, to perform another vitrectomy, this time through the pars-plana to release residual proliferation tissue and therefore facilitate retinal reattachment.

We will not deal with the post-operative results and the problems related to the posterior structures because they go beyond the subject we are examining; however, we will indeed be considering the problems related to the cornea. Our study is very limited because we only dealt with three cases with a 6 to 12 months follow-up.

The corneal problme we had to face was the following: can the cornea of an infant of a few months undergo an auto-transplantation and then, after some months, undergo another surgical trauma caused by a posterior closed vitrectomy? The surgical trauma of the first operation produced by the incision and the suture of the cornea did not cause any alteration of corneal transparency. Indeed, it is interesting to note that already during the immediate post-operative course, the corneal edema was very limited and certainly smaller than the one we observed in adult patients submitted to cornea transplantation. Probably, this means that the endothelial pump is more effective.

Also after the second operation, vitrectomy through the pars-plana, we did not have any problems with corneal transparency in spite of the vitrectomy performed on eyes which had become aphakic as a result of the previous surgery; therefore, on these eyes, the corneal endothelium was in contact with the infusion liquids. Because of the age of the patients, we could not perform any instrumental study, so that our evaluation is based only on corneal transparency.

Corneal leukoma

Another particular situation is that of a corneal leukoma that hampers the observation of the posterior structures.

In case of pathology involving also the posterior segment and requiring vitrectomy techniques, we find it helpful to use the temporary Landers Keratoprosthesis. This acrylic lens has a lateral thread and it is available in diameters of 6.2 and 7.2 mm.; the corneal aperture will consequently be 6.0 and 7.0 mm and the corneal button to be transplanted will have diameters of 6.5 and 7.5 mm.

Without describing in detail the surgical techniques, we will briefly say that, after having removed the pathological button of the cornea, the keratoprosthesis is placed in the corneal aperture and fixed with two sutures. Vitrectomy is then performed visualizing the internal structures through the above-mentioned lens. Once vitrectomy has been completed, the Landers keratoprosthesis is removed. At this point the transplant with the corneal donor button may be accomplished.

This technique allows an immediate operation in pathological situations involving the posterior segment, which otherwise would have to be operated some weeks after corneal transplantation. In fact, it is not possible to perform vitrectomy in an eye with a recently transplanted cornea because corneal edema hampers the focalization of the posterior structures. In these cases, an open sky vitrectomy can be performed; however, not all surgeons are in favour of or are familiar with this technique. It is well known that, if we postpone for a few weeks the surgery of these eyes which underwent penetrating trauma, we will usually have to face a process of vitreal organization caused by vitreoretinal proliferation. This may create some problems for the anatomical and functional recovery of the eye.

In conclusion, we may affirm that when facing this type of pathology, the use of a Landers lens is the most appropriate solution, even if vitrectomy may not be perfectly performed because the focalization of the posterior structures is more difficult, and also because, when operating, we do not achieve a good overall view of the structures.

Corneal bullous keratopathy

When vitrectomy involving the posterior segment is performed on a phakic eye through the pars-plana, the corneal endothelial cells will not be negatively affected. A possible secondary corneal lesion caused by the surgical manoeuvres heals during the immediate post-operative course. In this way, the situation is not worsened by vitrectomy even when dealing with pathological corneas.

The situation is different if vitrectomy through the pars-plana is performed on an aphakic eye. In this case, the infusion liquid comes into contact with the corneal endothelium and may cause an alteration of the endothelial cells. Such a lesion will be related to the vitality of the patient's endothelial cells, to the physiochemical properties of the infusion liquid, and to how long liquid and corneal endothelium remain in contact. Sometimes, particularly when dealing with corneas which already underwent trauma or have a limited cell population, we may be faced with bullous keratopathy as a consequence of an endothelial deficiency.

In these cases the only therapy is perforating keratoplasty. The surgical technique performed for this kind of pathology and the post-operative results are the same as for a bullous keratopathy provoked by other causes. When facing such a keratopathy it is better to operate soon to prevent the prolonged corneal edema that may cause neovascularization. In fact, as is well known, the percentage of rejection increases if the transplantation is performed on a vascularized cornea.

Another problem we had to deal with is the one related to corneal bullous keratopathy as a consequence of contact with silicone oil. If silicone oil injected during or after vitrectomy does not come into direct contact with the corneal endothelium, it will not cause any corneal alterations. This is also true if silicone oil is kept in the eye for a long period of time. Silicone oil was kept in the eyes of twelve patients for more than a year without coming into contact with the cornea and did not cause any change in corneal transparency. On the contrary, direct contact between the cornea and silicone oil may provoke endothelial deficiency perhaps due to mechanical trauma to the endothelial cells.

We have performed a corneal graft in three patients who were suffering from keratopathy provoked by silicone oil. The preoperative clinical picture showed a modest corneal bullous epitheliopathy, marked stromal edema with remarkable reduction of the transparency and folds of the Descemet membrane (Figs. 2 and 3). Naturally, silicone oil had been previously removed and replaced with air or saline solution. The surgical technique and the post-operative course were the same for all cases of corneal bullous keratopathy. We have a follow-up of 22, 19 and 17 months respectively. The corneal button of the first two patients maintained its transparency during the entire follow-up period, whereas the eye of the third patient, although there had not been any intra-

or post-operative complications, did show a relapse of the bullous keratopathy which began 11 months after surgery and reached its maximum 14 months after surgery. At that time the clinical picture was that of a typical bullous keratopathy.

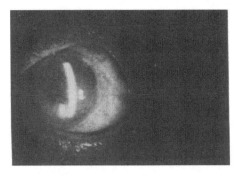 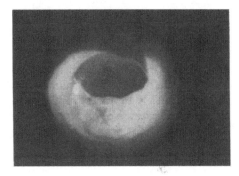

Figures 2 and 3. Preoperative and post-operative clinical picture of a keratopathy provoked by silicone oil.

We are unable to determine exactly the reason for this relapse, but since the eye did not show any alteration that might have explained this pathology, we are of the opinion that this depended on the state of the corneal button of the donor. However, this statement calls for further investigation.

Vitreous in the anterior chamber

A corneal keratopathy may be caused by vitreous in the anterior chamber. In these cases, an immediate anterior vitrectomy may prevent a possible corneal bullous keratopathy as an consequence of an endothelial lesion. If faced with this situation, when the cornea is still transparent, it is difficult to decide whether it is better to wait or to perform surgery in order to remove the vitreous in the anterior chamber. If it is possibile to perform a cell count, it will be better to proceed with surgery if under the endothelial microscope a progressive decrease in the number of endothelial cells is observed. A surgical procedure may be avoided if no such decrease is found. However, it is important to remember that the vitreous, with an open anterior hyaloid, is less harmful to the cornea than contact between the anterior hyaloid and the corneal endothelium. Obviously, another point to consider is the extent of the contact. When having to deal with a surgical procedure, we will decide whether it will be more appropiate to perform vitrectomy through the limbus or through the pars-plana.

We will be facing a different situation if the vitreous not only is in the anterior chamber, but also presents a certain tendency to fibrous organization. This may be the consequence of a corneal perforating lesion with incarceration of the vitreous, and lenticular and iridal residues in the cornea. In these cases, it will always be appropriate to perform surgery in order to prevent the possible complications caused by a fully developed vitreous organization: large corneal opacities, glaucoma as a result of the shallowing of the anterior chamber, hypotony provoked by the detachment of the ciliary body, retinal dialysis, traction retinal detachment and subatrophy of the bulb.

It is very important to determine the appropriate moment to proceed with surgery, because we usually have to deal with eyes which present very acute inflammation in process. If the time between trauma and vitrectomy is too long, the vitreous undergoes a process of organization and retraction; we already mentioned above the various consequences of this process. Immediate surgery on an eye congested by the recent trauma might create some problems. In our opinion it is better to wait a few days and to perform surgery a week after the trauma. Although the eye still suffers from strong congestion, the risk of new hemorrhages is reduced, and it is better to proceed with surgery, because otherwise, if the vitreous undergoes a process of retraction and organization, we will certainly be faced with further problems.

In these cases, we will not only have to perform anterior vitrectomy so as to release corneal adhesions, but will also have to remove the entire vitreous in order to prevent further proliferation.

CONCLUSION

The pathological situations discussed explain how, in particular cases, it is necessary for surgeons specialized in different ocular fields to work together. Indeed, in some situations such as cicatricial retrolental fibroplasia or corneal leukoma in an eye that is to be vitrectomized, the corneal surgeon will have to repair possible damage caused by posterior surgery. In other cases, that is, when the vitreous is in contact with the corneal endothelium or in the presence of vitreous strands incarcerated in a corneal lesion, vitreous surgery might prevent the formation of corneal opacities or even facilitate future corneal surgery.

LITERATURE

1. Tasman W (1979): Retinal detachment in retrolental fibroplasia. Albrecht von graefas Arch Klin Exp Ophthalmol 195-129.
2. Mc Pherson A and Hittner HM (1980): Scleral buckling in 2 and a half to 11 month old premature infants with retinal detachment associated with acute retrolental fibroplasia. Ophthalmology 86-819.
3. Kalina RE (1980): Treatment of retrolental fibroplasia. Surv Ophthalmol 89-651.
4. Lightfoot D and Irvine R (1982): Vitrectomy in infants and children with retinal detachment caused by cicatricial retrolental fibroplasia. Am J Ophthalmol 94-305.
5. Landers MB, Foulks GN, Landers DM et al (1981): Temporary keratoprosthesis for use during pars-plana vitrectomy. Am J Ophthalmol 91-615.
6. Carrol DM (1983): Instrument for placement of temporary keratoprosthesis during pars-plana vitrectomy. Am J Ophthalmol 95-718.
7. Groden LR, Arentsen JJ (1984): Penetrating keratoplasty following the use of a temporary keratoprosthesis during pars-plana vitrectomy. Ophthalmic Surg 15-208.
8. Muenzler WS, Narms WK (1981): Visual prognosis in aphakic bullous keratopathy treated by penetrating keratoplasty. A retrospective study of 73 cases. Ophthalmic Surg 12-210.
9. Burraquer J (1979): Keratoplasty in Fuchs' dystrophy and bullous keratopathy. Am J Ophthal 88-333.

10. Pollack FM (1979): Keratoplasty in aphakic eyes with corneal edema. Results in 100 cases with 10 years follow-up. Trans Am Ophthalmol Soc. 77-657.

11. Waring GI III, Welch SN, Cavanagh ND, Wilson LA (1983): Results of penetrating keratoplasty in 123 eyes with pseudophakic or aphakic corneal edema. Ophthalmology 90-25.

12. Benson WE and Machemer R (1976): Severe perforating injuries treated with pars-plana vitrectomy. Am J Ophthalmol 81-728.

13. Faulborn J, Atkinson A and Oliver D (1977): Primary vitrectomy as a preventive surgical procedure in the treatment of severely injured eyes. Br J Ophthalmol 61-202.

14. Ryan SJ and Allen AW (1979): Pars-plana vitrectomy in ocular trauma. Am J Ophthalmol 88-843.

15. Coleman DJ (1982): Early vitrectomy in the management of severely traumatized eyes. Am J Ophthalmol 93-543.

Basic and advanced vitreous surgery
G.W. Blankenship, M. Stirpe, M. Gonvers, S. Binder (eds.)
Fidia Research Series, vol. II,
Liviana Press, Padova © 1986

MANAGEMENT OF COMPLICATED CATARACTS USING VITRECTOMY INSTRUMENTS

John D. Gottsch, Walter J. Stark, Arlo C. Terry, M. Bowes Hamill, Peter A. Rapoza

The Wilmer Ophthalmological Institute, The Johns Hopkins Hospital, Baltimore, Maryland 21205, U.S.A.

Complicated congenital cataracts such as those associated with persistent hyperplastic primary vitreous (PHPV) were previously thought to be inoperable. However, utilizing the instrumentation and techniques developed for pars plana surgery (1, 2, 3) we are now able to successfully treat a variety of problems affecting the anterior segment. These techniques utilize a "closed eye" system which maintains the normal configuration of the globe and provides normal or elevated intraocular pressure during surgery. Modern instrumentation permits precise control for excising intraocular tissue, enabling one to remove lens material without damaging other tissues. Direct visualization of intraocular structures is provided by fiberoptic intraocular illumination. Other techniques such as intraocular diathermy may be used to dissect tissue planes. Herein we present the surgical techniques we have utilized in treating PHPV, our postoperative results, and our views on the surgical management of uncomplicated congenital cataracts.

SURGICAL MANAGEMENT

In advanced cases of PHPV, the cataract is removed and the retrolenticular fibrovascular mass excised, relieving traction on the ciliary body and creating a clear pupillary space. A limbal approach provides adequate access to the retrolenticular membrane and is preferred in micro-ophthalmic eyes because the area of the pars plana is narrow or non-existent. An incision is made through the limbus with a Ziegler knife and the anterior lens capsule is incised. Next, a 20 gauge infusion needle is placed in the anterior chamber nasally, and the vitrectomy instrument is introduced temporally (Figure 1). The soft lens material is then removed by aspiration or excision before any attempt is made to excise the pupillary membrane or formed vitreous.

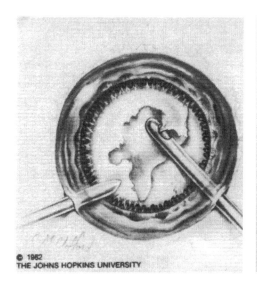 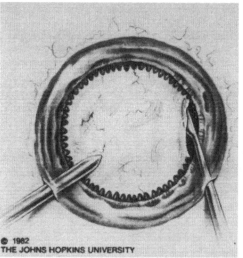

Figure 1. Vitrectomy instrument and 20-gauge infusion needle inserted through separate watertight limbal incisions. Soft lens material removed by aspiration before excision of vascularized retrolenticular membrane.

Figure 2. If the retrolenticular membrane is not firmly attached to the ciliary processes for 360°, a discission knife can be used to create an incision between the ciliary processes and the membrane.

Certain cases of PHPV have a "clear zone" in which the membrane is not firmly adherent to the ciliary processes. Excision should begin in such an area if present (Figure 2). In cases where such a zone is not present, an incision in the membrane is created using 20 gauge intraocular scissors (Figure 3). The edge of this incision provides access to the membrane (Figure 4), and the membrane is removed, sparing firm attachments to the ciliary proccesses (Figure 5).

By raising the infusion bottle and elevating intraocular pressure, bleeding from transected vessels in the membrane can usually be controlled. Large vessels can be sealed using intraocular, (bimanual) bipolar diathermy (Figure 6). The cut end of the hyaloid artery is cauterized between the Ocutome tip and the infusion needle (Figure 7). In order to hold back the remaining vitreous, air is injected through the infusion needle while the instruments are removed from the eye. The limbal incisions are closed using interrupted 10-0 nylon sutures, and the air is partially replaced with balanced salt solution.

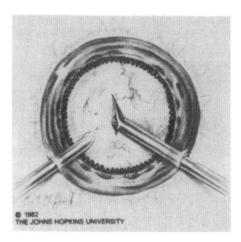

Figure 3. The membrane is incised at its thinnest part using 20-gauge intraocular scissors.

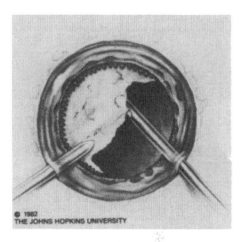

Figure 4. The membrane is then excised under direct visual control. The height of the infusion bottle is adjusted to maintain a normal or slightly elevated intraocular pressure.

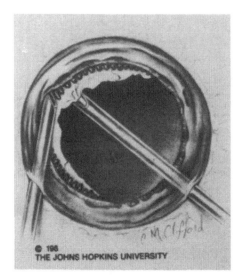

Figure 5. The infusion needle can be used to retract iris to improve visualization of peripheral membrane. The membrane cannot be completely excised in areas where it is firmly intermeshed with the ciliary processes.

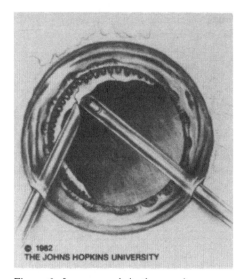

Figure 6. Large vessels in the membrane can be closed using bimanual, bipolar diathermy. The vascularized tissue is positioned between the instrument tips, and diathermy is applied.

RESULTS

Over the past nine years seven eyes of seven patients with persistent hyperplastic primary vitreous have been operated on at the Wilmer Institute using the techniques

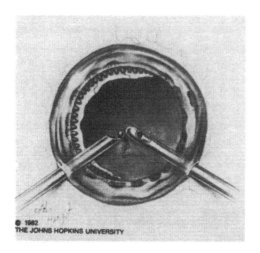

© 1982
THE JOHNS HOPKINS UNIVERSITY

Figure 7. The cut end of the persistent hyaloid artery can also be treated by bipolar diathermy using the same technique. A small bubble may appear when the diathermy is applied.

and instruments described above (Table 1). A limbal approach was used in all cases except one. Follow-up ranged from 3 to 9 years, with a mean follow-up of 6 years. Only one of the seven cases of PHPV was bilateral, and in this patient only one eye was operated upon.

Table 1. *Clinical data and results in seven patients*

Case No.	Age at Surgery	Intraoperative Complications/ Results	Postoperative Complications	Initial Refractive Error	Most recent Visual Acuity	Length of Clear Pupillary Space
1	14 mos	None; clear pupil	none	+ 14	20/60	8 yrs.
2	6 wks	None; clear pupil	pupillary membrane and RD* at 2 mos repaired	+ 34	LP	5 yrs.
3	5 mos	None; clear pupil	none	+ 23	5/200	4 yrs.
4	17 days	None; clear pupil	none	+ 13	20/200	4 yrs.
5	4 1/2 mos	None; clear pupil	pupillary membrane at 3 mos, repaired	+ 13	HM	4 yrs.
6	2 mos	None; clear pupil	none	+ 16	HM	3 yrs.
7	5 1/2 weeks	Tractional RD* noted at time of surgery and repaired; clear pupil	none	+ 18	LP	2 yrs.

*RD = Retinal detachment

The typical picture of PHPV consisting of micro-ophthalmia, shallowing of the anterior chamber, cataract, vascularized retrolenticular membrane, and persistent hyaloid artery were present in all seven cases. In five of the seven cases a clear pupillary space was achieved with one surgical procedure. Two eyes required a secondary discission, and one eye required a second procedure to repair a retinal detachment. All seven eyes were considered surgical successes with encouraging visual results in two children.

The child with bilateral PHPV was operated on at 14 months of age. She now attends a regular school and has 20/60 (Jaeger 4) vision with mild nystagmus of the operated eye, while her other eye has light perception vision. Another child operated on at 17 days of age has 20/200 vision. The other children have hand motion to count fingers vision, but in 3 of the 5 eyes with poor vision there were pre-existing macular or optic nerve abnormalities.

DISCUSSION

Aspiration of congenital cataracts was reintroduced by Scheie (1), and later modified by Maumenee (2) and others (3, 4). This one-stage aspiration technique with complete removal of all soft lens material is the preferred method of managing uncomplicated congenital cataracts. Most cases of uncomplicated congenital cataracts can be managed in one operation using an automated infusion-aspiration system and the operating microscope.

In children 7 years of age or older, the posterior lens capsule should be left intact. Younger children should have a primary discission in order to prevent an opacified capsule which almost always develops in patients with congenital cataracts operated on at an early age. Children in the amblyogenic age range should receive a permanently clear pupillary space if possible in one operation. Older children are more apt to tolerate a YAG capsulotomy if necessary.

In an otherwise healthy child who presents with classical PHPV (unilaterial leukocoria, varying degress of micro-ophthalmia, cataract, shallow anterior chamber, large radial iris vessels and a retrolenticular membrane) early surgical intervention is recommended for preservation of the globe. The natural history of PHPV is one of progressive cataract formation with shallowing of the anterior chamber, resulting in angle closure glaucoma. Spontaneous intraocular hemorrhage, retinal detachment, or phthisis may result from progressive traction on the ciliary body and peripheral retina. As a result of glaucoma and hemorrhage, the eye is usually lost at an early age (1, 6, 8). Relative contraindications to surgery are longstanding, intractable glaucoma or hemorrhage, severe micro-ophthalmia or minimal signs of PHPV with no evidence of progressive change. All children in this series met the criteria for surgical intervention.

Complicated cataracts include those with vascularized pupillary membranes, small fibrotic pupils, subluxed lenses, and PHPV. These cases usually require more extensive surgery than simple aspiration. Infusion and aspiration capabilities are required, and controlled excision of intraocular tissues under direct observation is vitally important. The instruments designed for pars plana vitreous surgery provide these capabilites and offer significant advantages over conventional techniques. Using vitrectomy instrumentation and "closed eye" techniques, a clear pupillary opening was achieved in five cases with one operation, while in two additional eyes a secondary discission was required. Due to the anatomical abnormalities associated with PHPV including a narrow pars plana, thick vitreous gel, anterior retinal insertion, and incarceration of retinal tissue within the retrolenticular membrane, the preferred site of entry is anteriorly through the limbus. The only eye in this series that subsequently developed a retinal detachment had been operated on via the pars plana approach.

All operations were considered anatomic successes, and all globes retained clear media, attached retinas and normal intraocular pressures. The minimum follow-up was 2 years, with a mean follow-up of 6 years. Early surgery and aphakic correction may result in useful vision, even with a unilateral cataract and micro-ophthalmia (9). Postoperatively our complicated cataracts were treated with contact lens correction and intermittent patching of the better eye. One child was dependent upon his post surgical 20/60 vision because of poor vision in the other eye. Because both eyes were micro-ophthalmic with retrolenticular vascularized membranes, salvaging the eye was the primary objective since the natural course of PHPV usually results in loss of the eye. Limited amblyopia therapy was employed with patching of the fellow eye for 15-30 minutes per day. Perhaps with more intensive occlusion therapy, better vision could have been achieved.

The limitations and disadvantages of vitrectomy instrumentation and techniques include reliance on complex and costly instrumentation, operative complications occurring as a result of excessive traction on tissues, use of excessive amounts of intraocular irrigating solution, and wide variation in intraocular pressure during surgery. The long-term effects of these surgical methods are not known, but follow-up of our patients suggests that early surgical intervention in advanced cases of PHPV is indicated.

ACKNOWLEDGMENTS

This work was supported in part by the Women's Committee of the International Medical Eye Bank of Maryland.

REFERENCES

1. Machemer R, Parel JM, Beutner H (1972): A new concept for vitreous surgery: 1. Instrumentation. Am J Ophthalmol 73:107.
2. Michels RG, Stark, WJ (1976): Symposium: Pars plana vitrectomy: Vitrectomy technique in anterior segment surgery. Trans Am Acad Ophthalmol Otolaryngol 81:382-390.
3. Taylor HR, Michels RG, Stark WJ (1979): Vitrectomy methods in anterior segment surgery. Ophthalmic Surg 10:22-58.
4. Scheie HG (1960): Aspiration of congenital or soft cataracts: A new technique. Am J Ophthalmol 50:1048-1056.
5. Maumenee AE (1969): Aspiration techniques for congenital cataracts. In Welsh RC, Welsh J (eds.): The new report on cataract surgery. Miami: Miami Educational Press, 419-423.
6. Von Norden GK, Ryan SJ, Maumenee AE (1970): Management of congenital cataracts. Trans Am Acad Ophthalmol Otolaryngol; 74:352-359.
7. Parks MM, Hiles DA (1967): Management of infantile cataracts. Am J Ophthalmol; 63:10-19.

8. Beller R, Hoyt CS, Marg E. Odom JV (1981): Good visual function after neonatal surgery for congenital monocular cataracts. Am J Ophthalmol 91:559-565.

9. Reese AB (1949): Persistence and hyperplasia of primary vitreous; retrolental fibroplasia - two entities. Arch Ophthalmol 41:527-552.

10. Smith RE, Maumenee AE (1974): Persistent hyperplastic primary vitreous: results of surgery. Trans Am Acad Ophthalmol Otolaryngol 78:OP 911-925.

11. Federman SL, Shields, Altman B, Koller A (1982): The surgical and non-surgical management of persistent hyperplastic primary vitreous. Ophthalmology 89:20-24.

Basic and advanced vitreous surgery
G.W. Blankenship, M. Stirpe, M. Gonvers, S. Binder (eds.)
Fidia Research Series, vol. II,
Liviana Press, Padova © 1986

PARS PLANA LENSECTOMY

G. Scuderi, E. Balestrazzi, V. Picardo, E. Moreno, and F. Crescenzi

University of Rome "La Sapienza", Institute of Ophthalmology, Roma

Until the beginning of the 1970's, the types of treatment commonly used in soft cataract surgery were:
— optical iridectomy
— discission
— linear extracapsular extraction (various techniques)
— intracapsular extraction (particular cases).

None of these treatments was devoid of immediate or delayed complications, and the functional results were not always excellent, although satisfactory results were sometimes obtained in the anatomy.

More recently some authors (Scuderi, 1969) had suggested extracapsular extraction planned in one step, in place of the discission and aspiration of the masses in more steps, by means of a mechanical instrument, consisting of a single cannula for simultaneous irrigation and aspiration of cataractous masses, connected to a pump whose negative pressure could be externally controlled step by step (Scuderi-Ranieri apparatus).

This instrument, however, though it had considerable success and offered various technical advantages compared to the old methods, with time also showed some of its limits, mostly due to the use of the anterior approach method. With such techniques, it was not unusual to have:
— more or less intense irido-ciliary reactions
— secondary keratoendotheliosis (due to the presence of vitreous in A.C.)
— secondary cataracts
— pupillary irregularities
— retinal detachment

An important step forward in soft cataract surgery techniques has thus lately been made (1970) thanks to the application of vitreous surgery methods and equipment to lenticular surgery (soft cataracts).

The instrument used, the vitreotome, is a device comprising a cutting, irrigation and aspiration mechanism which can function in one or two probes.

The technique is lensectomy via pars plana, conceptually deriving from vitrectomy which allows operating on congenital and traumatic forms, in cases of soft lens and in the cases of association of lenticular pathology and vitreoretinal disorders. Today, this technique represents the most widely used method in soft cataract surgery.

Table 1. *Advantages of Pars Plana Lensectomy*

— easy and complete approach to soft cataracts
— preservation of the anatomic integrity of the cornea and anterior segment.
— vitreous kept in physiological site
— possible release of A.C. and pupillary field from the vitreous in particular cases (traumatic and ectopic cataract)
— preservation of normal pupillary motility and integrity
— lack of prolonged ciliary inflammatory reaction, photophobia, lacrimation, perikeratic hyperaemia
— early mobilization of the patient
— short post-operative bed rest
— optimal esthetic and functional results
— early possibility of applying corneal lenses

The equipment at our disposal is: simple models with mechanical movement and manual aspiration, or more sophisticated instruments which are endowed with numerous computer-controlled functions. This has become a widespread technique thanks to its undeniable and obvious advantages (see Table 2), which make it more desirable than other equally modern techniques.

Table 2.

Advantages of Lesectomy and Vitrectomy (young patients, traumatic pathology)
— removal of lens with "closed eyeball" and simultaneous vitrectomy
— use of the same surgical wound
— direct and immediate sight of the posterior segment of the eyeball once lensectomy has been performed.

Contraindications to Lensectomy
— hard nucleus lentis
— other contraindications suggested by the surgeon's experience

Generally, whatever the type of equipment used, it is possible to perform a lensectomy by using a single probe for cutting, infusion and aspiration, or rather through two separate paths, one for cutting and aspiration, the other for infusion, or by using more probes and more paths.

It is furthermore possible to constantly regulate the intraocular pressure, by means of an electronic system connected to a pre-adjustable pressure transducer, which allows changing the tone even during the operation itself.

SURGICAL TECHNIQUE

The surgical technique used in the Eye Clinic II, Rome University does not differ, as far as general preparation is concerned, from the techniques employed for operations on the eyeball.

The patient is given general anesthesia under controlled hypotension, with a good pharmacological mydriasis (sometimes retrobulbar administration of 0.5% Marcaina to enhance mydriasis). The use of the surgical microscope is recommended.

The technique can be synthetized in the following stages:

— small conjunctival flap in the upper temporal sector +

— continuous overcast suture on the conjunctival margin, in black silk 5-0, thus allowing the surgeon to move the eyeball in all directions

— preventive U-shaped suture 4 mm from the limbus, on the pars plana

— small sclerotomy

— introduction of the knife (small Graefe, Beaver blade, discission needle) and discission of the nucleus and cortex lentis

— introduction of the scleral conformer

— extraction of the latter and introduction of the vitreotome tip, until it can be visualized in the pupillary field

— beginning of lensectomy, starting from the nucleus lentis and then proceeding to the anterior layers, the equator lentis and finally to the posterior capsule which is kept *in situ*, until the operation has reached an advanced stage in order to avoid the fall of small lenticular fragments into the vitreous

— anterior vitrectomy

— A.C. irrigation where necessary

— extraction of the vitreotome

— routine ophthalmoscopic examination of the retina and its periphery so as to reveal possible retinorhexis or rhegmatogenous areas to be treated simultaneously.

— suture of the sclerotomy

— suture of the conjunctiva

— retrobulbar of betametazone deposit

— local medication with atropine and antibiotics

— binocular bandaging for 24 hours

CLINICAL CASE-STUDY

The total number of lensectomies performed at our Institute during the period taken into consideration is 71, subdivided as follows:

lensectomies: 52
lensectomies + retinal detachment: 7
lensectomies + vitrectomies + retinal detachment: 4
lensectomies + vitrectomies: 4
lensectomies + corepraxies: 3
lensectomies + vitrectomies + foreign body extraction: 1

A) Lensectomies for congenital cataract: 34 cases

congenital cataract: 23
secondary congenital cataract: 10
complicated congenital cataract: 1

Pre-operative vision:

— not determinable due to age or not determined: 9 cases
— up to 1/10: 12 cases
— 2/10 to 4/10: 7 cases
— 5/10 to 7/10: 6 cases
— 8/10 to 10/10: none

Post-operative vision:

— not determinable due to age or not determined: 9 cases
— up to 1/10: 5 cases
— 2/10 to 4/10: 3 cases
— 5/10 to 7/10: 7 cases
— 8/10 to 10/10: 10 cases

In 32 operations out of 34 there were no intra-operative or post-operative severe complications.

In one case, a new operation (via pars plana) was performed after one year, for the removal of some capsular residues. In one case, after lensectomy + circular buckling + cryotherapy, a retinal detachment took place, which was presently treated. (The patient was suffering from secondary congenital cataract, severe bilateral myopia and retinal degenerations).

B) Lensectomies for traumatic cataract: 24 cases

traumatic cataract: 17
secondary traumatic cataract: 5
complicated traumatic cataract: 2

Pre-operative vision:

— not determined: 4 cases
— up to 1/10: 19 cases

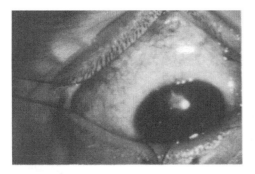

Figure 1. Right eye: soft cataract. The eye before the operation.

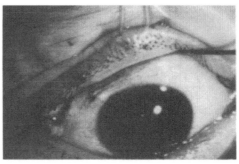

Figure 2. Right eye: the eye at the end of the operation (pars plana lensectomy).

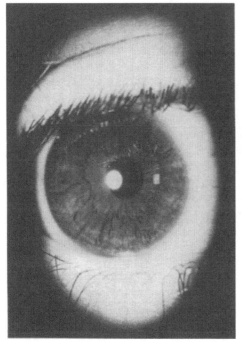

Figure 3. The same eye two months after the operation.

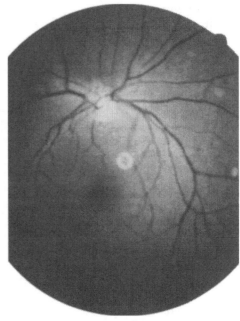

Figure 4. The ophthalmoscopical view of the fundus.

— 2/10 to 7/10: 1 case
— 8/10 to 10/10: none

Post-operative vision:

— not determined: 4 cases
— up to 1/10: 4 cases

— 2/10 to 4/10: 2 cases
— 5/10 to 7/10: 5 cases
— 8/10 to 10/10: 9 cases

No intra-operative or post-operative complications were observed

C) Lensectomies for severe myopia: 3 cases

(transparent lens - high anisometropia)

Pre-operative vision:

— 1/10: 2 cases
— 2/10: 1 cases

Post-operative vision:

— light perception: 1 case (lensectomy + cryotherapy were performed and a retinal detachment occurred)
— 1/10: 1 case
— 9/10: 1 case

In one case a retinal detachment occurred (see above). In the other two cases no intra-operative or post-operative complications occurred;

D) Lensectomies for complex pathology: 10 cases

lensectomies: 2
lensectomies + vitrectomy + retinal detachment: 4
lensectomies + vitrectomies: 2
lensectomies + retinal detachment: 1
lensectomies + vitrectomies + foreign body extraction: 1

Pre-operative vision:

— not determined: 1 case
— lower than 1/10: 9 cases

Post-operative vision:

— not determined: 1 case
— no perception of light: 3 cases
— up to 1/10: 1 case
— 2/10 to 4/10: 5 cases
— 5/10 to 7/10: no cases
— 8/10 to 10/10: no cases

In 4 cases anatomic recovery was achieved. In one case, vision after the operation was 1/10. In 4 cases a relapse of the retinal detachment occurred. All patients who underwent lensectomy were previously submitted to an accurate and complete pre-operative study, both of the eyes to be operated on and of the contralateral eyes, in addition to echography examination and determination of visual evoked potentials. Thanks to these tests, we were able to perform sufficiently aimed operations, encouraged by a whole series of clinical data which were precious for surgery.

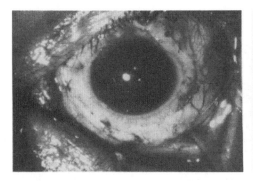

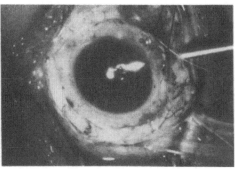

Figure 5. Left eye: eye with pupillary seclusion, secondary cataract, retinal detachment. The circular buckling is visible in the inferior temporal sector.

Figure 6. The same eye during the operation: the vitreotome is performing the sector iridectomy and the lesectomy.

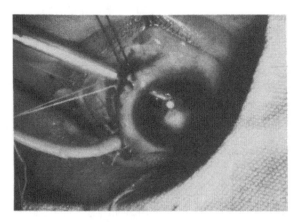

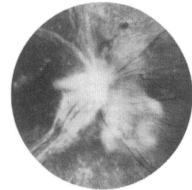

Figure 7. Retrolental fibroplasia + Ph.V. + hard nucleus cataract. Two ways vitrectomy.

Figure 8. The fundus of the same young patient.

This has enabled us to avoid unexpected findings during the operation, due to the presence of vitreoretinopathy of variable nature (post-traumatic, hemorrhagic).

When a posterior vitrectomy was expected in surgery, according to semiological data, whether or not associated with an operation for retinal detachment, a silicone circular buckling was preventively placed on the eyeball, before proceeding to sclerotomy and to the lensectomy stage.

If the ophthalmoscopic examination, routinely carried out at the end of lensectomy, revealed retinal areas of rhegmatogenous degeneration or retinorhexis, in the absence of retinal detachment, we performed localized and/or circular buckling. The post-operative course was generally easy, with low conjunctival and perikeratic reactions, a well formed anterior chamber, and the patient was mobilized already during the first day and discharged after 8-10 days.

The results obtained were always excellent from the anatomical point of view and variable as far as functional aspects were concerned considering the type of pathology treated (see Tables 3,4 and 5).

Table 3. *Intra-operative complications*

— sudden and transitory myosis, associated or not with shallow anterior chamber
— rare, sharp endo-ocular tone variations, always easily controlled by the computer system
— accidental picking of the iris
— fall of small cataractous masses in the vitreous body
— hemorrhagic opacity of the vitreous (in some cases of complex pathology)

Table 4. *Early post-operative complications*

— transitory hyphema
— pupillary irregularities
— hemorrhagic opacity of the vitreous (in some cases of complex pathology cases)

Table 5. *Delayed post-operative complications*

— vitreous opacity (in complex pathology cases, only in the case of posterior vitrectomy)
— retinal detachment
— cystoid macular oedema
— persistence of light pupillary irregularities (preserved motility)

CONCLUSIONS

The aim of this study was to verify the advantages of lensectomy via pars plana with respect to the previous anterior approach methods, and its main indications.

We have examined the case-records of lensectomy operations via pars plana, whether or not combined with vitrectomy, performed at the Eye Clinic II, Rome. 71 operations during the period from January 1978 to June 1984, and classified them according to type (congenital and traumatic cataract, cataract with transparent lens for cases of severe anisometropia associated with vitreoretinal pathology).

We evaluated the results on a short and long-term basis, with a follow-up of 6 months to 6 years, by examining all records and by periodically checking all the patients. On the basis of these tests, an improvement of vision, above 5/10 in 50% of the cases, occurred with some patients reaching even 10/10, however, depending on pre-existing pathology and absence of relevant complications both during the operation and in the short and long-term post-operative period.

From these studies, it became clear that pars plana lensectomy is the operation of choice in soft cataract microsurgery, not only in cases of simple pathology but even more in complex pathology, where it permits operation on the lens and on the retina at the same time, with a more favourable prognostic outlook.

A particular indication is moreover found in congenital cataracts, where the favourable post-operative course makes it easier to follow young patients and allows an early optical correction and a reduction in percentage of the incidence of amblyopia resulting from deprivation.

REFERENCES

1. Scuderi G, Recupero SM (1924): Congenital cataract - surgical problems. Docum Ophtalmol Proc Serie 21:209-230.
2. Girard, Bokobza, Biojout, Pasticier, Forest (1982): Broutage du cristallin par la parsa plana. Résultatas à court et à moyen terme. J Fr Ophtalmol 5, 6-7; 433-436.
3. Hoyt CS, Nickel B (1982): Aphakic cystoid macular edema... Arch Ophtalmol 100, 746-749.
4. Cardia L, Sborgia C, Giummarra C (1983): La lensectomia via pars plana nella cataratta congenita traumatica e giovanile. Cl Oculistica, Pat Ocul 1, 87-92.
5. Haut J (1978): Extraction des cataractes congénitales au moyen du vitreotome où brouter. J Fr Ophtalmol 1:469-470.
6. Krieglstein GK, Duzanec Z, Leydhecher W (1980): Cataract surgery: Types and frequencies of complications. Albrecht von Graefes Arch Klin Ophtalmol 214:9-13.

Basic and advanced vitreous surgery
G.W. Blankenship, M. Stirpe, M. Gonvers, S. Binder (eds.)
Fidia Research Series, vol. II,
Liviana Press, Padova © 1986

LENS AND VITREOUS COMPLICATIONS

E. Dal Fiume, G. Tassinari, C. Forlini

Divisione Oculistica, Ospedale Civile, Ravenna

Often the necessity of surgery of the vitreous gel and therefore the use of surgical techniques of vitrectomy are the consequence of surgery of the lens and of its pathology. The objective of this paper is to analyze the surgical techniques that must be used in every specific situation. We will examine among the causes of vitreous pathology after surgical intervention:

a) contact between cornea and vitreous (cornea vitreous touch)
b) vitreous incarceration with persistent aphakic cystoid macular edema
c) lens material in the pupillary area and pupillary membranes attached to the anterior vitreous
d) aphakic pupillary block glaucoma
e) traumatic cataract with opacity of posterior capsule and modification of anterior vitreous

Among the indications for vitreous surgery because of pathology of lens we will examine:

a) subluxated cataract
b) lens luxated in the vitreous
c) malignant glaucoma

a) Cornea vitreous touch

The contact between cornea and vitreous following cataract surgery as a result of rupture of the anterior hyaloid is one of the more frequent causes of Bullous Keratopathy. Vitreous gel causes a metaplastic change in the endothelial cells and loss of endothelial cells leading to edema of the overlying stroma and epithelium. In the most severe cases a corneal transplant is necessary. The vitreous gel is removed via the pars plana because removal from the anterior is more traumatic for the anterior segment, which is already in an inflammatory condition, and for a cornea with an unbalanced metabolism. The surgical technique used is total removal of the vitreous gel whether in the anterior chamber or in the vitreous chamber. We believe this type of intervention to be useful if the corneal touch is large and a pre-existing lesion of the endothelial cells is present.

In operated patients recovery of transparency of the cornea with improved vision has been seen only in cases of immediate surgery before the damage of the endothelial cells and the stroma became irreversible.

b) Vitreous incarceration with persistent aphakic cystoid macular edema

This is one of the more frequent complications of cataract surgery with loss of vitreous. Vitreous remains incarcerated in the wound, the pupil remains dislocated towards the point of incarceration and in the following months cystoid macular edema is seen with severe reduction in vision to 1/1200. The reason why macular edema is present is still a subject of discussion.

Traction of vitreous on the iris causes retinal vasculitis probably induced by prostaglandins of the iris and, at the level of peripheral capillary circulation, leakage of fluid that accumulates in the external plexiform layer causes the formation of cystoid cavities. The pars plana technique is used to remove the vitreous in the anterior chamber. Since the vitreous is often intimately attached to the iris and to the wound, it is necessary to use the bimanual technique entering the anterior chamber by way of the limbus with a 22 gauge needle with infusion or with a Barraquer spatula in order to break the adhesion formed by the vitreous in the anterior chamber. The surgery is completed by performing an anterior vitrectomy.

c) Presence of lens materials on the pupil and pupillary membranes attached to anterior vitreous

This situation can occur after cataract surgery due to a complication during the removal of the lens or even after inflammatory events during the days following surgery, or both. Fibrous and adherent membranes are formed by fibrin and lens material that close the pupil, thus preventing the recovery of sight, which must therefore be removed surgically. The preferred method for these cases is again the pars plana vitrectomy. Many times the vitrectomy instrument is not able to cut and remove these membranes and so it is necessary to use the bimanual technique: cutting the membrane with a Ziegler knife and if this is not sufficient, a vitreous scissor is used and the residual membrane is removed with the vitreophage. At times it is also necessary to use bipolar endodiathermy because these membranes are always the site of neovascularization.

d) Aphakic pupillary block glaucoma and malignant glaucoma

They represent two different entities but with a common pathogenetic basis: aqueous humor produced by the ciliary body remains in the vitreous chamber moving forward the anterior vitreous and the lens that close the pupil and the peripheral iridectomy. Sometimes in aphakic pupillary block glaucoma it is sufficient to perform argon laser iridotomy so as to reopen a passage between the anterior and posterior chambers. If this by itself is not sufficient, pars plana vitrectomy is necessary. The vitreous gel in the anterior chamber and most of the central vitreous are removed to prevent postoperative rehydration of the vitreous from closing the pupil again. In those cases in which there is a long-standing aphakic pupillary block, some authors, such as Michels, recommend the injection of air into the anterior chamber through the scleral incision in order to separate corneal endothelium from the vitreous and the iris.

e) Traumatic cataract

In cases of traumatic cataract it may be necessary to perform vitrectomy when a posterior capsule opacity and vitreous alteration are present. The cataract is removed through the anterior chamber by traditional techniques. The aspiration technique (if the nucleus is soft) or phacoemulsification is used if an anterior capsule break is present; if a posterior capsule opacity or a posterior capsule break are present, vitrectomy is done through the limbus: the posterior lens capsule is excised and a shallow anterior vitrectomy is performed.

f) Subluxated cataract

Vitrectomy is mandatory when there is a subluxated lens with vitreous in the anterior chamber. The following technique is used: a shallow anterior vitrectomy is performed and a limbal incision and extraction of the lens with a cryoprobe are used. During the operation, if the lens is extremely mobile and its complete luxation into the vitreous is possible, it is necessary to immobilize the lens with a needle introduced through the pars plana on the opposite side.

g) Lens luxated in the vitreous

It is extremely dangerous to remove the lens luxated in the vitreous with the vitrectomy instrument because of the possibility of causing a shock to the retina. Lens removal is always performed through the limbus. A double Flieringa ring is applied and a limbal incision is made to remove the lens. A pars plana vitrectomy is performed to excise the vitreous gel including the posterior cortical vitreous. The lens is grasped with the vitrectomy instrument and positioned in the anterior chamber. The pupil becomes contracted using acetylcholine and the lens is removed with a cryoprobe. In addition to this technique used by Michels, we remove the lens with a cryoprobe directly from the vitreous cavity after having performed a vitrectomy as previously described. A fluid/gas exchange is possible after complete vitrectomy, using a continuous infusion system. The lens is removed by the cryoprobe through the anterior chamber. This surgical technique appears to cause less shock to the posterior segment of the eye.

Basic and advanced vitreous surgery
G.W. Blankenship, M. Stirpe, M. Gonvers, S. Binder (eds.)
Fidia Research Series, vol. II,
Liviana Press, Padova © 1986

MANAGEMENT OF EPITHELIAL CYSTS AND INGROWTH

Walter J. Stark, Peter A. Rapoza, Arlo C. Terry, M. Bowes Hamill, John D. Gottsch, Ronald G. Michels

The Wilmer Ophthalmological Institute,
The Johns Hopkins Hospital, Baltimore, Maryland, 21205, U.S.A.

Epithelial invasion of the anterior chamber is a rare, but often devastating complication of penetrating ocular trauma and anterior segment surgery. In 1830, MacKenzie reported the presence of a semitransparent cyst in the anterior chamber of an eye following trauma. Rothmund, in 1872, speculated that implantation of epithelium at the time of surgery or penetrating trauma resulted in the development of anterior chamber cysts. Collins and Cross (1892) presented the initial description of the histopathology of epithelial cysts in eyes enucleated following cataract surgery. The cysts they observed were lined by laminated epithelium similar to that of the cornea. Pupillary block glaucoma was noted in one of the eyes. During 1937, Perera proposed a classification of epithelial invasion dividing it into three types of lesions: 1) "pearl" tumors of the iris, 2) post-traumatic cysts of the iris (epithelial cysts), and 3) epithelization of the anterior chamber (epithelial ingrowth).

EPITHELIAL PEARL TUMORS

Rare cases of "pearl" tumors have been reported to occur following intraocular surgery or penetrating trauma. Clinically, they appear as solid pearly white tumors or opaque white cysts on the surface of the iris. No connection to an entry wound has been demonstrated. Pearl tumors may develop from implantation of skin or a hair follicle into the anterior chamber (Maumenee and Shannon, 1956). They usually grow slowly to a size less than 3 mm in diameter. Occasionally, however, a pearl tumor may fill the entire anterior chamber and even extend into the posterior chamber. Uveitis may be present.

Histologically, pearl tumors are encapsulated lesions consisting of layers of stratified or cuboidal epithelium. The central core is composed of concentric layers of keratinized cells or a necrotic, amorphous mass of keratinized epithelium and cholesterol crystals. Hair follicles or a foreign body may be present within the tumor.

The natural history of pearl tumors is generally benign. Asymptomatic eyes should be examined at regular intervals to watch for a change in size, the presence of an inflammatory reaction, or the rare occurrence of a secondary glaucoma. Generally, no treatment is required. En bloc resection of the lesion with a sector iridectomy may be necessary to control persistent uveitis or secondary glaucoma.

EPITHELIAL CYSTS

The true incidence of epithelial invasion is unknown due to its low frequency of occurrence, difficulty of clinical recognition, and the lack of distinction between epithelial cysts and ingrowth in much of the literature. The reported incidence of histologically proven epithelial invasion following cataract surgery ranges from 0.09% (Bernardino et al., 1969) to 0.11% (Theobald and Hass, 1948). Maumenee (1964) reviewed reports of several series of eyes enucleated after cataract surgery and found that approximately 16% had evidence of epithelial invasion. Eldrup-Jorgensen (1968) noted that 36% of enucleated eyes found to have epithelial invasion following cataract extraction contained epithelial cysts while 64% had evidence of epithelial ingrowth. Bettman (1969) found epithelial invasion in 12 of 739 eyes enucleated for complications of intraocular surgery. Five had epithelial cysts and seven demonstrated evidence of epithelial ingrowth.

The majority of cases of epithelial cyst formation have followed poor surgical wound closure. Hypotony, fistula formation, and incarceration of intraocular tissues are thought to be predisposing conditions. After finding plaques of stratified squamous epithelium on iridectomy specimens, Ferry (1971) postulated that instruments used to handle intraocular tissues following manipulation of extraocular epithelium might be responsible for transferring epithelial implants into the anterior chamber. Although the literature abounds with declarations that epithelial invasion occurs less frequently with limbus than with fornix-based conjunctival flaps (Bernardino et al., 1969), no conclusive evidence supports this presumption (Maumenee et al., 1970).

Attempts to study epithelial invasion in an animal model have generally been disappointing (Gundersen, 1938; Dunnington, 1951; Cogan, 1955; Regan, 1958). Free implants of conjunctival or corneal epithelium were usually reabsorbed or did not proliferate. Growth seemed to require contact with iris stroma, persistent production of secondary aqueous, an inturned conjunctival flap, or a large gaping wound often with incarceration of intraocular tissues.

Histologically, epithelial cysts are thin-walled epithelium-lined structures containing serous fluid with protein, cholesterol, and cellular debris. The cysts range in size from one to several millimeters in diameter. Electron microscopy demonstrates that epithelial cells are connected by desmosomal junctions, exhibit microvillous processes, and contain numerous cytoplasmic filaments, but few mitochondria (Eiferman and Rodrigues, 1981).

Clinically, early signs of epithelial cyst implantation include slight pupillary distortion or displacement of an iris pillar towards the cyst. Cysts appear as translucent or shimmering gray structures usually located adjacent to the entry site (Figure 1). A fistula is often present, frequently resulting in hypotony. Anterior chamber inflammation persisting beyond the usual postoperative period is frequently reported (Calhoun, 1949).

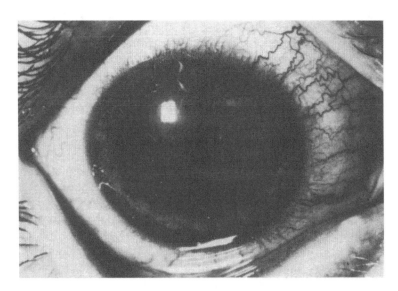

Figure 1. Moderate-sized epithelial cyst in the anterior chamber.

The natural history of epithelial cysts varies from no growth to a rapid increase in size with spread into the posterior chamber and subsequent development of glaucoma due to pupillary block and/or obstruction of the angle (Stark and Bruner, 1982). Epithelial cysts must be distinguished from primary iris cysts which usually contain more pigment within their walls and cause less iris atrophy. Epithelial cysts may be confused with parasitic cysts, but the latter are extremely rare, occurring almost exclusively in third world countries.

Management of epithelial cysts includes periodic examinations for the presence of 1) an increase in size, 2) uveitis, 3) corneal edema, and 4) secondary glaucoma. Visual acuity may be affected due to tumor obstruction of the visual axis. Presence of one of the above complications (unresponsive to medical management) is an indication for surgical treatment. A number of treatment modalities have been used in the past including repeated aspiration of cystic fluid, iodine injection, electrolysis and diathermy. More recently, these techniques have been replaced by photocoagulation, aspiration combined with cryodestruction, and surgical excision.

Cleasby (1971) successfully treated four cases of epithelial cyst with xenon arc photocoagulation. Okun and Mandell (1974) treated three eyes with multiple photocoagulation sessions collapsing the cysts. Maumenee and Shannon (1956) performed total or subtotal excisions of epithelial cysts in ten patients. Fluid was first aspirated from the cyst with a narrow gauge needle introduced into the cyst at its point of contact with the posterior cornea. A groove was made so that the cyst could be grasped with forceps and extracted. The cornea overlying the cyst was curetted or swabbed with a cotton-tip applicator dipped in 70% alcohol. All the iris to which the cyst had been adherent was excised via a basal iridectomy. Visual acuity improved or stayed the same in five eyes. Hogan and Goodner (1960) aspirated fluid from epithelial cysts, then applied diathermy via the aspirating needle to treat six eyes. Four cysts were completely destroyed, one eye experienced a recurrence requiring surgical excision, and one case had too short a follow-up period to evaluate the results of treatment. In all cases, vision remained the same or improved. Ferry and Naghdi (1967) altered surgical excision by removing the cyst with a cryoprobe introduced into the cyst itself. Sugar (1967) advocated posterior lamellar resection of the cornea for removal of epithelial cysts of the anterior chamber.

Current surgical management of epithelial cysts at the Wilmer Ophthalmological Institute combines cryotherapy and surgical excision by vitrectomy techniques as described by Bruner et al. (1981). In aphakic eyes, a closed eye technique is preferred with the infusion cannula being introduced via the limbus or pars plana. Contents of the epithelial cyst are evacuated through a small gauge needle which enters the cyst where it is attached to adjacent cornea or sclera. An attempt is made not to violate the wall of the cyst within the eye. Opposite to the aspirating needle a small diameter vitrectomy probe is placed through the limbus or pars plana to perform an anterior vitrectomy. When necessary, radial incision through the iris adjacent to the cyst will allow further collapse of the cyst against the internal eye wall. Air is injected into the anterior chamber via the infusion cannula while fluid is aspirated by the vitrectomy instrument. The air bubble flattens the collapsed cyst against the internal wall of the eye and insulates other ocular structures from transcorneal or translimbal cryotherapy which is applied using a freeze-refreeze technique (Figure 2). The freezing effect is limited to the peripheral 2 mm of cornea. The air bubble is replaced by a sterile physiologic solution at the conclusion of the case.

An open sky approach is preferred for phakic eyes with clear lenses and for aphakic eyes when it appears that the cyst can be completely removed without rupture. A limbal based conjunctival flap is prepared and a small gauge needle is placed into the cyst through the adjacent limbus to aspirate the cystic fluid. Air is injected into the anterior chamber through a separate needle in order to collapse the cyst and displace the lens posteriorly. Adhesions between the cyst and cornea are lysed and a limbal groove is prepared through which the cyst is prolapsed. Holding the cyst with smooth forceps, it is excised with sharp scissors exercising great care not to rupture the cyst wall (Figure 3). The adjacent iris is removed to lessen the chance of leaving residual epithelium in the eye. The groove is permanently closed and air injected into the anterior chamber in order to move the lens posteriorly and provide thermal insulation during transcorneal or translimbal application of cryotherapy. Partial anterior vitrectomy is performed in aphakic eyes if the cyst wall ruptures during an open sky excision.

Seven patients were treated utilizing the above techniques with no recurrence in six eyes. Final visual acuity of 20/50 or better was reported in three cases. A fourth eye was a surgical success, but vision remained poor secondary to amblyopia. Two eyes developed clinically significant cystoid macular edema and one eye developed epithelial ingrowth postoperatively. Corneal edema followed further surgical treatment of the epithelial ingrowth. No eyes developed glaucoma.

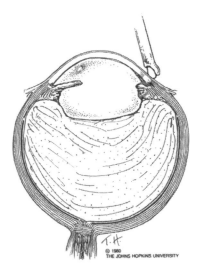

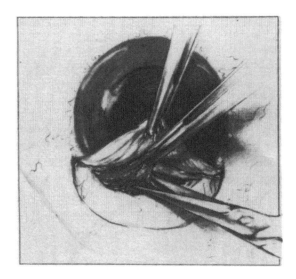

Figure 2. Following aspiration of cystic contents and anterior vitrectomy, air is injected into the anterior chamber to insulate intraocular structures while the collapsed epithelial cyst is treated with transcorneal or translimbal cryotherapy.

Figure 3. Enbloc excision of epithelial cyst and adherent iris.

Eiferman and Rodrigues (1981) have managed an epithelial cyst occupying the superior one-third of the iris and anterior chamber in an eye with a corneal scar and corneal edema by means of eccentric penetrating keratoplasty combined with iridocyclectomy. The patient sustained blunt trauma to the eye postoperatively causing wound dehiscence and graft failure, but there has been no evidence of recurrence of the epithelial ingrowth cyst.

EPITHELIAL INGROWTH

Histologic specimens from eyes with epithelial ingrowth demonstrate a layer of epithelium on the posterior corneal surface, trabecular angle, iris, and occasionally lens capsule or vitreous. The sheet of cells may be one or several layers thick. The advancing edge of the ingrowth is seen most clearly because it tends to be thicker than the remainder of the epithelial sheet.

Growth along the iris and trabecular angle is usually more widespread than along the avascular cornea (Christensen, 1960). Jensen et al. (1977) found that this epithelium induces major anatomic modifications of underlying intraocular structures such as endothelial cell degeneration, and trabecular meshwork disorganization which may progress to total sclerosis of the meshwork with intractable glaucoma. A fistula is present in up to one-half of eyes with epithelial ingrowth, clinically manifested as hypotony with a positive Siedel sign (Stark et al., 1978). Electron microscopy has revealed that the cellular sheets have the characteristics of surface epithelium including frequent hemidesmosomes and a well developed basal lamina (Jensen et al., 1977).

Symptoms suggestive of epithelial ingrowth in the post-traumatic or postoperative eye include persistent pain, tearing, and photophobia. An updrawn pupil, persistent irititis, or hypotony may indicate the presence of epithelial ingrowth. The advancing edge of an epithelial sheet on the posterior surface of the cornea eventually confirms the diagnosis (Figure 4). The membrane itself is transparent, but its thickened, wavy leading edge is readily identified, especially by retroillumination.

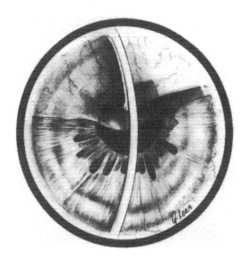

Figure 4. Epithelial ingrowth involving the posterior surface of the cornea, surperior iris, and vitreous face.

Initially, the advancing membrane has a convex edge leading away from the site of origin of the ingrowth. The edge becomes concave due to preferential growth of the epithelial sheet along the corneal limbus where it is supported by the limbal vasculature. Once the membrane grows into the trabecular angle and across the iris, it contracts, resulting in massive peripheral anterior synechiae. Deep corneal vascularization may develop. Rapidity of progression of the disease cannot be judged by observing the advance of the leading edge along the cornea as this does not correlate with activity over the angle or iris (Maumenee, 1964).

The natural history of epithelial ingrowth is varied. Persistent iritis and fistula formation often occur. Secondary glaucoma occurs unless a patent fistula is present. Mechanisms of glaucoma include: 1) epithelium lining the trabecular meshwork, 2) dense anterior synechiae closing the angle, 3) pupillary block, and 4) blockage of the angle by desquamated epithelium (Stark and Bruner, 1982). If left untreated, intractable glaucoma, massive epithelial invasion, and eventual loss of the eye will occur.

The differential diagnosis of epithelial ingrowth includes: 1) glassy membrane on the posterior surface of the cornea and anterior surface of the iris consisting of newly formed Descemet's membrane (usually in eyes with a history of iritis), 2) anteriorly shelved corneal section for cataract extraction, 3) vitreo-corneal touch, 4) invasion of the anterior chamber by connective tissue and blood vessels, and 5) detachment of Descemet's membrane. In the latter four conditions, the anterior surface of the iris is at most only slightly involved by the process. A detachment of Descemet's membrane may be distinguished by observing the inward curling at this inferior edge. (Maumenee, 1957).

The diagnosis may be further established by a positive Siedel test confirming the presence of a fistula, photocoagulation of the epithelial ingrowth overlying the iris resulting in white burns (Maumenee, 1968), scraping or biopsy of the posterior corneal membrane, or by specular microscopy.

Early attempts to treat epithelial ingrowth included irradiation by an external beam (Perera, 1937, Pincus, 1950) and radium plaque (Vail, 1936).

The most reliable means for eradication of epithelial ingrowth is surgical excision. Maumenee (1964) successfully treated epithelial ingrowth in 26 eyes by curetting the posterior corneal surface and excising the involved iris. Seven eyes maintained vision of 20/80 or better, thirteen developed corneal edema, three incurred retinal detachments, and three were enucleated for painful glaucoma.

A variation of the above technique utilized argon laser photocoagulation to delineate the extent of the ingrowth, and cryotherapy to devitalize remnants of epithelium adhering to the posterior corneal surface (Maumenee, 1970). Of forty eyes treated in this fashion, 27% retained vision of 20/50 or better and had normal intraocular pressure or glaucoma readily controlled on topical medication. There were no recurrences.

Brown (1973) altered Maumenee's technique by exposing and excising angle tissues which might otherwise have served as a source of recurrence. No recurrences were reported, and the glaucoma which developed in each of the three eyes was controlled medically. Postoperative visual acuity was only reported in two of the patients: 20/80 and 20/400.

Friedman (1977) utilized a more radical en bloc resection of the cornea and sclera with contiguous iris, ciliary body, and vitreous excision (when necessary) followed by replacement with a free-hand corneoscleral graft. In three patients with 7 to 44 months follow-up, visual acuity ranged from 20/50 to 20/100 with intraocular pressure controlled on acetazolamide and no evidence of recurrence.

Stark et al. (1978) modified Maumenee's techniques by using vitrectomy instrumentation to excise involved tissues and by introducing an intraocular air bubble as thermal insulation to protect uninvolved tissues during transcorneal and transcleral cryotherapy. Preoperative argon laser photocoagulation was used to define the extent of epithelial ingrowth on the anterior surface of the iris (Figure 5). Five-hundred micron size spots are placed along the advancing edge of epithelium so that one-half of each spot turned brown indicating uninvolved iris tissue. Two percent fluorescein dye is applied to the eye, and external pressure is exerted to identify potential fistulas. If found, fistulas are closed by preparation of anteriorly hinged one-half thickness scleral flaps.

Using a pars plana approach, a sclerotomy is performed 4 mm posterior and parallel to the limbus in the superior temporal quadrant. The vitrectomy instrument, is inserted through the sclerotomy and into the pupillary space. Involved vitreous and iris are ex-

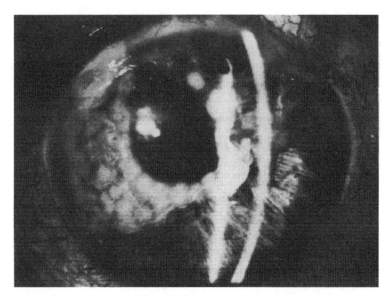

Figure 5. Argon laser photocoagulation delineates the extent of epithelial ingrowth over the iris.

cised using the oscillating cutting mode to minimize traction on the iris root (Figure 6). Hemostasis is maintained with bipolar diathermy and by temporarily increasing the intraocular pressure (Michels and Rice, 1977). The anterior one-half of the vitreous gel is excised to provide for a large air bubble used during cryodestruction. Air is inserted via a fluid-gas exchange prior to withdrawing the vitrectomy instrument, or by means of a needle attached by a three-way stopcock to an aspiration syringe and a syringe filled with air. The vitrectomy instrument is removed and the sclerotomy closed with multiple sutures.

At this stage, a hinged scleral flap is used to close the fistula. The fundus is examined by indirect ophthalmoscopy and scleral buckling is used to eliminate vitreous traction where present. Transcorneal and transscleral cryotherapy are applied to devitalize remnants of the epithelial ingrowth remaining on the posterior corneal surface, in the anterior chamber angle, and on the ciliary body (Figure 7). Presence of a bubble in the anterior chamber allows each freeze to persist longer and provides improved control over the size of each cryo-application. The full-thickness freeze is advanced just beyond the edge of the epithelial sheet. The air bubble is replaced with a physiologic solution.

Ten cases of epithelial ingrowth involving at least one-third of the cornea, iris, and anterior chamber were treated with the above technique with a mean follow-up of 33 months. Postoperative visual acuity was improved in eight of the eyes with four achieving 20/40 or better. Only two eyes required medications to normalize intraocular pressure. Penetrating keratoplasty was performed on four eyes with postoperative corneal edema. Cystoid macular edema accounted for the decrease in visual acuity in three of the six eyes with vision of less than 20/40. The remaining eyes had decreased vision secondary to hypotony, a periretinal membrane or optic nerve damage from previous

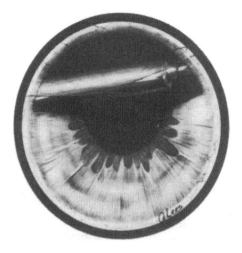

Figure 6. Vitrectomy instrumentation is used to excise areas of the iris and vitreous covered by epithelial ingrowth.

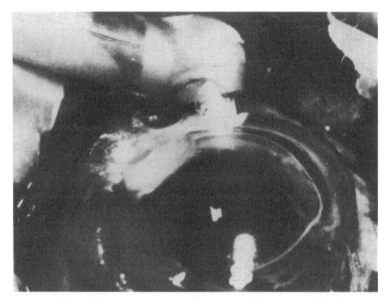

Figure 7. Transcorneal and transscleral cryotherapy is applied to destroy epithelial ingrowth on the cornea, in the angle, and on the ciliary body. An air bubble insulates non-involved intraocular structures from the effects of the freeze.

glaucoma. One eye had residual epithelial ingrowth. Long-term follow-up of a larger series showed that only 25% of eyes maintained visual acuity of 20/40 or better (Stark, 1981). Due to hypotony occurring in two eyes, the cryotherapy technique was altered to a single application rather than the freeze-refreeze method initially employed.

Early recognition of epithelial ingrowth and prompt surgical treatment can result in a higher success rate, as less of the eye is involved and less extensive therapy is required (Stark et al., 1978). Due to the poor prognosis in far advanced cases of epithelial ingrowth, it may be preferable to avoid radical surgery in patients with good visual function in the fellow eye. Cyclocryotherapy can be used to treat secondary glaucoma unresponsive to medical management. If the involved eye is the patient's only eye, prompt surgical treatment is recommended (Stark and Bruner, 1982).

ACKNOWLEDGMENTS

This work was supported in part by the Women's Committee of the International Medical Eye Bank of Maryland. Reprint requests to Walter J. Stark, M.D., the Wilmer Institute, Maumenee Bldg., Room 327, Johns Hopkins Hospital, Baltimore, Maryland 21205.

REFERENCES

1. Bernardino VB, Kim JC, and Smith TR (1969): Epithelization of the anterior chamber after cataract extraction. Arch Ophth 82:742-750.
2. Bettman JW, Jr (1969): Pathology of complications of intraocular surgery. Am J Ophth 68:1037-1050.
3. Brown SI (1973): Treatment of advanced epithelial downgrowth. Tr Am Acad Oph 77:618-622.
4. Bruner WE, Michels RG, Stark WJ, and Maumenee AE (1981): Management of epithelial cysts of the anterior chamber. Ophth Surg 12:279-285.
5. Calhoun FP, Jr (1949): The clinical recognition and treatment of epithelization of the anterior chamber following cataract extraction. Tr Am Oph Soc 47:498-553.
6. Christensen L (1960): Epithelization of the anterior chamber. Tr Am Ophthal Soc 58:294-300.
7. Cleasby GW (1971): Photocoagulation or iris-ciliary body epithelial cysts. Trans Am Acad Oph Oto 75:638-642.
8. Cogan DG (1955): Experimental implants of conjunctiva into the anterior chamber. Am J Ophth 39:165-172.
9. Collins ET, and Cross FR (1982): Two cases of epithelial implantation cyst in the anterior chamber after extraction of cataract. Trans Oph Soc UK. 12:175-180.
10. Dunnington JH (1951): Healing of incision for cataract extraction Am J Ophth 34:36-45.
11. Eiferman RA, and Rodrigues MM (1981): Squamous epithelial implantation cyst of the iris. Ophthalmol 86:1281-1285.
12. Eldrup-Jorgensen P (1969): Epithelization of the anterior chamber. A clinical and histological study of a Danish material. Acta Ophth 47:328-338, 1969.
13. Ferry AP (1971): The possible role of epithelium-bearing surgical instruments in the pathogenesis of epithelization of the anterior chamber. Annals of Ophthalmol 3:1089-1093.
14. Ferry AP, and Naghdi MR (1967): Cryosurgical removal of epithelial cyst or iris and anterior chamber. Arch Ophth 77:86-87.
15. Friedman AH (1977): Radical anterior segment surgery for epithelial invasion of the anterior chamber: Report of three cases. Tr Am Acad Oph Oto 83:216-223.
16. Jensen P, Minckler DS, and Chandler JW (1977): Epithelial ingrowth. Arch Ophth 95:837-842.
17. Gundersen T (1938): Results of autotransplantation of cornea into the anterior chamber: Their significance regarding corneal nutrition. Trans Am Oph Soc 6:207-212.
18. Hogan MJ, and Goodner EK (1960): Surgical treatment of epithelial cysts of the anterior chamber. Arch Ophth 64:286-291.

19. MacKenzie W (1830): A practical treatise on disease of the eye. Longman, Rees, Orme, Brown, and Green. London.

20. Maumenee AE (1957): Symposium. Postoperative cataract complications. Epithelial invasion of the anterior chamber, retinal detachment, corneal edema, anterior chamber hemorrhages, changes in the macula. Trans Am Acad Oph Oto, 61:51-68.

21. Maumenee AE (1964): Treatment of epithelial downgrowth and intraocular fistula following cataract surgery. Tr Am Oph Soc 62:153-166.

22. Maumenee AE (1968): Complications of cataract surgery. Highlights of Ophth 11:120-132.

23. Maumenee AE, Paton D, Morse PH, and Butner R (1970): Review of 40 histologically proven cases of epithelial downgrowth following cataract extraction and suggested surgical management. Am J Ophth 69:598-603.

24. Maumenee AE, and Shannon CR (1956): Epithelial invasion of the anterior chamber. Am J Ophth 11:929-942.

25. Michels RG, and Rice TR (1977): Internal-external bimanual bipolar diathermy for treatment of bleeding from the anterior chamber angle. Am J Ophth 83:873.

26. Okun E and Mandell E (1974): Photocoagulation as treatment of epithelial implantation cysts following cataract surgery. Tr Am Ophth Soc 72:170-183.

27. Perera CA (1937): Epithelium in the anterior chamber of the eye after operation and injury. Trans Am Soc Oph Oto 42:142-164.

28. Pincus MH (1950): Epithelial invasion of anterior chamber following cataract extraction: Effect of radiation therapy. Arch Ophth 43:509-519.

29. Regan EF (1958): Epithelial invasion of the anterior chamber. Arch Ophth 60:907-927.

30. Rothmund A (1872): Ueber cystern der regenbogenhaut, Klin Mbl Augenheilk 10:189-223.

31. Stark WJ (1981): Management of epithelial ingrowth and cysts. Dev. Ophth 5:64-73.

32. Stark WJ, and Bruner WE (1982): Epithelial ingrowth and fibrous proliferations. In: The Secondary Glaucomas, edited by Ritch R and Shields HB, CV Mosby Co, St Louis.

33. Stark WJ, Michels RG, Maumenee AE, and Cupples H (1978): Surgical Management of epithelial ingrowth. Am J Ophth 85:772-780

34. Sugar H (1967): Further experience with posterior lamellar resection of the cornea for epithelial implantation cyst. Am J Ophth 64:291-299.

35. Theobald GD, and Hass JS (1948): Epithelial invasion of the anterior chamber following cataract extraction. Trans Am Acad Oph Oto 52:470-485.

36. Vail D (1936): Epithelial overgrowth into the anterior chamber following cataract extraction: Arrest by radium treatment. Arch Ophth 15:270-282.

Basic and advanced vitreous surgery
G.W. Blankenship, M. Stirpe, M. Gonvers, S. Binder (eds.)
Fidia Research Series, vol. II,
Liviana Press, Padova © 1986

VITRECTOMY IN THE MANAGEMENT OF DISLOCATED CRYSTALLINE LENSES

Harry W. Flynn, Jr., M.D.

The Bascom Palmer Eye Institute, Department of Ophthalmology,
University of Miami School of Medicine, Miami, Florida.

The indications for surgical removal of the dislocated crystalline lens are controversial and the benefits of lens removal must be weighed against possible complications of surgery (1-4). Because retained non-encapsulated crystalline lens fragments are poorly tolerated, surgical intervention is usually necessary (4). Posterior dislocation of the lens nucleus after attempted extracapsular cataract extraction is the most common lens indication for vitreous surgery. Since severe intraocular inflammation and glaucoma often result, the retained lens nucleus and cortical material must be removed from the eye. Other considerations for surgical removal of the dislocated crystalline lens or retained lens fragments include the presence of a dislocated lens in the visual axis causing a major disturbance in vision or a poor view of the fundus in an eye with retinal detachment.

A traditional surgical approach employs needles passed across the anterior chamber or pars plana region to trap the lens nucleus in the anterior chamber after face-down positioning (1, 5). An open-sky approach can then be used to remove the lens from the anterior chamber with the patient returned to the supine position on the operating table. Although this technique can be attempted, it is technically very difficult and has a high risk of complications. Often the dense anterior vitreous gel prevents anterior positioning of the posteriorly dislocated lens.

In any surgical approach to a dislocated crystalline lens, vitreous loss will occur and vitrectomy instrumentation is essential. The exact surgical approach to the dislocated crystalline lens is determined by the hardness of the lens nucleus and by the ability to prolapse the lens nucleus into the anterior chamber (4, 6). Soft crystalline lenses may be readily aspirated into the vitrectomy or fragmenting instrument. However, a hard lens nucleus may be much more difficult to aspirate or fragment in the vitreous cavity and limbal extraction may be necessary. In addition to removal of the hard lens nucleus, cortical lens material may be mixed with formed vitreous and a more complete vitrectomy may be necessary.

VITRECTOMY APPROACHES TO THE DISLOCATED CRYSTALLINE LENS

Four basic surgical approaches using vitrectomy instrumentation will be discussed in this report. These approaches are the following:
1. Open-sky vitrectomy with limbal cryoextraction of the hard lens nucleus (or the entire crystalline lens in elderly patients).
2. Pars plana vitrectomy with instrument delivery of the hard lens nucleus into the anterior chamber for limbal cryoextraction.
3. Pars plana vitrectomy with aspirating and crushing of softer lens material using a two-instrument approach.
4. Pars plana vitrectomy with fragmentation of the relatively soft lens nucleus.

1. OPEN-SKY VITRECTOMY WITH LIMBAL CRYOEXTRACTION (Figure 1)

This approach is commonly used in elderly patients with dislocation of the entire hard lens nucleus into the vitreous cavity during extracapsular cataract extraction. Attempts to fragment or crush the hard lens nucleus in the vitreous cavity are often very time consuming, unsuccessful, or prone to secondary complications. The open-sky approach may be the most efficient way to remove the entire hard lens nucleus using the pre-existing limbal incision.

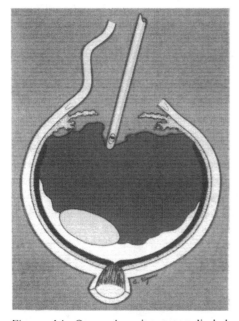

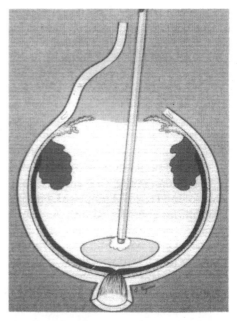

Figure 1A. Open sky vitrectomy limbal cryoextraction. A limbal incision is used to lift the cornea. An open-sky vitrectomy is performed without infusion in order to approach the dislocated hard lens nucleus.

Figure 1B. Open sky vitrectomy limbal cryoextraction. The intravitreal cryoprobe is used to extract the lens nucleus from the vitreous cavity. The eye is reformed with balanced salt solution. The limbal wound is closed in the standard fashion.

A limbal peritomy is performed and a limbal incision or the previous cataract incision is extended to a full 180°. The anterior vitreous gel is excised with the vitrectomy instrument, removing as much vitreous as possible in front of the retained lens nucleus. Any residual lens cortex is also removed. The lens nucleus is contacted by the intravitreal cryoprobe or by a suction needle and the lens nucleus is delivered from the eye through the limbal incision. Retraction of the iris is necessary to protect the pupillary margin from inadvertent freezing by the cryoprobe. The plastic sheath on the intravitreal cryoprobe will help avoid contact with the iris. After the vitreous cavity is filled with a balanced salt solution, the limbal incision is closed with standard nylon sutures.

Major concerns using this technique are scleral collapse and retinal detachment. A Flieringa ring is necessary in younger patients or in patients with high myopia. Because the intravitreal cryoprobe may adhere to formed vitreous gel and therefore exert traction on the retinal periphery, removal of the vitreous gel in front of the dislocated lens is essential.

REPORT OF CASES

Case Report 1

This 75-year-old man had unplanned extracapsular cataract extraction with loss of the hard lens nucleus into the vitreous cavity, left eye, on August 9, 1982. An anterior vitrectomy was performed, removing cortical lens material and anterior vitreous, but the lens nucleus could not be retrieved. An anterior chamber intraocular lens was inserted and the eye was closed with interrupted nylon sutures. Postoperatively, the patient had progressive inflammation, glaucoma and pain in the left eye.

The patient was seen in consultation on September 20, 1984, at which time a visual acuity of 20/25, right eye; hand motions, left eye, was present. The tension by applanation was 6 right eye and 42 left eye. Slitlamp examination of the left eye showed mild epithelial corneal edema with heavy cell and flare in the anterior chamber. The intraocular lens was well positioned, and multiple dilated iris vessels were observed. The dislocated lens nucleus could be seen in the inferior vitreous cavity.

The patient was taken to surgery on September 22, 1982, at which time an open sky approach was used to remove both the intraocular lens and the dislocated hard lens nucleus. The limbal cataract wound was opened and the anterior chamber IOL was removed first. Next, an open-sky vitrectomy without intraocular irrigation was performed and the lens nucleus was extracted, using the intravitreal cryoprobe. Following instillation of balanced salt solution, the limbal incision was closed with interrupted 10-0 nylon sutures.

The patient had a gradual resolution of intraocular inflammation, but continued to have mild corneal epithelial and stromal edema. The best corrected visual acuity on February 14, 1983 was 20/80 left eye. The tension by applanation was 21 on Timoptic 0.5% drops twice daily.

114

Case Report 2

This 72-year-old white man had a steel wire strike his right eye in 1968, causing traumatic lens dislocation. The lens remained in the inferior pupillary axis, but with a contact lens he had achieved good visual acuity. The patient had chronic glaucoma treated with Pilocarpine 2% three times daily and Eppy-N 2% twice daily to the right eye. The patient also complained of a superior altitudinal field defect in the right eye which prompted referral.

His examination on December 19, 1979 revealed a visual acuity best corrected to 8/200 right eye and 20/20 left eye. The slitlamp examination showed a mature white dislocated cataract in the inferior pupillary axis behind the iris. There was diffuse vitreous inflammation causing a hazy view of posterior segment details, but an inferior retinal detachment could be identified.

The patient was taken to surgery on January 7, 1980, at which time an open-sky vitrectomy and cryo-extraction of the dislocated cataract was performed. After closure of the limbal incision with multiple interrupted nylon sutures, a scleral buckling procedure was performed.

The postoperative course showed return of intraocular pressure to normal, and complete retinal reattachment was achieved. The most recent visual acuity in the right eye was 20/60 with contact lens on November 30, 1983.

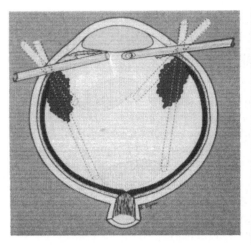

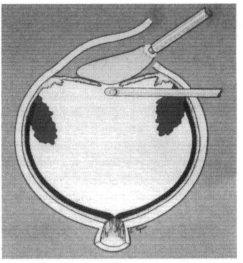

Figure 2A. Pars plana vitrectomy limbal cryoextraction.
A pars plana approach is used to remove remaining lens cortex from the central vitreous cavity. The hard lens nucleus is brought forward using two instruments. One instrument is maintained in the pars plana to secure the nucleus in the AC. (Infusion cannula not shown).

Figure 2B. Pars plana vitrectomy limbal cryoextraction.
While the assistant holds the pars plana instrument in place, the surgeon opens the limbal incision and uses a cryoprobe to remove the lens nucleus. (Infusion cannula not shown).

2. PARS PLANA VITRECTOMY WITH INSTRUMENT DELIVERY OF THE HARD LENS NUCLEUS INTO THE ANTERIOR CHAMBER (Figure 2)

This approach is a variation of the first technique in that a limbal incision is required to remove the hard nucleus. A standard three sclerotomy vitrectomy approach is used with an infusion cannula in the inferior temporal quadrant 3.5 mm posterior to the limbus and additional sclerotomies made in the superior temporal and superior nasal quadrants, also 3.5 mm posterior to the limbus. A pars plana vitrectomy is performed to remove the vitreous gel and retained cortical lens fragments from the anterior chamber and vitreous cavity. The vitrectomy instrument (or intraocular forceps) is used to deliver the nucleus into the anterior chamber. The position of the nucleus is maintained in the anterior chamber by the vitrectomy instrument or intraocular forceps. A limbal incision is made by the surgeon, while the assistant holds the pars plana instrument. The lens nucleus is delivered from the eye with the cryoprobe or a lens loop.

Case Report 3

This 86-year-old man had attempted intracapsular cataract extraction performed on the left eye on July 18, 1983. During the operative procedure, there was unplanned rupture of the capsule, followed by dislocation of the lens nucleus into the vitreous cavity. A partial anterior vitrectomy was performed by way of the limbus but the lens nucleus could not be retrieved. Postoperatively the patient had progressive intraocular inflammation, glaucoma, and pain in the left eye.

The patient was initially examined by referral on August 31, 1983, at which time a best corrected visual acuity of 20/20 right eye and 10/200 left eye was recorded. The slitlamp examination showed residual lens cortex in the anterior chamber and vitreous strands adherent to the internal aspect of the cataract incision. The intraocular pressure was 24 in the left eye. The posterior segment examination showed a darkly brunescent lens nucleus in the inferior vitreous cavity surrounded by cortical debris.

Surgical removal of the hard lens nucleus was performed on September 1, 1983. A pars plana approach was used to first remove the residual lens cortex and vitreous strands in the anterior chamber, as well as to remove the majority of lens cortical fragments in the vitreous cavity. An intraocular foreign body forceps was used to grasp the hard lens nucleus, which was brought forward into the anterior chamber.

The previous limbal cataract incision was opened and the lens nucleus was extracted with the intravitreal cryoprobe. A small piece of lens nucleus fell posteriorly during the initial cryoextraction. A second open-sky cryoapplication was necessary to retrieve this small piece of hard lens nucleus.

The patient had decreasing inflammation during the postoperative period. The visual acuity with correction has improved to 20/80 but the intraocular pressure has remained elevated (IOP 24 on Timoptic 0.5% drops twice daily). The cornea shows mild, persistent epithelial and stromal edema. No visible cystoid macular edema is present in the left eye.

3. PARS PLANA VITRECTOMY WITH ASPIRATING AND CRUSHING OF SOFTER LENS MATERIAL USING A TWO-INSTRUMENT APPROACH
(Figure 3)

This technique can be used in younger patients with softer nuclei. The approach can also be used in patients with only a small portion of retained lens material, such as a small nuclear fragment lost after phacoemulsification. Using the standard three sclerotomy vitrectomy approach, the lens material can be directly aspirated into the vitrectomy instrument with assistance from the fiberoptics light pipe. Larger pieces of lens material can be crushed and aspirated using the two instruments.

Figure 3. Pars plana vitrectomy crush, aspirate lens.
A two instrument approach is used to remove fragments of retained lens materials. These fragments can be crushed between the two instruments and aspirated into the vitrectomy instrument. (Infusion cannula not shown).

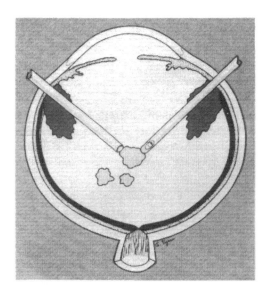

Case Report 4

This 62-year-old patient was referred with lens-induced uveitis and glaucoma in the right eye. The patient reported a traumatic injury to the right eye in 1937 while playing football. The patient had worn a contact lens with improved vision, but noted a gradual loss of vision over the six-month period prior to his examination here on February 17, 1982.

The best corrected visual acuity was recorded as 20/100 right eye and 20/20 left eye. The slitlamp examination of the right eye showed moderate cell and flare in the anterior chamber with marked inflammation in the anterior and mid-vitreous. The tension by applanation was 33 in the right eye and 21 in the left eye. The posterior segment examination showed a mature white lens freely floating in the vitreous cavity, lying near the surface of the retina.

The patient was taken to surgery on February 22, 1982, at which time a pars plana approach was used on the right eye. The lens was removed by the vitrectomy instrument, using an aspirating and crushing technique.

Postoperatively, the inflammation gradually subsided, and the intraocular pressure returned to normal. The visual acuity improved to 20/60 in the right eye on May 14, 1984. Atrophic changes in the retinal pigment epithelium were noted in the macula.

4. PARS PLANA VITRECTOMY WITH FRAGMENTATION OF THE LENS NUCLEUS (Figure 4)

This approach also uses the standard three sclerotomy approach but the fragmentating instrument is used to break up the lens material. The fragmenting instrument must be used in anterior or mid-vitreous in order to avoid retinal damage from the instrument or from hard pieces of lens material pushed against the retina. Vitrectomy is also necessary in these cases to remove portions of the vitreous gel around the dislocated lens and residual small pieces of lens material. This technique is the most efficient and the least time-consuming way of removing lenses with relatively soft nuclei.

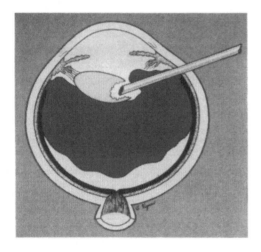

Figure 4. Pars plana fragmentation vitrectomy.
The fragmenting instrument is used to remove the soft lens nucleus and much of the lens cortex. Remaining fragments of lens mixed with vitreous can be removed with the vitrectomy instrument. (Infusion cannula not shown).

Case Report 5

This 41-year-old lady was involved in an automobile accident on December 30, 1982, at which time she suffered a right orbital floor fracture, multiple lid lacerations, and traumatic subluxation of the lens in the right eye. On March 18, 1983, she had a best corrected visual acuity of 20/50 right eye and 20/20 left eye. The slitlamp examination of the right eye showed vitreous extending around the superior temporal edge of the lens and mild posterior subcapsular opacity in the lens. Observation was recommended, and the patient again returned for follow-up on September 23, 1983. The best corrected visual acuity in the right eye had dropped to 20/200 because of the presence of a dense posterior subcapsular and cortical cataract. Vitreous now was herniated through the pupil into the anterior chamber.

The patient was taken to surgery on September 26, 1983, at which time a pars plana approach was used. The lens was aspirated using the fragmentation instrument. Residual cortex and vitreous were removed with the vitrectomy instrument. Postoperatively, the visual acuity in the right eye was corrected to 20/20 with contact lens wear. The last follow-up information on the patient was May 17, 1984.

CONCLUSION

Dislocated crystalline lenses may be well tolerated in the posterior segment without the need for surgical intervention. Selected cases of dislocated lenses may require surgical intervention. This report describes four current approaches using vitrectomy instrumentation for the removal of dislocated lenses in complicated cases.

REFERENCES

1. Calhoun FT, Hagler WS (1960): Experience with the Jose Barraquer method of extracting a dislocated lens. Am J Ophthalmol. 50:701-714.
2. Barraquer J (1972): Surgery of a dislocated lens. Trans Am Acad Ophthalmol Otolaryngol. 78:44-59.
3. Maumenee AE, Ryan SJ (1969): Aspiration technique in the management of a dislocated lens. Am J Ophthalmol. 68:808-811.
4. Michels RG, Shacklett DE (1977): Vitrectomy technique for removal of retained lens material. Arch Ophthalmol. 95:1767-1772.
5. Agnew CR (1885): An operation for a double needle bident for the removal of a crystalline lens dislocated into the vitreous chamber. Trans Am Ophthalmol Soc. 4:69-76.
6. Peyman GA, Raichand M, Goldberg MS, Ritacca D (1979): Management of subluxated and dislocated lenses with the Vitreophage. Br J Ophthalmol. 63:771-778.

Basic and advanced vitreous surgery
G.W. Blankenship, M. Stirpe, M. Gonvers, S. Binder (eds.)
Fidia Research Series, vol. II,
Liviana Press, Padova © 1986

VISCOMICROSURGERY: THE USE OF A NEW FRACTION OF THE SODIUM SALT OF HYALURONATE

Riccardo Neuschüler, Vito Gasparri and Diego Girardi

Divisione Oculistica, Ospedale Fatebenefratelli, Isola Tiberina, Roma

Balazs (1950) first had the idea of using hyaluronic acid in ocular surgery. He was struck by the notable morphological similarity of this substance to the vitreous. The first preparation, extracted from the bovine eye, and with a low molecular weight (Etamucin) was, in fact, used as a substitute for the vitreous; but because of the serious reactions that it caused, its use was only tentative.

Balazs (1972) then experimented with hyaluronic acid combined with collagen liquid, but the results were still unsatisfactory. Later on, he used pure high molecular weight hyaluronic acid extracted from the human umbilical cord, but this product continued to cause problems of inflammation.

The principal use, therefore, of hyaluronic acid was as a substitute for the vitreous, but perhaps because of the imperfect method of extraction, which yielded a somewhat impure preparation, results were poor.

If hyaluronic acid had not begun to be used in the late 1970s in surgery of the anterior segment, it would perhaps have been completely forgotten. It was used by chance as a lubricant to help in the implant of the artificial crystalline lens, a use which led to an even better use, in the U.S.A., in cataract surgery — that of the routine implant of intraocular lenses.

The diffusion of the use of hyaluronic acid and its progressive modification and refinement resulted in the product called Healon (1970), a high molecular weight extract from cock's crest.

It is important to note what exactly hyaluronic acid is and where it comes from. From the biological point of view it belongs to the glycosaminoglycans; it is extracted from animal connective tissue, especially pig-skin, from the aorta of the bovine heart, from the bovine eye, from the human umbilical cord, and finally, from the cock's crest. The length of its molecular chain can vary notably in its original state, and for this reason hyaluronic acid extracted as such is seen as heterogeneous from the physical point of view in that it can contain material with a molecular weight of from 30,000 to 2,000,000, and even more, with different properties.

As has been said, the product now most widely used is Healon, which has a high molecular weight of about 1,000,000; its noteworthy and progressive diffusion has been accompanied by an observation of its complications, above all, a significant and menacing increase in the postoperative intraocular pressure (IOP) — to the point that it must be removed from the operating field after it has served its purpose.

The principal use of hyaluronic acid until now, therefore, has been as a lubricant, and hence as protection of the ocular membranes during the implant of an artificial crystalline lens; and, more tentatively as a substitute for the vitreous. In any case, the attempt has been made to produce preparations of high molecular weight in order to increase its viscous and protective properties.

By further careful study of hyaluronic acid, about which we so far know little, it would seem to be possible to produce another, better version devoid of the secondary complications of the original product, especially regarding the pathological changes of IOP.

It has been seen, moreover, that the fractions of hyaluronic acid of lower molecular weight (30,000-80,000) have the striking property of favouring the recovery of the tissues. The beneficial effect of preparations based on hyaluronic acid with low molecular weight is known in certain pathologies of tissue recovery, for example torpid ulcers and arthrotic degeneration of the connective tissues in the articular capsule.

We therefore began to try preparations of different molecular weights, and we found that the most useful fraction was that of a molecular weight between 500,000 and 650,000, which, while retaining excellent viscous and protective properties is nevertheless free from the well known pathological consequences on IOP, and also has the reparative and stimulating qualities of preparations of lower molecular weight.

On the basis of these findings, the concept of viscomicrosurgery has gradually been developed, progressively gaining greater importance. In practice, it means a new type of substance which is absolutely harmless for the various structures of the eye of which it is in fact a normal component, especially of the vitreous. Hence, it is helpful for practical surgery in various ways.

All this could only be obtained with a preparation which has the right viscosity and the highest protective power, and that can be left in the operated eye — rapidly metabolized by the enzymes present in the eye (hyaluronidase); not easily aggregated with blood or cataract masses, absolutely free from any kind of IOP complications.

All the experiments and studies of the various possibilities of the use of hyaluronic acid in ocular surgery have been carried out by FIDIA Pharmaceutics, using their refined method of extraction from cock's crest so as to obtain a final product called IAL.

IAL has to the greatest degree the ideal prerequisites required by the ophthalmic surgeon in order to perform viscomicrosurgery:
- The biological compatibility of the substance with the human eye so as not to cause any inflammatory reaction
- It does not increase IOP
- It constitutes a mechanical tampon to reestablish or maintain normal anatomical relationships; it counterbalances, if necessary, the vitreal force.
- It does not cause corneal edema

— It is effective in a relatively short time
— It does not interfere with normal physiological mechanisms such as pupillary mobility or the circulation of aqueous humor
— It has a protective effect on the endocular structures
— The use of the product is simple and helps in surgical manipulation
— It has a good refractive index
— It stabilizies the anterior chamber in order to perform surgical micromanipulation
— It has a surprising cicatrizing effect in surgical diastasis and serious corneal lesions
— It prevents irido-corneal synechiae
— It has excellent mechanical hemostatic effects on the anterior chamber
— The security afforded by the product has permitted surgery under local anesthesia in that the viscous substance maintains the anterior chamber even during possible movements of the patient
— No untoward effects have appeared during or after the operation
— It has a constant myotic effect following its introduction in the anterior chamber, perhaps due to a mechanical effect.
— It does not increase postsurgical astigmatism
— 14-18 hours after surgery pupillary mobility is normal
— Its introduction is easy with the common cannula needle
— It easily and homogenously fills all the desired anatomical spaces
— It does not tend to move from the position where it has been placed
— At the level of a surgical suture it does not interfere with the various suture materials.
— It does not mix with the vitreous body and can be easily separated from it
— It remains in the anterior chamber for an average of 7-12 days.

More specifically, the application, the type of operation, and the true usefulness of IAL are indicated in Table 1.

From this table, the important use of IAL in vitreoretinal surgery has intentionally been omitted. If this substance has not succeeded, either as a retinal tampon in comparison with silicone oil or as a vitreous substitute, it has nevertheless become an excellent tool as a delicate surgical instrument.

The removal of epiretinal membrane, especially in serious diabetic retinopathy which demands vitrectomy, has always been a big technical problem, solved by surgeons in various ways. To have at one's disposal a substance like IAL, that can be used to separate membranes, to tampon haemorrhages, to open virtual spaces and thus to create delicate planes of cleavage with excellent transparency and without the presence of blood of fibrin, in fact to separate these substances from the margins of the operating field is, for the surgeon of the vitreous, a considerable technical advance and instrument.

Stirpe-Orciuolo, in fact, have devised an appropriate syringe which functions at various pressures and by means of a fine needle can apply to the desired areas the manifold actions of IAL, a surprisingly effective aid to vitreoretinal surgery.

Table 1

Application	Type of operation	Utility
Intravitreous	Retinal Detachment	Mechanical tampon to stabilize the surgical result
Intravitreous	Repair surgery after trauma	To correct and maintain ocular volume
Anterior Chamber	Cataract Extraction	To maintain the depth of the a.c., to prevent the protrusion of the vitreous through the pupil and to protect the corneal endothelium
Anterior Chamber	Implant of IOL	To maintain the depth of the a.c., to prevent the protrusion of the vitreous through the pupil and to protect the corneal endothelium
Anterior Chamber	Corneal Transplant	To reconstruct the a.c. and to protect the cornea
Anterior Chamber	Trabeculectomy for glaucoma	To avoid the collapse of the a.c. and to protect the cornea
Extraocular (between the cornea and the microscope lens)	Closed Vitrectomy	To protect the corneal epithelium
Extraocular (instillation)	Cataract Extraction	To protect the corneal epithelium and the conjunctiva
Extraocular (instillation)	Normal ocular surgery and keratitis	To maintain vital epithelium if there is a risk of drying.

Even from its first tentative uses, one can see the great potential use of hyaluronic acid to solve technical problems which until now were not easily mastered.

In IAL, FIDIA Pharmaceutics has developed a new application of hyaluronic acid, and, because of the noteworthy properties of this product, has made the development of viscomicrosurgery possible, applicable not only in the anterior segment but also in the more delicate field of vitreoretinal operations.

LITERATURE

Algvere P (1971): Intravitreal implantation of a high-molecular hyaluronic acid in surgery for retinal detachment. Acta Ophthamol 49: 975-976

Balazs EA, Freeman MI, Klön R, Meyer-Schwickirath G, Regnault E, Sweeney DB (1972): Hyaluronic acid and replacement of vitreous and aqueous humor. Secondary Detachment of the Retina. Mod Probl Ophthal 10: 3-21.

Binkhorst CD (1981): Advantages and disadvantages of intracamerular Na-hyaluronate (Healon) in intraocular lens surgery. Documenta Ophthalmologica, 50, (2): 233-236

Body BF (1981): What is Healon? Is it really the most important substance to come along in cataract surgery since alphachymotrypsin? What is its contribution to penetrating keratoplasty, intraocular lens implant surgery and dry eyes? Highlights of Ophthalmology, 9, (12): 1-5

Comper WD, Laurent TC (1978): Physiological function of connective tissue polysaccharides. Phys Rev, 58, (1): 255-315

Dessì P (1976): Relazione tossicologica per il Ministero della Sanità. Istituto Farmacocinetica e Tossicologia dell'Università di Bologna. datata 13/7/1976.

Edmund J (1974): Vitreous substitute in the treatment of retinal detachment. Limitations and Prospects for Retinal Surgery. Mod Probl Ophthal, 12: 370-377

Gnad HD (1979): Partial vitreous substitution with Ringer's solution or sodium hyaluronate. Ophthalmic Res, 11: 108-122

Graue EL, Polack FM, Balazs EA (1980): The protective effect of Na-hyaluronate to corneal endothelium. Exp Eye Res, 31: 119-127

Kanski JJ (1975): Intravitreal hyaluronic acid injection. A long-term clinical evaluation. Brit J Ophthal 59: 255-256

Klöti R (1972): Hyaluronsäure als Glaskörpersubstituent. Ophthalmologica, 165: 351-359

Miller D, O'Connor P, Williams J. (1977): Use of Na-hyaluronate during intraocular lens implantation in rabbits. Ophthalmic Surgery, 8, (6): 58-61

Norm M (1981): Preoperative protection of cornea and conjunctiva. Acta Ophthalmologica, 59: 587:594

Pape LG, Balazs EA: Final report on the use of Healon in glaucoma visco-surgery. Personal communication.

Polack FM, Demong T, Santaella H (1981): Sodium hyaluronate (Healon) in Keratoplasty and I01 implantation. Ophthalmology, 88: 425-431

Pruett RC, Schepens CL, Swann DA (1979): Hyaluronic acid vitreous substitute. A six-year clinical evaluation. Arch Ophthalmol, 97: 2325-2330.

Razemon PMM, Turut P, Capier MJ (1972): L'acide hyaluronique dans les traumatismes délabrants du globe. Bulletin des sociétés d'Ophthalmologie de France, 72, (11): 105-107

Regnault F, Bregeat P (1974): Treatment of severe cases of retinal detachment with highly viscous hyaluronic acid. Limitations and Prospects for Retinal Surgery. Mod Probl Ophthal, 12: 378-383.

Richter W (1974): Non immunogenicity of purified hyaluronic acid preparations tested by passive cutaneous anaphylaxis. Int Arch Allergy. 47: 211-217

Richter AW, Ryde EM, Zatterstrom EO (1979): Non immunogenicity of a purified sodium hyaluronate preparation in man. Int Archs Appl Immun 59: 45-48.

Stanifer R, Kretzer F, Mehta R (1981): Effect of Healon on intraocular pressure, corneal thickness, and endothelial morphology in the rabbit. Investigative Opthalmology & Visual Science, 20, (3 Suppl.): 230.

Basic and advanced vitreous surgery
G.W. Blankenship, M. Stirpe, M. Gonvers, S. Binder (eds.)
Fidia Research Series, vol. II,
Liviana Press, Padova © 1986

USE OF THE NEODYNIUM YAG LASER
FOR THE ANTERIOR SEGMENT SURGEON

Walter J. Stark, Arlo C. Terry, John D. Gottsch, M. Bowes Hamill, Peter A. Rapoza

The Wilmer Ophthalmological Institute, The Johns Hopkins Medical Hospital, Baltimore, Maryland, 21205, U.S.A.

RETROLENTICULAR MEMBRANES

The most recent data available from the FDA indicate that 70% of the intraocular lenses currently being implanted in the United States are of the posterior chamber variety. Anterior chamber lenses account for nearly 30% of the lenses being implanted in the United States, but at least half of these are implanted secondarily, so that over 80% of lenses implanted primarily are posterior chamber lens implants.

The increasing popularity of posterior chamber lens implants necessitates extracapsular cataract extraction, and in our experience the posterior capsule opacifies in at least half of patients over a period of 2 to 5 years following surgery. A growing interest in the management of retrolenticular membranes, particularly the opaque posterior capsule, has occurred as a result of the shift towards extracapsular surgery.

Standard vitrectomy techniques may be used to excise retrolenticular membranes such as the opaque posterior capsule, but the Neodynium YAG laser is equally effective and less invasive. The laser has therefore emerged as the modality of choice for cutting thin membranes such as the opaque posterior capsule, and vitrectomy techniques are now reserved for the occasional membrane which is too thick for the laser to disrupt.

Our experience in using the YAG laser for posterior capsulotomy has been very encouraging: visual acuity has improved by one or more Snellen lines in 90%, by three or more lines in 63%, and by six or more lines in 33% of eyes treated. Visual acuity after capsulotomy has been better than the best visual acuity recorded between extracapsular cataract extraction and laser treatment in one-third of cases.

The most common complication encountered following laser capsulotomy has been a post-treatment elevation in intraocular pressure which has occurred in two-thirds of the eyes treated (Figure 1). In 7% of cases, pressures greater than 40 mm Hg were

126

detected. The increase in intraocular pressure was detectable within 3 hours after treatment in 90% of those eyes in which the intraocular pressure rose to 30 mm Hg or greater (Figure 2).

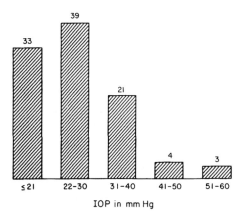

Figure 1. Maximum detected intraocular pressure in 100 eyes following Neodynium YAG laser discission of the posterior capsule.

Figure 2. Time at which maximum intraocular pressure was detected in 100 eyes after Neodynium YAG laser discission of the posterior capsule.

The close proximity of the posterior chamber intraocular lens to the posterior capsule results in damage to the intraocular lens at the time of capsulotomy in up to 40% of our cases. This damage, which appears as pits and/or cracks in the implant, appears to be visually insignificant provided the damage is minimal. However, we have recently seen a number of laser-damaged implants referred from other sources with damage severe enough to reduce visual acuity. Significant damage to the implant may be avoided by aiming slightly posterior to the posterior capsule and then moving slowly anteriorly until the capsule is cut.

Because of the potential release of toxic substances from laser-damaged intraocular lenses, we are currently in the process of examining a number of lenses produced by different manufacturers in order to evaluate this possibility.

Rupture of the vitreous face with forward displacement of vitreous into the anterior chamber has occurred in about half of eyes without implants. One of these eyes, (highly myopic) subsequently developed a rhegmatogenous retinal detachment 10 weeks after laser treatment, while another developed corneal edema 3 weeks after treatment. In order to reduce the chances of rupturing the anterior hyaloid face when no intraocular lens is present, we focus the laser beam slightly anterior to the capsule and then move slowly posteriorly.

An average of 33 bursts were used to create a clear pupillary opening in the first 100 eyes we treated with the YAG laser, but as we have become more experienced we have been able to achieve the same results with considerably fewer bursts. In addition, the recent acquistion of a Coherent YAG laser has added the capability of a multiple burst mode allowing us to excise floppy membranes using less total energy and fewer applications. We have found the optics in the slit lamp of the Coherent laser to be superior to those of the American Medical Optical laser.

VITREOUS STRANDS

Aside from cutting retrolenticular membranes, we have found the Neodynium YAG laser to be useful in cutting vitreous strands incarcerated in the wound following intracapsular cataract extraction. Energy settings required to cut vitreous strands are usually 3-4 times higher than those required for posterior capsulotomy, and use of an Abraham contact lens is essential. The number of applications required varies widely depending on the number and size of vitreous strands present. Large amounts of vitreous incised generally cannot be incised using the laser, and conventional vitrectomy techniques are required in these cases.

ACKNOWLEDGMENTS

This work was supported in part by the Women's Committee of the International Medical Eye Bank of Maryland.

Basic and advanced vitreous surgery
G.W. Blankenship, M. Stirpe, M. Gonvers, S. Binder (eds.)
Fidia Research Series, vol. II,
Liviana Press, Padova © 1986

SURGICAL MANAGEMENT OF SELECTED INTRAOCULAR LENS COMPLICATIONS

Walter J. Stark, Arlo C. Terry, Mario Stirpe*, Ronald G. Michels, M. Bowes Hamill, John D. Gottsch, Peter A. Rapoza

The Wilmer Ophthalmological Institute, The Johns Hopkins Hospital, Baltimore, Maryland, 21205, U.S.A., *Fondazione Oftalmologica 'G.B. Bietti', Piazza Sassari 5, Roma, Italia

The total number of cataract operations performed annually in the United States is not known with certainty, but it is estimated that 75% of cataract operations performed in the United States are associated with implantation of an intraocular lens (IOL) (1). As lens designs and surgical techniques improve, fewer IOL-related complications are being encountered. By way of this communication we discuss the surgical management of selected intraocular lens complications.

THE SUBLUXED POSTERIOR CHAMBER IMPLANT

Although uncommon, subluxation is probably the most frequent complication seen in association with posterior chamber lens implants. Optical symptoms caused by the edge of the optic within the pupillary space can usually be alleviated by using miotics, but occasionally surgical repositioning of the implant becomes necessary. A modification of the McCannel iris fixation suture provides the best means for refixation of such a lens (2).

In an eye with a widely dilated pupil, a peripheral clear corneal tract is created using a Ziegler knife at the position desired for the displaced haptic. The anterior chamber is then filled with sodium hyaluronate and a second limbal incision is made two to three clock hours from the initial incision. The implant is rotated into the desired position using a bent thirty gauge needle introduced through the second incision.

Following constriction of the pupil with acetylcholine, a 10-0 prolene suture attached to an Ethicon CIF-4 needle is passed through the second limbal incision, down through the iris, beneath the lens haptic, up through the iris and out through the cornea near the limbus in the adjacent quadrant (Figure 1). The needle is removed from the suture, and a hooked thirty gauge needle is introduced through the first incision and used to retrieve both ends of the suture (Figure 2). The prolene suture is tied externally and cut, after which it is allowed to retract into the anterior chamber. Usually, fixating one haptic is suffcient to secure the implant, but occasionally it is necessary to suture the other haptic to the iris in a similar fashion.

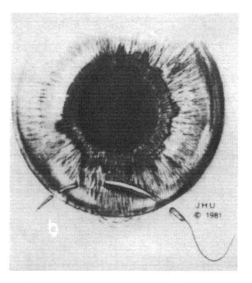

Figure 1. Ethicon CIF-4 needle attached to 10-0 Prolene suture, is passed through limbus, down through the iris, beneath the IOL haptic, up through iris, and out through limbus.

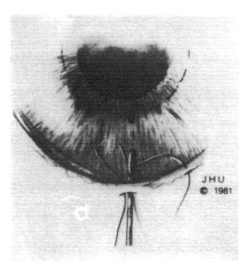

Figure 2. Hook-tip bent needle is used to retrieve ends of 10-0 Prolene suture.

REMOVAL OF THE POSTERIOR CHAMBER LENS IMPLANT

In over 2000 posterior chamber implant cases, we have not removed a single implant, and referred cases requiring removal of posterior chamber implants are rare. However, when removal of a posterior chamber implant becomes necessary it can be accomplished through a 7 mm superior limbal incision in a widely dilated pupil. Most often, the intraocular lens haptics have become firmly fixed, and both haptics are cut prior to grasping the optic of the implant centrally and removing it through the superior opening. The severed haptics are usually left in place because of firm adhesions to the posterior lens capsule and/or ciliary body.

We have found that the most common indication for removal of a posterior chamber implant is dislocation into the vitreous cavity. We attempt to avoid this in our patients by placing both haptics in the ciliary sulcus because we believe that dislocation is more likely to occur following placement of both haptics within the capsular bag.

Retrieval of an implant from the vitreous cavity always requires vitrectomy. Divided system instrumention is used with an infusion cannula, a fiber optic illuminator, and a vitrectomy probe. The vitrectomy probe is inserted through a separate scleral incision located 3 mm posterior to the limbus.

Prior to beginning the vitrectomy, a 7 mm limbal groove is prepared superiorly with three preplaced sutures. A vitrectomy probe is then used to excise vitreous gel until the intraocular lens is completely freed from surrounding vitreous. The vitrectomy probe is withdrawn and intraocular forceps are inserted through the same scleral opening. The forceps are used to grasp the optical portion of the implant, and the IOL is elevated into the pupillary plane with one haptic loop in the anterior chamber. The IOL is held in this position while the fiber optic illuminator is withdrawn. The limbal incision is then completed into the anterior chamber and enlarged to 7 mm. The anterior edge of the corneal incision is elevated, and the implant is delivered through the wound. Following closure of the limbal incision, the vitrectomy probe and fiber optic illuminator are reintroduced to remove any vitreous that may have prolapsed into the anterior chamber during removal of the implant.

REMOVAL OF THE ANTERIOR CHAMBER IMPLANT

Persistent uveitis, malposition, or chronic endothelial cell loss may require the removal of an anterior chamber intraocular lens. Although the need to remove an anterior chamber lens seldom arrises, in our experience conditions requiring the removal of an implant are more common with anterior chamber lenses than with the posterior chamber variety.

Removal of a closed-loop anterior chamber lens presents a special problem because the haptics often become firmly imbedded within the base of the iris (Figure 3) or ciliary body (3) (Figure 4).

Attempted removal of such an implant may be complicated by uncontrollable bleeding, creation of an iridodialysis, or even avulsion of the iris at its root. This type of lens, however, may be removed without difficulty by converting it to an open-loop and sliding it out through a 6 mm superior limbal incision (4).

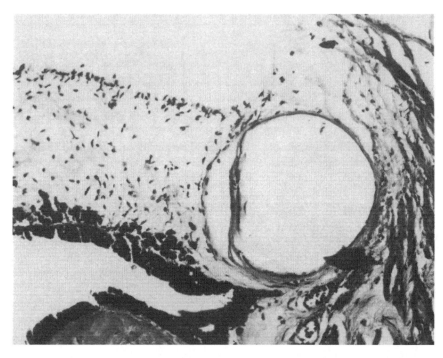

Figure 3. Superior haptic embedded in base of iris (reprinted with permission of Ophthalmology).

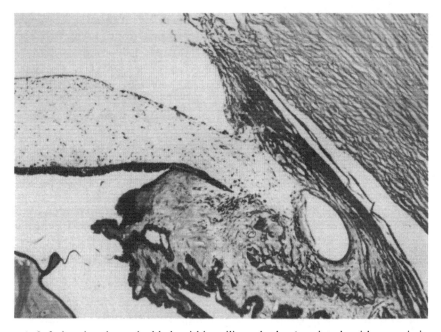

Figure 4. Inferior haptic embedded within ciliary body (reprinted with permission of Ophthalmology).

A 6 mm incision is made and the anterior chamber is immediately filled with Healon. Right angle intraocular scissors are then used to sever one arm of the inferior haptic, following which Wescott scissors are used to sever both arms of the superior haptic. The amputated superior haptic will then glide through the enveloping tissue tract with little resistance. Finally, the optic of the implant is grasped centrally and cautiously removed through the superior opening (Figure 5).

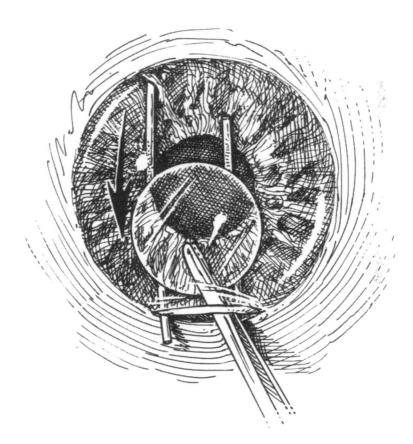

Figure 5. Grasping optic firmly with tying forceps, the implant is carefully pulled through superior opening (Reprinted with permission of Ophthalmic Surgery).

Alternately, an additional 3 mm limbal incision may be made inferiorly adjacent to one arm of the inferior haptic. The inferior haptic is then cut through this incision and the implant is removed as described above. This additional incision is necessary when removing closed-loop anterior lenses with PMMA haptics, because the delicate intraocular scissors may be damaged in attempting to cut through the rigid PMMA haptic.

134

ACKNOWLEDGMENTS

This work was supported in part by the Women's Committee of the International Medical Eye Bank of Maryland.

REFERENCES

1. Stark et al (1983): Trends in Cataract Surgery and Intraocular Lenses in the United States. Am J Ophthalmol 96:304-310.
2. Stark WJ, Bruner WE, Martin NF (1982): Management of Subluxed Posterior-Chamber Intraocular Lenses. Ophthalmic Surg 13 (2): 130-133.
3. McDonnel PJ, Green WR, Maumenee AE., et al (1983): Pathology of intraocular lenses in 33 eyes post mortem. Ophthalmol 90:386-403.
4. Terry AC, Stark WJ (1984): Removal of Closed-Loop Anterior Chamber Lens Implants. Ophthalmic Surg 15(7):575-577.

Basic and advanced vitreous surgery
G.W. Blankenship, M. Stirpe, M. Gonvers, S. Binder (eds.)
Fidia Research Series, vol. II,
Liviana Press, Padova © 1986

CLOSED VITREOUS SURGERY FOR COMPLICATIONS OF INTRAOCULAR LENS IMPLANTATION
I. INDICATIONS

C.P. Wilkinson, M.D.

Dean A. McGee Eye Institute and the Department of Ophthalmology,
University of Oklahoma Health Sciences Center, Oklahoma City, Oklahoma.

Modern closed vitrectomy techniques have provided a means of managing complications of cataract surgery in ways which are far superior to those which were popular prior to the revolutionary work of Machemer (1). The advantages of these techniques include the precise control of tissue excision (using microscopic visualization, efficient cutters, and optimal illumination), the maintenance of normal globe configuration, and the ability to perform a variety of accessory techniques, such as intraocular diathermy, scissors excision, and fragmentation. Complications of intraocular lens implantation can arbitrarily be divided into anterior and posterior indications for subsequent vitreous surgery (Tables 1 and 2). The goals of vitreous surgery in this setting include the removal of opaque or otherwise abnormal tissue, the elimination of certain traction forces, and the reduction of inflammation.

PROBLEMS ASSOCIATED WITH VITREOUS IN THE ANTERIOR CHAMBER

The most obvious indications for closed vitreous surgery are complications related to the presence of vitreous in the anterior chamber. These problems include: 1) vitreo-corneal contact with subsequent endothelial decompensation; 2) severe vitreous opacifications; 3) vitreous incarceration in the cataract wound associated with either chronic and

Table 1. *Anterior indications for vitreous surgery following intraocular lens implantation*

Vitreous in the Anterior Chamber
    Vitreous Touch Syndrome
    Vitreous Opacification
    Vitreous Incarceration in Cataract Wound
        Chronic CME
        Malposition of IOL
    Vitreous Wick Syndrome

Reduced Media
    Pupillary Membranes Unacceptable for YAG Capsulotomy
    Retained lens material
    Vitreous Opacification
    Vitreous Hemorrhage, Hyphema

Secondary Open-Angle Glaucoma
    Blood-Induced
    Retained Lens Material
        Phacogenic Uveitis
        Phacolytic
    Implant-Induced Inflammation

Pseudophakic Pupillary Block Glaucoma

Endophthalmitis

Repositioning/Removal of IOL

Epithelial Ingrowth

Table 2. *Posterior indications for vitreous surgery following intraocular lens implantation*

Certain Retinal Detachments
    Opaque Media (See Table 1)
    Traction Retinal Detachments
    Giant Tears
    Certain Posterior Breaks
    Massive PVR

Macular Pucker
Other (arbitrarily placed in Table 1)

---

severe cystoid macular edema or with malposition of the implant; 4) the "vitreous wick syndrome" with externalized vitreous gel. Vitreous touch alone does not represent a definite indication for vitreous surgery, but if evidence of subsequent endothelial decompensation can be documented clinically or with serial ultrasonic pachymetry, closed vitrectomy techniques provide a safe means of eliminating the harmful effects of vitreous touch, and subsequent chronic corneal edema can be avoided (2). Occasionally vitreous in the anterior chamber is relatively opaque, thereby reducing central visual acuity and causing symptoms similar to those associated with posterior subcapsular cataract, in which miosis reduces vision further. Fluorescein angiography should be performed before recommending vitreous surgery for this indication, as cystoid macular edema is frequently associated with some opacification of the vitreous gel. The precise levels of visual acuity which represent indications for subsequent vitrectomy are arbitrary. Vitreous incarceration in the cataract incision is known to be associated with a more severe natural course than is observed in eyes without the anterior segment changes. In pseudophakic eyes the role of vitreous surgery in relieving chronic cystoid macular edema associated with vitreous traction forces between the limbal wound, iris, and vitreous base remains unproven at the present time, although the procedure is being evaluated in a prospective study of aphakic cases (3). When vitreous incarceration in the cataract wound causes significant distortion or displacement of an intraocular lens, the excision of these sheets may allow the implant to resume a normal position. Vitreous gel externalized through a wound dehiscence is an unusual condition following modern suture techniques, but it represents a distinct indication for immediate vitrectomy combined with adequate closure of the fistula.

REDUCED MEDIA

Complications of cataract surgery with subsequent implantation include a variety of conditions in which a reduction in the media is observed post-operatively. These include: 1) pupillary membranes; 2) retained lens material; 3) vitreous opacification (mentioned above); 4) intraocular hemorrhage. Opaque membranes posterior to an intraocular lens usually result from cellular proliferation upon the membrane or from cellular contraction forces which distort the membrane. These are much more common following extracapsular surgery, but occasionally inflammatory pupillary membranes are observed on both sides of the implant following intracapsular procedures. Vitrectomy techniques permit excision of the opaque tissues in the pupillary area and a restoration of clear media. The YAG laser has replaced vitreous surgery in many of the cases with isolated pupillary membranes, but closed vitrectomy techniques may remain the method of choice in thick membranes in close apposition to the intraocular lens, in patients who cannot keep their heads immobile, in certain vascularized membranes, and in eyes in which the pupillary membranes are associated with vitreous opacification. Although retained lens material is a rather common complication of extracapsular cataract extraction, relatively few eyes with large amounts of lens material are subsequently implanted. Nevertheless, the occasional severe case of retained lens material in association with intraocular lenses remains a significant indication for subsequent closed vitrectomy techniques to prevent phacogenic uveitis, secondary open-angle glaucoma, reduced media, or a combination of all (4). Intraocular hemorrhage following lens implantation is more common than observed following simple cataract extraction, and this problem is more common in association with implants in which iris fixation was employed. It will probably become less common as an increasing percentage of posterior chamber lenses are used. Most of these intraocular hemorrhages spontaneously clear, but with severe and persistent hemorrhage, closed vitreous surgery may be the only method to allow a rapid restoration of clear media.

SECONDARY OPEN-ANGLE GLAUCOMA

Following implantation various forms of secondary open-angle glaucoma can occur, and if these cannot be managed medically, they represent indications for subsequent vitrectomy techniques. These include: 1) blood-induced glaucoma; 2) lens material-induced glaucoma; 3) glaucoma related to IOL-induced intraocular inflammation. Intraocular hemorrhage may cause a mechanical obstruction of the anterior chamber outflow channels with erythrocytic debris, pigment-laden macrophages, or devitalized red blood cells with rigid plasma membranes. If medical measures will not control the problem, even in the face of relatively clear media, closed vitreous surgery may allow one to remove the reservoir of erythrocytes as well as opaque vitreous gel. Similarly, lens material may cause phacogenic uveitis with a secondary glaucoma related to inflammation or a classical phacolytic glaucoma. Removal of the responsible material by closed vitrectomy techniques may allow the restoration of normal pressure as well as improvement in the media. Similarly, inflammation related to the presence of certain intraocular lenses may be associated with an open-angle glaucoma. Most of these cases can be medically controlled, although implant removal must be considered at time (see below).

PSEUDOPHAKIC PUPILLARY BLOCK GLAUCOMA

This complication is related to an abnormal direction of aqueous flow with anterior displacement of vitreous causing pupillary block in a closure of the anterior chamber angle. Corneal damage due to implant-endothelial touch may also occur. In cases in which laser iridectomy is not helpful, closed vitrectomy techniques may be used to excise a generous portion of the anterior vitreous for the restoration of normal aqueous flow.

ENDOPHTHALMITIS

Infective endophthalmitis represents a distinct indication for closed vitreous surgery if the intraocular inflammation is sufficient to eliminate an excellent view of the retina. Vitrectomy techniques provide suitable material for microscopic examination and culture studies. They may also have a beneficial effect in the reduction of retinal and uveal damage caused by bacterial toxins and proteolytic enzymes from leukocytes. Vitreous surgery may also improve intraocular penetration of subconjuctival systemic antibiotics and antifungal medications, and it provides a route for direct intracameral injections.

REPOSITIONING AND REMOVAL OF INTRAOCULAR LENSES

Dislocations of intraocular lenses are seen less frequently now that iris fixation implants are becoming less popular. An anteriorly or posteriorly dislocated IOL may cause difficult management problems, and occasionally closed vitrectomy techniques should be employed to reposition these implants. Implants dislocated anteriorly should always be repositioned, although this usually can be performed using movements of the bead and body as well as pharmacological manipulations of the pupil. Posterior dislocations frequently can be ignored, although many patients insist on a repositioning of the implant. Closed vitrectomy techniques aid in implant repositioning with intraocular forceps by providing optimal visualization of the vitreous-implant relationship and by reducing vitreous traction upon the peripheral retina. In certain eyes intraocular lenses cause serious problems including uveitis, hemorrhage, rubeosis, glaucoma, endothelial touch, and protracted course of cystoid macular edema. In some of these situations in which medical therapy is unsuccessful, removal of the intraocular lens may be indicated. As was the case with repositioning of implants, closed vitrectomy techniques aid in the removal of certain implants by reducing vitreous traction upon the peripheral retina.

EPITHELIAL INGROWTH

Epithelial invasion of the inner portion of the eye is a serious complication frequently leading to loss of visual function. Closed vitrectomy techniques are employed to excise involved iris tissue and vitreous as well as to provide a space for an anterior segment intraocular air bubble, which acting as a thermal insulator, increases the effect of transscleral and transcorneal cryotherapy in treating remaining epithelial cells on the endothelial surface, anterior chamber angle, and ciliary body (5).

POSTERIOR INDICATIONS

These indications are listed in Table 2, and they will not be discussed in detail. Vitreous surgery can be combined with other retinal reattachment methods in an effort to 1) improve visualization of the detachment; 2) eliminate vitreous and preretinal traction; 3) provide a fluid space in the vitreous cavity to assist in the creation of scleral buckle or placement of an intravitreal gas bubble; and 4) perform other manipulations such as unfolding the flap of a giant tear, performing transretinal drainage of subretinal fluid, and performing a simultaneous fluid gas exchange. These indications are identical to those problems occurring in eyes unassociated with intraocular lenses, and they will be discussed in more detail elsewhere in this publication.

SUMMARY

Modern closed vitrectomy techniques are of value in treating many complications associated with intraocular lenses. Although newer models of intraocular lenses are associated with a reduced incidence of severe complications, and although the YAG laser has replaced closed vitrectomy for certain indications, the use of closed vitrectomy techniques remains an important means of managing many of these severe problems.

REFERENCES

1. Machemer R, Beuttner H, Norton EWD et al. (1971): Vitrectomy: a pars plana approach. Trans Am Ophthalmol and Otolaryngol, 75:813-820.
2. Wilkinson CP, Rowsey JJ (1980): Closed vitrectomy for the vitreous touch syndrome. Am J Ophthalmol, 90:304-308.
3. Fung WE (Personal Communication)
4. Michels RG, Shacklett DE (1977): Vitrectomy techniques for removal of retained lens material. Arch Ophthalmol, 95:1767-1773.
5. Stark WJ, Michels RG, Maumenee AE et al. (1978): Surgical management of epithelial ingrowth. Am J Ophthalmol, 85:772-780.

Basic and advanced vitreous surgery
G.W. Blankenship, M. Stirpe, M. Gonvers, S. Binder (eds.)
Fidia Research Series, vol. II,
Liviana Press, Padova © 1986

CLOSED VITREOUS SURGERY FOR COMPLICATIONS OF INTRAOCULAR LENS IMPLANTATION II. TECHNIQUES

C.P. Wilkinson, M.D.

Dean A. McGee Eye Institute and the Department of Ophthalmology,
University of Oklahoma Health Sciences Center, Oklahoma City, Oklahoma.

As noted in I. Indications, many complications of intraocular lens implantation represent indications for subsequent closed vitreous surgery. The purpose of this report is to discuss methods in managing the indications listed in Table 1 of I. Indications.

Both limbal and pars plana approaches may be used as sites for infusion and for the introduction of the vitrectomy probe. The precise approach depends upon the type of intraocular lens, the location of the material to be excised, and the experience of the surgeon involved. Factors favoring a pars plana incision include the need for fiberoptic intraocular illumination, the necessity of removing large portions of posterior vitreous gel, and cases in which anticipated anatomical objectives cannot be accomplished by a limbal incision. For procedures in which tissue excision is limited to the anterior portion of the eye, I prefer using a needle of approximately 20 guage size for infusion rather than an infusion cannula sutured to the globe, as used in traditional posterior vitrectomies. The use of this longer needle involves less time and assures the surgeon that the infusion source is in its intended position. This bimanual approach facilitates movement of the globe, and infusion and cutting sites can be exchanged for a better approach to peripheral tissues. If intraocular illumination is required, one may employ a combination light pipe-infusion cannula. When limbal incisions are used, great care must be taken to avoid vitreous incarceration in the incision site. Air should be injected into the anterior chamber at the end of the case to keep the vitreous gel behind the pupillary plane as the instruments are withdrawn (1). In cases in which iris fixation of the implant has been employed and in which tissue excision is limited to the anterior portion of the eye, a limbal infusion site is recommended to maintain a deep anterior chamber and to prevent contact between the implant and cornea. In most other situations I use pars plana incisions 3 mm posterior to the limbus and approximately 160 degrees apart.

VITREOUS IN THE ANTERIOR CHAMBER

In cases in which the vitreous gel can be well visualized with the operating microscope and in which only a limited vitrectomy is necessary, a two incision technique, as noted above, is used. A pars plana approach is preferred for the introduction of the vitrectomy instrument unless the tissue to be excised cannot be reached by this route. Most pseudophakic eyes with vitreous in the anterior chamber have an associated posterior vitreous separation and a large core vitrectomy, penetrating the detached posterior hyaloid face, is usually performed in these circumstances. Intraocular illumination must be employed in cases in which the posterior hyaloid face has not shifted forward and in which opaque axial vitreous opacities are encountered, and a traditional three incision vitrectomy is usually required to achieve optimal goals. In cases with vitreous incarceration in the cataract incision, the vitreous gel may be very difficult to see, and intraocular illumination is recommended, even though the pathology is far anterior. In most cases a small knife or probe is introduced through the limbus to engage these vitreous strands and to displace them away from the iris and into the pupillary space where they may be more easily visualized (2).

REDUCED MEDIA

The recommended incisions for this group of indications depend upon the location and extent of opaque material to be excised. Thick and vascularized pupillary membranes can occur both anterior and posterior to implants, and their location dictates the site of introduction of the cutting instrument. As noted above, with iris fixation implants, a limbal incision is advised for infusion. When stiff non-pliable tissue must be excised, and when it cannot be easily engaged in the cutting port, the membrane must first be cut into small triangular sections which can be aspirated into the cutting port, and this may require the use of a small knife or intraocular scissors. Bipolar diathermy can be used to treat a vascularized membrane prior to cutting or to stop active bleeding following excision. In cases with extensive retained lens material posterior to the lens capsule, severe and diffuse vitreous opacification, or severe vitreous hemorrhage, intraocular illumination is desirable, and the use of three standard pars plana incisions for infusion, illumination, and a cutting source is recommended. If retained lens material is relatively soft, this can be easily removed from the eye with a conventional vitrectomy instrument. Firm pieces of lens nucleus are difficult to engage in the cutting port, and the use of an aspiration-fragmentation technique is recommended. If these pieces lie upon the retinal surface, they must first be aspirated into the midvitreous prior to activation of the ultrasonic fragmentor. This procedure may need to be repeated many times because of the tendency of the nuclear pieces to fragment and fly from the aspiration port when the needle is activated. If a posterior vitreous separation has not occurred this should be surgically created at the time of posterior vitrectomy when all axial opacities are removed. The removal of non-clotted blood from the retinal surface can be best accomplished using a blunt needle and flute handle (3).

SECONDARY OPEN ANGLE GLAUCOMA

The management of the removal of the material responsible for uncontrollable pressure elevation is similar to that discussed in the previous section. Care must be taken to eliminate as much of the offending substances as possible rather than simple axial opacities, because persistent peripheral material can continue to occlude the outflow channels post-operatively. In dealing with blood-induced glaucoma, one must always attempt to find a bleeding source, although in our experience the ability to detect such a site is unusual.

PSEUDOPHAKIC PUPILLARY BLOCK GLAUCOMA

This syndrome can usually be treated using an infusion needle and vitrectomy probe via the pars plana without intraocular illumination. Removal of the anterior and mid portions of the vitreous gel relieves the pupillary block, restores the normal flow of aqueous, and prevents recurrences of the syndrome.

ENDOPHTHALMITIS

The precise value of vitrectomy in the therapy of endophthalmitis remains controversial. I recommend excision of vitreous gel in cases in which the retina cannot be easily visualized with the indirect ophthalmoscope, in cases in which the clinical course worsens in eyes initially treated with intraocular and systemic antibiotics, and in eyes in which symtoms of endophthalmitis have been present for more than 72 hours. Removal of the intraocular lens is not advised. Unlike the cases discussed above, in these infected eyes I do not recommend approaching the retinal surface posteriorly, because the retina may be much more likely to bleed and tear when relatively minimal suction forces are applied to it. Intravitreal antibiotics or antifungal medications are of course instilled at the time of vitreous surgery.

REPOSITIONING/REMOVAL OF INTRAOCULAR LENSES

Prior to repositioning displaced intraocular lenses in which more conservative measures are not successful, a large portion of the central vitreous gel should be excised. Porterior gel should be retained to protect the retina from injury should the implant be inadvertently dropped. Since the primary reason to excise vitreous gel is to reduce vitreoretinal traction, and since the vitreous gel is usually relatively clear, we recommend intraocular illumination during vitrectomy. The implant is grasped with foreign body forceps and repositioned in the iris plane or, with some dislocated posterior chamber lenses, in the ciliary sulcus. In certain iris fixated implants, suturing of the haptics to the iris may then be performed to insure future optimal fixation. If the implant is to be removed I recommend the use of a double Fleirenger ring to prevent collapse of the anterior chamber during the limbal incision. In this situation the implant is trapped in the anterior chamber by instilling Miochol prior to removal of the implant via a large limbal section.

EPITHELIAL INGROWTH

In this situation vitrectomy instrumentation is used to excise involved iris and vitreous gel. Prior to vitrectomy, photoacoagulation therapy is applied to the iris to determine the extent of epithelial involvment of this structure. Standard pars plana approaches are used to excise the involved iris and vitreous gel, and after a large portion of the latter has been excised an air bubble is instilled to provide thermal insulation, enhancing the ability of cryotherapy to destroy epithelial cells involving the cornea, angle, and cilliary body (4).

The management of complications associated with retinal disorders outlined in Table II Part I of this discussion are beyond the scope of this presentation, but these techniques are identical to those used in eyes without intraocular lenses and they will be discussed elsewhere in this publication.

REFERENCES

1. Michels RG (1981): Vitreous Surgery. St. Louis: CV Mosby Co., p 298.
2. Michels RG (1981): Vitreous Surgery. St. Louis: CV Mosby Co., p 313-314.
3. Charles S (1977): Fluid-gas exchange in the vitreous cavity. Ocutome Newsletter, 2 (2):1.
4. Stark WJ, Michels RG, Maumenee AE et al. (1978): Surgical management of epithelial ingrowth. Am J Ophthalmol, 85:772-780.

Basic and advanced vitreous surgery
G.W. Blankenship, M. Stirpe, M. Gonvers, S. Binder (eds.)
Fidia Research Series, vol. II,
Liviana Press, Padova © 1986

CLOSED VITREOUS SURGERY FOR COMPLICATIONS OF INTRAOCULAR LENS IMPLANTATION III. RESULTS AND COMPLICATIONS

C.P. Wilkinson, M.D.

Dean A. McGee Eye Institute and the Department of Ophthalmology, University of Oklahoma Health Sciences Center, Oklahoma City, Oklahoma.

Closed vitrectomy techniques have been useful in managing many complications of intraocular lens implantation. Over the past few years we have managed a consecutive series of 74 cases in which complications of intraocular lens implantation represented indications for subsequent closed vitreous surgery (Table 1). This report will discuss the anatomical and visual results and the complications observed in 48 consecutive cases unassociated with retinal detachment, macular pucker, or massive proliferative vitreo-retinopathy. Follow-up information was obtained a minimum of six months following surgery. It should be noted that this series does not include cases of infectious endophthalmitis, but during the same time period that this series was obtained, 28 cases of culture proven pseudophakic endophthalmitis were diagnosed and managed at our institution by J. James Rowsey, M.D. (personal communication-July 1984), and these will not be discussed in this presentation.

PUPILLARY MEMBRANES

Pseudophakic pupillary membranes were removed in 10 cases (Table 2). In eight of these the membrane was located behind the implant. The optical results were good in all cases, but visual results were limited by retinal disorders in four instances. These included cystoid macular edema in two, macular damage due to a prior retinal detachment in one, and an old venous occlusion in one. Complications of vitreous surgery included cystoid macular edema in two cases. In each of these normal visual acuity was documented following surgery, but this decreased in the following months due to the onset of CME. A retinal detachment not involving the macula occurred four months following vitreous surgery in one other case, but this was repaired without loss of vision.

Table 1. *Indications for vitreous surgery*

"Anterior"	
Pupillary Membrane	10
Hemorrhage	10
Reposition IOL	9
Vitreous Opacification	8
Remove IOL	5
Retained Lens Material	4
Pupillary-Block Glaucoma	2
	48
"Posterior"	
Retinal Detachment	
With massive PVR	21
With pupillary membrane	2
Macular Pucker	3
	26

Table 2. *Pupillary membrane visual results*

Pre-op Visions		Post-op Visions	
20/70	(2)	20/40 +	(6)
20/100-400	(4)	20/50-70	(3)
CF - HM	(1)	HM	(1)
LP	(3)		

INTRAOCULAR HEMORRHAGE

Severe intraocular hemorrhage associated with implantation was the indication for vitreous surgery in ten eyes (Table 3). The blood was successfully removed in all, but vision was limited by pre-existing posterior pathology in three. This included age related macular degeneration in two instances and optic atrophy in the third. Secondary open-angle glaucoma due to hemorrhage was controlled in all four cases in which it was present. Complications related to vitreous surgery were not observed.

IMPLANT REPOSITIONING/REMOVAL

Nine implants were repositioned using closed vitrectomy techniques, and five other intraocular lenses were removed (Table 4). Pre-operative visual acuities were excellent with aphakic corrections in the former group but were less than 20/40 in all cases in the latter. Implants were removed for uveitis unresponsive to medical therapy in three instances and for severe rubeosis in two. Complications in the repositioning group in-

Table 3. *Hemorrhage visual results**

Pre-op Visions		Post-op Visions	
HM	(3)	20/40 +	(4)
		20/50	(2)
LP	(7)	20/200	(3)
		CF - HM	(1)

* Glaucoma Controlled in 4/4

Table 4. *Reposition/removal visual results*

Post-op Visions	
20/40 +	(7)
20/50-70	(4)
CF - HM	(2)
LP*	(1)

* Due to inoperable retinal detachment. This represents the only case in the series with pre-op vision significantly lower than post-op.

cluded an iatrogenic retinal tear due to contact with a Copeland lens in a single case. This was initially successfully repaired, but massive proliferative vitreo-retinopathy developed five weeks following surgery, and the retina has remained detached. Cystoid macular edema occurred post-operatively in one other case. Visual acuities in the five eyes in which implants were removed were limited due to preexisting problems in four. The single complication in this group consisted of a vitreous hemorrhage which occurred following vitreous surgery in an eye with severe pre-operative rubeosis. The retina remains attached in all five eyes in this group.

VITREOUS OPACIFICATION

Significant vitreous opacification associated with intraocular lenses was the indication for surgery in eight eyes (Table 5). In four cases vitreous had prolapsed around the implant. In two this was associated with intracapsular surgery, and in two this occurred following extracapsular procedures. In one of the latter group a YAG capsulotomy had been performed prior to vitreous prolapse. The pre-operative visual acuities were better than those in most of the groups. Fluorescein studies revealed no cystoid macular edema prior to surgery in all cases. Visual results were good, and no complications of vitrectomy were observerd.

Table 5. *Vitreous opacification visual results*

Pre-op Visions		Post-op Visions	
20/40 +	(1)	20/30 +	(6)
20/50-80	(4)	20/40	(2)
20/100-400	(3)		

REMOVAL OF RETAINED LENS MATERIAL

Vitrectomy techniques were used to remove vitreous and retained lens material in four instances (Table 6). Visual acuity results were good, and glaucoma was cured in the two cases in which it existed pre-operatively. Complications were not observed.

Table 6. *Retained lens material visula results**

Pre-op Visions		Post-op Visions	
20/100	(1)	20/40 +	(3)
CF - HM	(2)	20/60	(1)
LM	(1)		

* Glaucoma controlled in 2/2.

PSEUDOPHAKIC PUPILLARY BLOCK GLAUCOMA

Pupillary block was eliminated by vitreous surgery in the two cases in which it was required. Pre-op visual acuities were poor in both eyes. Post-op vision was reduced to 20/400, due to persistent corneal edema, in one of these, but direct complications of vitreous surgery were not observed.

DISCUSSION

In all cases the original anatomical objectives for surgery were accomplished. Significant complications of vitreous surgery included the development of cystoid macular edema in six percent and retinal detachment in four percent of cases. Hopefully many of the cases with CME have exhibited spontaneous resolution. One of the two retinal detachments was successfully repaired without a loss of visual acuity, but the other eye is now blind. This eye is the only one in this series of 48 cases in which the post-operative vision was worse than that noted pre-operatively. Closed vitrectomy techniques provide an efficient and a relatively safe means of managing some of the important complications of intraocular lens implantation. YAG laser therapy has replaced vitreous surgery in dealing with some of these complications, particularly pupillary membranes, and it is hoped that the introduction of newer and safer models of intraocular lenses will further reduce the need for closed vitrectomy techniques following cataract extraction.

Basic and advanced vitreous surgery
G.W. Blankenship, M. Stirpe, M. Gonvers, S. Binder (eds.)
Fidia Research Series, vol. II,
Liviana Press, Padova © 1986

VITRECTOMY IN THE MANAGEMENT OF POSTERIORLY DISLOCATED INTRAOCULAR LENSES

Harry W. Flynn, Jr., M.D.

The Bascom Palmer Eye Institute, Department of Ophthalmology,
University of Miami School of Medicine, Miami, Florida.

Although natural history studies have not been reported, posteriorly dislocated intraocular lenses can be well tolerated in many cases. Standard spectacle or contact lens correction may be adequate to achieve visual rehabilitation in such an eye. The decision to surgically reposition a dislocated intraocular lens may be influenced by a number of factors. These factors are the severity of intraocular inflammation (including cystoid macular edema), the inability to tolerate or achieve visual correction using standard optical techniques, the visual requirements of the individual patient, and the status of the fellow eye.

The Food and Drug Administration Report (1) on intraocular lenses reviewed the frequency of lens dislocation, as well as other postoperative complications. Anterior chamber implants rarely dislocate posteriorly. Iris fixation IOLs are most frequently dislocated and repositioning is often necessary, especially when anterior dislocation occurred. Iris plane lenses, including both iris fixation types and iridocapsular types may achieve fixation by a McCannel suture (2) after repositioning. Posterior chamber lenses can be repositioned anterior to the zonular ring or in the ciliary sulcus, and a fixating suture may or may not be necessary (3).

A standard three sclerotomy pars plana vitrectomy approach is used when an intraocular lens is dislocated into the vitreous cavity (4). After the vitreous gel anterior to the dislocated IOL is removed, the vitrectomy instrument tip is withdrawn from the sclerotomy. Using a foreign body forceps introduced into the same sclerotomy and fiberoptics illumination through the opposite sclerotomy, the intraocular lens is grasped with foreign body forceps and brought forward in the eye. If remaining vitreous traction is present, the fiberoptics light pipe can be removed and further anterior vitrectomy can be performed. Next, the intraocular lens can be repositioned into the correct anatomical plane. If necessary, Acetylcholine can be used to achieve miosis, and fixation by a McCannel suture can be performed in selected cases.

Case Report 1

This 77-year-old lady had unplanned extracapsular cataract extraction with implantation of a flexible loop anterior chamber intraocular lens in the left eye on December 29, 1982. The intraocular lens was inadvertently placed posterior to the iris, and the intraocular lens fell into the mid-vitreous cavity at the time of initial surgery. No attempt was made to retrieve the dislocated intraocular lens. Postoperatively, unsuccessful attempts were made to fit the patient with a soft contact lens.

The patient was initially referred on June 10, 1983, at which time the best corrected visual acuity was 20/200 right eye and 20/60 left eye. The slitlamp examination of the right eye showed a dense nuclear sclerotic cataract. The left eye had residual capsular remnants in the superior portion of the pupillary axis. The intraocular lens was freely floating in mid-vitreous cavity but not touching the retina. The vitreous cavity showed moderate inflammation and there was prominent cystoid macular edema.

Repeat attempts to wear contact lens in the left eye were unsuccessful. Because of this inability to be visually rehabilitated and because of progressive vitreous inflammation, surgery was recommended to reposition the intraocular lens into the anterior chamber.

The patient was taken to surgery on July 11, 1983, at which time a pars plana vitrectomy was performed and the intraocular lens was repositioned into the anterior chamber using foreign body forceps. The postoperative course has been uneventful and on the latest follow-up examination of July 3, 1984, a best corrected visual acuity of 20/20-1 was achieved in the left eye. There was no obvious cystoid macular edema by Hruby lens examination, but fluorescein angiography has not been repeated.

Case Report 2

This 78-year-old lady had extracapsular cataract extraction and implantation of a posterior chamber intraocular lens in the left eye on June 15, 1983. No complications were observed at the time of this surgery. The patient had improved visual acuity postoperatively to 20/30 in the left eye, but vitreous was noted to extend anterior to the intraocular lens through a large break in the posterior capsule. The patient suddenly lost vision in the left eye on April 27, 1984, and the posterior chamber IOL was found to be dislocated posteriorly, with one haptic attached to the temporal edge of the posterior capsular ring. Vitreous herniation into the mid-portion of the pupil was present. Aphakic spectacles improved the vision to 20/40 in the left eye, but attempts to fit the patient with a soft contact lens for the left eye were unsuccessful.

Pars plana vitrectomy and repositioning of the posterior chamber intraocular lens in the left eye was performed on May 30, 1984. The IOL was held in position with a Jaffe hook while the anterior and mid-vitreous was removed by way of a pars plana vitrectomy. The intraocular lens was then brought forward with the intraocular foreign body forceps and the lens haptics were positioned anterior to the zonular ring. Two Jaffe hooks were used to dial the IOL into the ciliary sulcus until the implant became securely fixed. No fixation sutures were placed.

Postoperatively, the patient's visual acuity has improved to 20/20 in the left eye. The intraocular lens has remained in position, with the last follow-up visit on June 29, 1984.

CONCLUSION

Vitrectomy instrumentation can be used in selected cases of posteriorly dislocated intraocular lenses. Thoughtful case selection, together with long-term observation for posterior segment complications, is necessary in these patients.

REFERENCES

1. Stark WJ, Worthen DM, Holladay JT et al (1983): The FDA Report on Intraocular Lenses. Ophthalmology 90:311-317.
2. McCannel MA (1976): A retrievable suture idea for anterior uveal problems. Ophthalmic Surg. 7:98-103.
3. Stark WJ, Bruner WE, Martin NF (1982): Management of subluxed posterior chamber intraocular lenses. Ophthalmic Surgery. 13:130-133.
4. Stark WJ, Michels RG, Bruner WE (1980): Management of posteriorly dislocated intraocular lenses. Ophthalmic Surgery. 11:495-497.

Basic and advanced vitreous surgery
G.W. Blankenship, M. Stirpe, M. Gonvers, S. Binder (eds.)
Fidia Research Series, vol. II,
Liviana Press, Padova © 1986

PSEUDOPHAKIA: INCIDENCE OF CYSTOID MACULAR EDEMA

Walter J. Stark, David E. Denlinger, Arlo C. Terry, A. Edward Maumenee

The Wilmer Ophthalmological Institute, The Johns Hopkins Medical Institutions, Baltimore, Maryland, 21205, U.S.A.

Cystoid macular edema (CME) remains a significant cause of decreased visual acuity following cataract extraction. Fluorescein angiographically proven cystoid macular edema is reported to occur in greater than 50% of patients, causing decreased visual acuity in approximately 8% of cases (1-6). At the Wilmer Institute we are in the process of re-examining our incidence of cystoid macular edema following extracapsular cataract extraction with implantation of a posterior chamber lens implant. We are also attempting to determine whether eyes undergoing primary capsulotomy are more likely to develop clinically significant CME.

Clinically significant cystoid macular edema was defined as a reduction in Snellen acuity of one or more lines associated with biomicroscopic or fluorescein angiographic evidence of CME.

RESULTS

Clinically significant CME was detected in 2.3% of eyes undergoing extracapsular cataract extraction with the insertion of a posterior chamber lens. In a large majority of these cases, the CME resolved spontaneously so that only 0.12% of eyes were left with permanently reduced visual acuity.

Those eyes with CME had a statistically significant increased incidence of vitreous loss, vitreous prolapse, macular degeneration, persistent iritis, and retinal detachment. Eyes with branch vein occlusion or diabetic retinopathy showed no increased incidence of CME, but we have only recently begun to place implants in these eyes.

The decision regarding primary posterior capsulotomy is largely a matter of the surgeon's preference. One of us (AEM) performed a capsulotomy in a large majority of his cases, while the other (WJS) seldom did so. Nearly 2/3 of the eyes included in this study underwent primary posterior capsulotomy, and approximately 3% of these eyes developed clinically significant CME. The incidence of CME in eyes without a capsulotomy was 1.9%. The difference between these two groups was not statistically significant.

As reported previously, there was a higher incidence of transient and persistent CME associated with intracapsular extraction with iris fixation implants as compared with extracapsular extraction and posterior chamber lenses (Table 1). A comparison of the CME occurring in eyes with iris fixated implants as compared with those with posterior chamber implants showed that the CME in the latter group was earlier in onset and of shorter duration. These differences were found to be statistically significant.

Table 1. *Transient and persistent CME in eyes after ICCE and iris fixation implants as compared with ECCE and posterior chamber implants*

	ICCE, Iris Fixation (200 Eyes)	ECCE, Posterior Chamber (1700 Eyes)
CME by Fluorescein	10.0%	2.3 %
Persistent CME	1.0%	0.12%

On a national level, raw data provided by the FDA CORE study showed that posterior chamber lenses provided better visual acuity than iris fixated or anterior chamber lenses (Table 2). If eyes with pre-existing pathology such as abnormal corneas, glaucoma, macular degeneration, or amblyopia are excluded, vision in eyes receiving a posterior chamber lens was only slightly better than in those receiving an anterior or iris-fixated lens.

Table 2. *Visual results in CORE patients: Posterior Chamber (PC) vs. Anterior Chamber (AC) vs. iris fixation (IF) implants*

Lens Type	Number of Eyes	% $\geq 20/40$
PC	5363	87.3
AC	6686	83.9
IF	1428	83.3

One year following implantation, complications such as macular edema, secondary glaucoma, and corneal edema were present more frequently in eyes with anterior chamber and iris fixated lenses than in eyes with posterior chamber lenses (Table 3).

Table 3. *Sight-threatening complications present one year after implantation in CORE patients with posterior chamber (PC), anterior chamber (AC), and iris fixation (IF) implants*

	Posterior Chamber (6834 eyes)	Anterior Chamber (5411 eyes)	Iris Fixation (1045 eyes)
Macular Edema	1.0	2.4	1.7
Lens Dislocation	0.1	0.1	0.7
Secondary Glaucoma	0.3	1.2	1.1
Pupillary Block	0.1	0.2	0.0
Corneal Edema	0.6	1.3	1.1

ACKNOWLEDGMENTS

This work was supported in part by the Women's Committee of the International Medical Eye Bank of Maryland.

REFERENCES

1. Gehring JR (1968): Macular edema following cataract extraction. Arch Ophthalmol. 80:626-31.
2. Irvine AR, Bresky R, Crowder BM, Forster RK, Hunter DM, Kulvin SM (1971): Macular edema after cataract extraction. Ann Ophthalmol 3:1234-40.
3. Meredith TA, Maumenee AE (1979): A review of one thousand cases of intracapsular cataract extraction: I. Complications Ophth Surg 10(12):32-41.
4. Meredith TA, Maumenee AE (1979): A review of one thousand cases of intracapsular cataract extraction: II. Visual results and astigmatic analysis. Ophth Surg 10(12):42-5.
5. Meredith TA, Kenyon KR, Singerman LJ, Fine SL (1976): Peripheral vascular leakage and macular edema after intracapsular cataract extraction. Br J Ophthalmol 60:765-9.
6. Jaffe NS, Clayman HM, Jaffe MS (1982): Cystoid macular edema after intracapsular and extracapsular cataract extraction with and without an intraocular lens. Ophthalmology 89:25-9.

Basic and advanced vitreous surgery
G.W. Blankenship, M. Stirpe, M. Gonvers, S. Binder (eds.)
Fidia Research Series, vol. II,
Liviana Press, Padova © 1986

PSEUDOPHAKIC RETINAL DETACHMENTS

C. P. Wilkinson, M.D.

Dean A. McGee Eye Institute and Department of Ophthalmology,
University of Oklahoma Health Sciences Center, Oklahoma City, Oklahoma.

Pseudophakic retinal detachments have become much more common in recent years because of the increased popularity of intraocular lenses. This report will describe our experiences in managing a large consecutive series of pseudophakic eyes in which retinal detachment occurred following cataract extraction.

MATERIALS AND METHODS

From 1976 through December of 1983 we observed a series of 194 eyes in which retinal detachments were associated with intraocular lenses. In 154 eyes a primary scleral buckling procedure was performed following the diagnosis of pseudophakic detachment, and these cases will be discussed in this report. Forty eyes were excluded from this study because of a variety of reasons, including the need for a primary vitrectomy (14 eyes), a history of an unsuccessful buckling procedure elsewhere (8 eyes), the presence of focal detachments which were treated without buckling (8 eyes), detachments occurring after additional anterior segment surgery (6 eyes), and detachments detected following the removal of intraocular lenses (4 eyes).

The majority of the 154 consecutive cases in which primary buckles were employed could be divided into three groups: 1) extracapsular cataract surgery and implantation with iridocapsular fixation (EC/IC)--73 eyes; 2) extracapsular cataract surgery and posterior chamber implant (EC/PC)--24 eyes; 3) intracapsular surgery with iris fixation implant (ICCE)--48 eyes. Anterior chamber lenses were employed in only nine of the eyes in this series. In five cases intracapsular surgery had been performed, and the anterior chamber implant was placed primarily in four. In four of the nine eyes in the anterior chamber group, extracapsular surgery had been performed, and implantation was performed primarily in three. Because of the small number of anterior chamber lenses, these nine eyes were deleted from a statistical analysis of other clinical factors.

RESULTS

In the vast majority of extracapsular eyes, a capsulotomy had been performed. The time of retinal detachment following implantation is recorded in Table 1. Posterior chamber lenses have been used only recently in our community, and perhaps the apparent earlier onset of detachments in this group will change with time. The status of the macula is recorded in Table 2. Approximately three-fourths of eyes had macular involvement, and significant differences in the three groups were not observed. The incidence of significant pre-operative proliferative vitreo-retinopathy (PVR) (1) is recorded in Table 3, and these differences were particularly striking if eyes are included in which a primary vitrectomy was required because of massive PVR (Table 4).

Table 1. *Time of retinal detachment*

Group	6 mo.	6-12 mo.	1-2 yr.	2 yr +
EC/IC (73)	34%	20%	19%	27%
EC/PC (24)	42%	16%	29%	13%
ICCE (48)	28%	15%	36%	21%

Table 2. *Macular involvement*

Group	Macula Involved
EC/IC (73)	85%
EC/PC (24)	67%
ICCE (48)	75%

Table 3. *Pre operative PVR (1)*

Group	PVR
EC/IC (73)	23%
EC/PC (24)	13%
ICCE (48)	27%

Table 4. *Pre operative PVR (1)**

Group	PVR
EC/IC (74)	24%
EC/PC (25)	16%
ICCE (57)	39%

* Includes eyes in which a primary vitrectomy was required because of massive PVR.

The major grouping of surgical procedures employed are recorded in Table 5. In most cases an encircling procedure with drainage was performed. Cryotherapy and silicone exoplants were employed in all cases. Segmental buckling combined with no drainage was used infrequently in all groups. Six eyes were lost to follow-up prior to an examination six months or more following their surgery. All of these eyes were in the EC/IC group. In all six of these eyes the retina was attached when last observed, but the cases are excluded from an analysis of post-operative results. Two eyes in the EC/PC group have not been followed six months, and they are not included in the analysis of results. A single case in the ICCE group in which a primary vitrectomy was required for massive PVR is not included in an analysis of results because the patient died eight days following therapy.

Table 5. *Surgical procedures*

Group	Circlage + Drain	Segmental without drainage
EC/IC (73)	90%	7%
EC/PC (24)	96%	0%
ICCE (48)	73%	8%

The anatomical results related to the type of implant are recorded in Tables 6 and 7. Well over 90% of eyes were successfully reattached. One-hundred percent of the nine cases in which anterior chamber lenses had been employed were also successfully repaired. The reattachment rates for the initial buckling procedures were a bit lower than those recorded in Table 6. There were six primary failures in the 67 EC/IC eyes, and two of these were successfully repaired with reoperations. There was one primary failure in the EC/PC group, and this was ultimately repaired using vitrectomy techniques. There were four primary failures in the 48 ICCE eyes, and two were subsequently repaired. The success rate of the closed vitrectomy procedures in the ten eyes in which massive PVR was encountered pre-operatively was 50%. All failures in all groups were due to this important problem.

Visual results in the series of successful primary buckles are recorded in Table 8. Approximately 52% of eyes achieved 20/50 or better post operatively. There was a trend for somewhat lower visual acuities in the ICCE group. Approximately 14% of eyes without macular involvement and with good visual acuity experienced a drop of vision to less than 20/50. This was due to macular pucker (2 eyes), CME (1 eye), and recurrent detachment (1 eye).

Table 6. *Anatomical results*

Group	Anatomical Success
EC/IC (67)	94%
EC/PC (22)	100%
ICCE (48)	96%

Table 7. *Anatomical results**

Group	Anatomical Success
EC/IC (68)	92%
EC/PC (23)	96%
ICCE (56)	91%

* Includes eyes in which a primary vitrectomy was required because of massive PVR.

Table 8. *Visual results*

Group	Post Op Visions			
	20/50 +	20/60-100	20/400	Less
EC/IC				
Macula On (9)	8	1	—	—
Macula Off (54)	26	12	11	5
Total (63)	34 (54%)	13	11	5
EC/IC				
Macula On (7)	6	1	—	—
Macula Off (15)	9	2	3	1
Total (22)	15 (68%)	3	3	1
ICCE				
Macula On (12)	10	—	2	—
Macula Of (34)	9	9	13	3
Total (46)	19 (41%)	9	15	3

DISCUSSION

The precise incidence of retinal detachment following intra-ocular lens implantation remains unknown. There is increasing evidence (2) that an intact posterior lens capsule reduces the rate of retinal detachment following extracapsular cataract surgery, but many intact capsules require subsequent capsulotomy, either surgically or with the YAG laser. The incidence of retinal detachment following extracapsular cataract surgery and posterior capsulotomy approaches that following intracapsular procedures (3). At the present time there is little data demonstrating conclusively that the rate of retinal detachment following intraocular lens implantation in pseudophakic eyes is lower than that following cataract surgery of a similar type in which implantation has not been employed.

Pseudophakic detachments appear clinically similar to the aphakic variety in terms of the time of detachment, the configuration of the detachment, and the characteristics of the responsible retinal breaks (4). Surgical procedures for pseudophakic detachments are more difficult than for aphakic eyes because of significant problems in visualizing the peripheral retina. Nevertheless, the anatomical success rate in this series corresponds closely to data that have been published following the repair of aphakic retinal detachments (3). All of the failures in this series were due to massive proliferative vitreoretinopathy (1), and the majority of these failures exhibited preretinal membranes prior to surgery. The visual acuities in this group of eyes compare favorably with previously published data regarding aphakic (2) and pseudophakic (5) detachments.

In this series the incidence of pre-operative severe PVR was higher in the intracapsular-iris fixation group of cases than in either of the extracapsular groups. Hopefully the decline in popularity of iris fixation implants will be associated with a reduced incidence of massive PVR, the process responsible for the vast majority of surgical failures. Although it is possible that the tendency for the iris fixation lenses to be associated with reduced vision post-operatively may be due to associated inflammatory complications of these implants, we were unable to document this in this study. As is the case following most retinal reattachment surgery, the visual outcomes were less satisfactory than the anatomical, and an improvement in visual results represents a major goal for the future.

REFERENCES

1. The Retina Society Terminology Committee (1983): The classification of retinal detachment with proliferative vitreoretinopathy. Ophthalmology, 90:121-125.
2. Jaffe NS, Clayman HM, Jaffe MS (1984): Retinal detachment in myopic eyes after intracapsular and extracapsular cataract extraction. Am J Ophthalmol, 97:48-52.
3. Wilkinson CP (1979): Retinal detachment after phacoemulsification. Am J Ophthalmol, 87:628-631.
4. Wilkinson CP (1981): Retinal detachments following intraocular lens implantation. Ophthalmology, 88:410-413.
5. Hagler WS (1983): Pseudophakic retinal detachment. Trans Am Ophthalmol Soc, 80:45-59.

Basic and advanced vitreous surgery
G.W. Blankenship, M. Stirpe, M. Gonvers, S. Binder (eds.)
Fidia Research Series, vol. II,
Liviana Press, Padova © 1986

IOL AND VITREO-RETINAL COMPLICATIONS

M. Stirpe, P. Lischetti and S. Fruscella

Fondazione Oftalmologica 'G.B. Bietti', Piazza Sassari, 5, Roma

An eye in which an intraocular lens has been implanted has the same potential risk as a phakic eye for contracting vitreo-retinal disease; in addition, there is the general risk of aphakia.

It must be added that a lens implanted in the posterior chamber after extracapsular cataract extraction does not substantially increase the risk of vitreo-retinal complications; a lens implanted in the anterior or posterior chamber after intracapsular cataract extraction, however, is a greater risk than simple aphakia. Furthermore, once a vitreo-retinal complication arises, the presence of an intraocular lens is bound to make the surgical approach more difficult and may create further complications. However, a well positioned lens should be left in place as long as possible. Re-opening the anterior chamber may lead to a state of corneal edema, and thus add to the difficulty of posterior exploration during surgery, or may cause oozing of blood, which is difficult to control.

The problem of vitreo-retinal complications associated with IOL has two aspects:
1) Possibility of vitreo-retinal complications caused by the presence of an IOL;
2) Obstacles to the resolution of vitreo-retinal complications owing to the presence of an IOL.

COMPLICATIONS

Vitreo-retinal complications caused by the presence of an IOL

These complications are direct, that is, caused by the mechanical effect of the lens, or indirect, that is, caused by an inflammatory stimulus or by extravasation of blood due to the presence of the lens.

Direct complications may result from the dislocation of the lens, due to vitreal fibers becoming entangled with the loops of the IOL after intracapsular cataract extraction.

Even if intracapsular cataract extraction has been completed with the hyaloid membrane perfectly intact, spontaneous rupture of this membrane is often observed subsequently. If this happens in the presence of an IOL, vitreal fibers become entangled with the loops and subsequently contract. This leads to traction on the peripheral and even on the posterior retina if the vitreous is not detached posteriorly or is only partially detached posteriorly (Fig. 1). On the other hand, this complication is not encountered with lenses implanted in the posterior chamber after extracapsular extraction unless the surgeon has risked implanting the lens in a non-intact capsula.

Obstacles to the resolution of vitreo-retinal complications owing to the presence of an IOL

The presence of an IOL obliges the surgeon who must resolve a posterior complication to proceed with the utmost caution during surgical manoeuvres. During surgery for retinal detachment, special attention must be given to the extraction of subretinal fluid; this must be extracted gradually, so as to avoid any decrease of pressure, and to prevent both the possibility of blood extravasation into the anterior chamber and the dislocation of the lens. However, the most frequent obstacles are those which in the presence of an IOL add to the difficulty of posterior exploration of the eye. These obstacles are often connected with the type of implanted lens and with certain complications that emerge during surgery or become evident in the postoperative stage. The following obstacles most frequentely interfere with the exploration of the fundus:

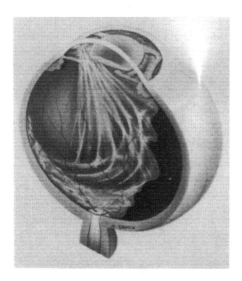

Figure 1. Vitreal fibers entangled with the loops of the IOL and vitreo-retinal traction.

a) *Insufficient dilatation of the pupil*

This may be caused:
1) by the necessity of not dilating the pupil beyond a certain degree for fear of causing the lens to become dislodged (these limits were usually imposed by the types of lenses used in the past)
2) by posterior adhesions to the loops
3) by synechiae between iris and lens

b) *Reflections caused by the lens or by the posterior capsule during indirect ophthalmoscopy*

These are especially disturbing to the surgeon if the pupil has not been dilated sufficiently or if the dioptric media are not particularly transparent.

c) *Area of focal variability*

This area corresponds to the passage between the margin of the implanted lens and the aphakic area.

d) *Persistence of precipitates on the surface of the lens*

e) *Presence of peripheral cortical residues, capsular thickening, retrolental membranes*

f) *Further obstacles* not different from those encountered in common aphakic eyes are: Postoperative alterations of the cornea, residual blood trapped in the anterior vitreous cortex, and vitreal opacities secondary to inflammatory processes.

Some difficulties caused by the presence of the implanted lens, such as those due to reflections or to the area of focal variability, are not easily resolved since they are connected with the structure and shape of the implanted lens. Others must be solved by choosing the simplest way. For example, in case of severe posterior adhesions, it may be more convenient to perform a sectorial iridectomy so as to permit sufficient exploration (Fig. 2).

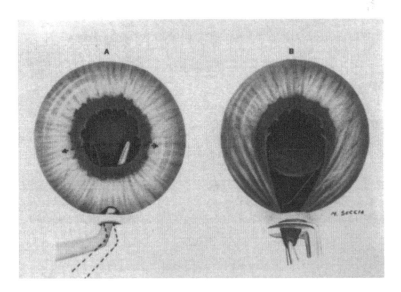

Figure 2. Sectorial iridectomy in cases of severe posterior adhesions: (a) sectorial separation of adhesions by introducing a microspatula through a peripheral iridotomy; (b) sectorial iridectomy.

If the capsule has become opaque in pseudophakia, the surgeon cannot remove it without running the risk of having the lens fall into the vitreous chamber. He must therefore decide in each case if the removal of the intraocular lens is more desirable than inadequate retinal exploration. Before the surgeon decides to remove the lens, he should first attempt to open the fibrous capsule. This can be done by bimanual use of a hooked needle and a sickle-shaped microblade moved from the center towards the periphery (Figs. 3-4).

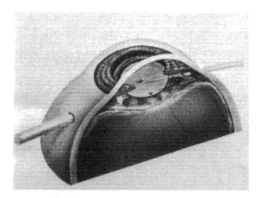 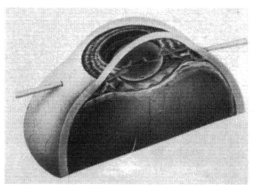

Figure 3. An opening is made in the capsule with a sickle-shaped microblade, introduced through the pars plana; the optic fibers provide posterior illumination.

Figure 4. Bimanual use of a hooked needle and sickle-shaped microblade.

Surgery for simple retinal detachment is performed according to traditional techniques.

Vitrectomy techniques are applied

1) For the removal of retrolental opaque membranes. In many cases nowadays, however, YAG laser is a useful alternative.

2) In case of dislocation of the IOL: a lens originally implanted in the posterior chamber after extracapsular removal of the cataract and which subsequently has become dislodged into the vitreous chamber must be removed (Fig. 5). A lens originally implanted in the anterior or posterior chamber with preiridial loops after intracapsular removal of the cataract and which subsequently has shifted into the vitreous chamber can be repositioned (Figs. 6-7). In either case, vitrectomy has to be performed. The vitreous must be removed so as to free the lens completely from all connections with the vitreous substance.

3) In case of posterior blood extravasation: if there appears to be no possibility of spontaneous albeit slow resolution; or in case of extensive contact of blood clots with the posterior portion of the implanted lens (after intracapsular operations); or with the capsule containing the implanted lens (after extracapsular operations) (Fig. 8).

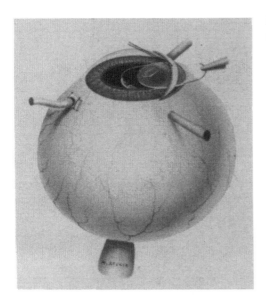

Figure 5. Extraction of dislocated IOL originally implanted in the posterior chamber.

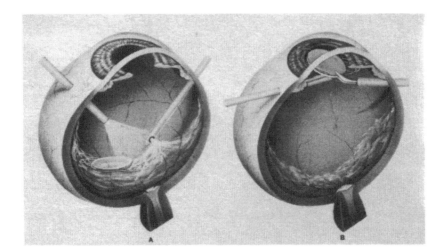

Figure 6. a) Dislocation of the IOL; b) Repositioning of the IOL with preiridial loops.

4) In special conditions of retinal detachment:
   a) traction detachment of the retina with or without breaks;
   b) macular holes;
   c) giant breaks with retinal eversion;
   d) retinal detachment with PVR.

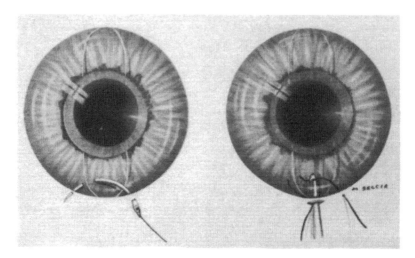

Figure 7. Suture of the IOL to the iris (Stark technique).

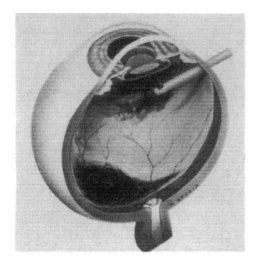

Figure 8. Removal of clotted blood from under the posterior capsule.

As for internal tamponade in vitreo-retinal surgery: air may be used in pseudophakic eyes with or without posterior lens capsule; SF_6 and silicone oil can be used in pseudophakic eyes with posterior lens capsule.

Basic and advanced vitreous surgery
G.W. Blankenship, M. Stirpe, M. Gonvers, S. Binder (eds.)
Fidia Research Series, vol. II,
Liviana Press, Padova © 1986

PARS PLANA VITRECTOMY FOR THE TREATMENT OF VITREAL HEMORRHAGE

V. De Molfetta, A. Battistini, E. Fiorentini, G. Boilo, P. Vinciguerra, S. Zenoni

Divisione Oculistica, Ospedale Civile, Monza

Surgical treatment of vitreous hemorrhage by vitrectomy via pars plana follows some general lines but is subject to change according to the anatomo - pathologic situation present in individual cases as a consequence of the hemorrhage.

Referring to the most typical cases of vitreous hemorrhage with vitreous collapsed but adhering in one or more places to the retinal surface, the surgical steps are as follows.

1. Introduction of instruments through one or more sclerotomies according to various authors at 4 mm from the limbus. The vitreophage and the endoilluminator are brought to the center of the vitreous chamber right behind the posterior surface of the lens, from which they remain separated by a thin sheet of vitreous.
   In this way it is possible by the degree of visibility of the instruments themselves through a thin sheet of vitreous to draw some conclusions about the intensity of the vitreous hemorrhage and about the opportunity to save from vitrectomy a little sheet of cortical vitreous in order to protect the posterior surface of the lens during vitrectomy.

2. The vitreophage is then set in action, keeping its mouth at the highest opening in the center of the anterior vitreous body, at a very high speed (140 beats/sec) and with a low degree of aspiration, so that it causes slight traction on the peripheral vitreous body during vitrectomy.

3. Vitrectomy is then extended from forward to backward, always inside the collapsed vitreous bag. In this way the interior of the vitreous bag is emptied, leaving the posterior cortical vitreous intact, at a certain moment the latter becomes half-transparent, allowing the surgeon to observe the retro-hyaloid field and to appreciate its contents.

4. An opening is made in the posterior hyaloid usually at the equator and in the inferior area or in the zone that shows the greatest collapse on echograph. In order to make this opening the vitreophage's mouth is turned outside, vitrectomy speed is kept at its minimun and aspiration is markedly intensified.

5. After opening the posterior hyaloid one could suddenly be faced with the problem of the "blood pool" treatment. In fact, as a consequence of the aspiration the blood flows down quickly from the retrohyaloid space dimming the surgical field. At this point, one should temporarily interrupt the vitrectomy and aspirate the retro-hyaloid blood with a Charles' needle, making use of the pressure gradient between vitreous hollow, infusion fluid and outside room.

6. After freeing the surgical field of the vitreous from the blood of the "blood pool", vitrectomy is carried out removing the peripheral vitreous proceeding from backward to forward towards the vitreous base always at 360° until one is close to the base itself, especially in the superior area, to allow sufficient vision of the peripheral retina. The posterior vitreous is then removed up to its adhesion(s) to the retina, which are isolated from one another but not removed in order not to damage the retina itself. Of course, in this way all strands of posterior hyaloid extending between two or more vitreo-retinal adhesions are removed. If these (as is almost always the case) consist of fibro-vascular membrane, once vitrectomy has been completed endodiathermy of the sectioned vessels will have to be carried out.

This is the treatment of the most frequent situation of vitreous hemorrhage. Some changes are to be made, as has already been said, for different anatomo-pathological conditions:

1. In the case of completely detached hematic vitreous vitrectomy is very simple and will be done by just keeping the instruments behind the lens in the anterior part of the vitreous chamber. The lens itself, free from any adhesion, will move towards the opening of the vitreophage.

2. In the case of detached vitreous with detached retina (trauma) echography must be used to identify an area where there is no or only slight retinal detachment and vitreous collapse is most marked, and the vitreous cortex is opened at this point. Vitrectomy will then be performed while keeping the detached retina under control.

3. If the vitreous is still adhering to the retina and vitrectomy is too urgent to be postponed (vitreous adhering to detached retina-traumata) vitrectomy will surely be difficult. A small area will have to be found of vitreous detached from the retina or its detachment must be provoked by traction upon the cortex in the parapapillary area. At this point we think it advisable to introduce with a long, thin needle some Healon into the retro-hyaloid area, which will unglue the hyaloid from the retina making the vitrectomy easier.

Echographic aspects can be divided as follows by topographic criteria:
1) Complete posterior vitreous detachment with vitreous collapse without adhesions to the retina
2) Partial vitreous detachment with vitreo-retinal adhesion and possibly localised tractional retinal detachment
3) Collapsed and detached vitreous associated with extensive retinal detachment

If the first type of the echographic aspect persists, surgery can be programmed so as to allow it to be performed in the most favorable conditions. Finding a situation with vitreoretinal adhesions without any tractional detachment suggests more frequent controls considering imminent surgery. Finally, the echographical finding, of a tractional retinal detachment or of one that is not only tractional, suggests immediate surgery.

The presence of blood in the vitreous is always a pathological sign. The causes of vitreous hemorrhage can be:
1) increased venous pressure with consequent rupture of retinal vessels. This condition can be accessory to a thrombosis with central vein occlusion, to hematological disorders or to subarachnoid hemorrhage.
2) hypertension
3) neovascularization (diabetes, venous occlusion, immunologic disorders)
4) retinal breaks (caused by vitreoretinal traction)
5) direct bulbar contusion (acute modification of the eye with rupture of a vessel due to the stretch)

EVOLUTION OF VITREOUS HEMORRHAGES

We have to distinguish between an isolated hemorrhage occurring for the first time and relapsing hemorrhages; the first will be reabsorbed in two different ways:
— hemolysis
— phagocytosis

The latter especially if hemorrhage is abundant and the vitreous is scarcely fluid. Once spread into the vitreous, the blood produces structural changes caused especially by hemoglobin. Given the pathological action of hemoglobin we must consider the action of leukocytes which on coming into contact with the vitreous gel, can transform into fibroblasts causing the formation of cicatricial vitreal strands. Platelets which aggregate in the presence of the gel produce vitreous opacities.

It has been demonstrated that the destruction of the vitreous structure is proportional to the hemorrhage: the more extensive and recurrent the hemorrhages the greater the number of fibrovascular strands formed.

It is a common observation that while the first hemorrhages have good chances of a spontaneous reabsorption, (even a total one), for later ones this becomes more and more difficult up to the moment when reabsorption is impossible because the vitreous has become organised in fibroblastic strands. In addition to the cytotoxic and fibroblast effects, the mechanical effect of traction caused by fibrous strands on the retina is equally important: the latter can have two consequences:
— tractional retinal schisis
— continuous stimulus to neovascularization that can finally lead to proliferating retinopathy.

LOCALISATION OF VITREOUS HEMORRHAGES

The hemorrhage can be
— anterior, especially if caused by trauma with ciliary body wound
— it can involve all the vitreous gel, with different intensity: from vitreous flare to a true thickening that completely obscures the retina, dark or bright red according

to whether the hemorrhage is recent or an old one

— it can be in the retrovitreal area

The different temperature between the retina posteriorly and the vitreous cortex anteriorly can make the red globules form an adhesion on the posterior cortex to the vitreous. If there are some posterior breaks in the posterior vitreous edge it is possible to see the blood spread into the vitreous gel dimming it to a greater or lesser degree through them.

The retrovitreal blood does not coagulate and it is not invaded by fibroblasts.

FUNCTIONAL TESTS PRIOR TO SURGERY

They can be useful in order to give surgical indications in cases of vitreous hemorrhage.

This is of course the case in patients whose visual acuity is inferior to 1/10 and whose retina cannot be explored. The semeiotic procedure is based on three types of examination. The research with light projections made on the eight meridians is useful. If light perception is absent or wrong a retinal lesion must be suspected on the corresponding meridian.

If there is no light perception vitrectomy must not be carried out. We made an analysis on 109 patients suffering from vitreous hemorrhages caused by different etiologies evaluating their light perception.

In 72 patients having light perception on 8 meridians we had the highest percentage (63%) of the useful visual recovery. In the remaining patients, positive results diminished in relation to the number of meridians with light perception.

The ERG is not decisive for the preoperative prognosis, although it is important when examined together with other elements. We are studying the relationship between preoperative ERG and functional results. In 35 cases studied up to now we recorded dynamic ERG with a red-orange stimulus. In the case with extinguished ERG we used a bright flash stimulus. In 18% of the cases we found a good correlation between visual acuity obtained after the vitrectomy and ERG.

Basic and advanced vitreous surgery
G.W. Blankenship, M. Stirpe, M. Gonvers, S. Binder (eds.)
Fidia Research Series, vol. II,
Liviana Press, Padova © 1986

PARS PLANA VITRECTOMY IN CHRONIC UVEITIS

Klaus Heimann

Department for Vitreo Retinal Surgery
University Eye Clinic, Cologne, FRG

Therapy of chronic uveitis is an unsatisfactory chapter in ophthalmology. Recurrent, long-lasting opacities of the vitreous, secondary cataract and cystic edema of the macula mostly varying in intensity give rise to reductions of vision which are very depressing for the patients. Vascular proliferations, formation of epiretinal membranes or a retinal detachment can occur in addition.

Formerly, surgical operations on such eyes were only performed reluctantly, since a deterioration of the result was very frequently observed postoperatively with renewed flaring up of the intraocular irritation.

The reason for this was that the vitreous could not be removed surgically in such eyes, so that it had a negative effect on the future course, e.g. due to the development of posterior synechias and an occluded pupil after cataract extraction. The astonishingly irritation-free postoperative course, e.g. after repair of retinal detachments in chronic uveitis by means of pars plana vitrectomy has led to a radical change in our views here. For this reason (Heimann et al., 1981), we have gone over the performing lensectomy and vitrectomy systematically in cases of chronic uveitis, after Diamond and Kaplan (1978) had similar experience.

SURGICAL GOALS AND INDICATIONS

Removal of the opaque vitreous and the secondary cataract are the goals of the surgical technique in order to improve vision, but also to render the further course of the chronic uveitis less disadvantageous. It can be assumed that part of the immunological process occurs in the vitreous (Klöti, 1981), and with removal of the vitreous the focus of inflammation becomes smaller and the inflammatory cells in vitrectomized eyes can be transported away more rapidly. It is, therefore, also to be recommended that the vitreous be removed simultaneously in patients with a complicated cataract (Figs. 1 and 2).

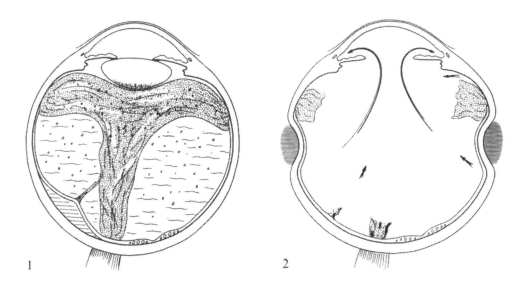

Figures 1 and 2. Objectives of pars-plana-vitrectomy in chronic-uveitis are: 1) Removal of secondary cataract, infiltrated vitreous and transvitreal and epiretinal strands. 2) In the post-operative course the intraocular fluid circulation is improved. CME remains.

A reduction of the visual acuity to at least 0.1 is regarded as an indication for surgery. Since it is not uncommon that young or middle-aged people can be affected by this chronic disease, surgery can also be performed in the presence of better visual acuity, when for example the ability to work is to be restored. Removal of epiretinal proliferations, ischemic vasoproliferative retinopathy and prophylaxis or treatment of a secondary retinal detachment are further indications. Occasionally, it is also desirable to obtain vitreous material for further diagnostic procedures, e.g. in toxocariasis.

SURGICAL PROCEDURE

Preoperatively, the patient is first given intensive local treatment with steroids. If there is a secondary cataract, it must be removed intracapsularly in order to insure a sufficient circulation of chamber fluid in the region of the vitreous cavity and the anterior chamber after operation. Vitrectomy itself does not give rise to any appreciable technical difficulties, since in most cases the vitreous displays a total posterior detachment and has shrunk together. If epiretinal surgery is necessary, it is carried out in accordance with the familiar principles.

POSTOPERATIVE COURSE

In the postoperative phase, it is astonishing how well the operation is tolerated by these eyes. Nevertheless, local steroid administration is to be recommended. Freedom from recurrence will of course not be attained. However, fresh recurrence of inflammation can be caused to regress within a few days by local steroid therapy. General therapy with all its disadvantages is then no longer necessary. If there is danger of rubeosis iridis due to retinal vasculitis, a panretinal photocoagulation should be carried out after surgery. The main problem of the postoperative phase remains the therapy-refractory cystic edema of the macula, however, in many cases, this prevents recovery of visual acuity to normal levels.

RESULTS

In our own patients (86 cases), an improvement compared to the initial finding could be achieved in 89%. Deteriorations mostly occurred due to retinal detachment in peripheral necrotizing retinochorioditis.

Vitrectomy in chronic uveitis thus remains one of the most successful indications for pars plana vitrectomy. It does not only enable marked improvements to be achieved in visual acuity, but the clinical picture has a mitigated course and it thus leads to an appreciable reduction of subjective symptoms.

REFERENCES

1. Diamond JG, Kaplan HJ (1978): Lensectomy and vitrectomy for complicated cataract secondary to Uveitis. Arch Ophthalmol 96:1798-1804.
2. Heimann K, Tavakolian U, Paulmann H, Morris R, (1981): Pars plana-Vitrektomie zur Behandlung der chronischen Uveitis. Ber Dtsch Ophthalmol Ges 78:249-251.
3. Klöti R. (1981): Vitrektomie bei chronischer Uveitis und anderen entzündlichen Eintrübungen des Glaskörpers. Ber Dtsch Ophthalmol Ges 78:233-241.

Basic and advanced vitreous surgery
G.W. Blankenship, M. Stirpe, M. Gonvers, S. Binder (eds.)
Fidia Research Series, vol. II,
Liviana Press, Padova © 1986

GIANT RETINAL TEARS

Ronald G. Michels, M.D.

The Vitreoretinal Service, Department of Ophthalmology,
Johns Hopkins University School of Medicine, Baltimore, Maryland

Giant retinal tears with an inverted retinal flap are difficult to treat successfully (Fig. 1). The principle of unfolding the inverted flap by preoperative (1, 2) or intraoperative (2, 3) positioning of the patient and/or by use of an intravitreal bubble and postoperative rotation of the patient (4, 5) has been widely accepted. However, only since development of modern vitreous surgery methods has it been possible to effectively unfold the inverted retinal flap in the majority of cases. Vitreous surgery provides capabilities to: 1) relieve vitreoretinal traction and traction due to epiretinal tissue, and 2) to create a large fluid-filled space in the vitreous cavity that permits effective use of an intraocular bubble to unfold the retinal flap during (6, 7) or after surgery (7, 8).

SURGICAL TECHNIQUE

A 360° conjunctival peritomy is made near the limbus, and traction sutures are placed beneath each rectus muscle (Fig. 2). Transcleral cryotherapy is applied to the peripheral retina or to the bare pigment epithelium in areas where the retina is highly detached or where the pigment epithelium is exposed anterior to the folded retinal flap. Two rows of contiguous cryotherapy applications are made for 360°, extending from the ora serrata posteriorly to near the equator. In the area of the giant retinal tear, and for about 3 mm beyond the ends of the tear, the anterior cryotherapy applications are applied straddling the ora serrata (Fig. 3). This is done to treat the elevated anterior edge of the retinal tear. Treatment is extended posteriorly to the equator throughout the limits of the retinal flap.

Preparations are made for a broad encircling scleral buckle to extend from the ora serrata to the equator. A scleral buckle in this location does not compress the vortex veins, although the necessary width of the buckle varies from case to case, depending on the size of the globe. Usually a silicone rubber exoplant of 7 mm width is used, and

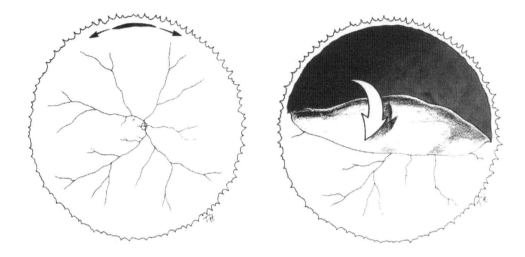

Figure 1. Giant retinal tear with inverted retinal flap. *A*, retinal tear begins along posterior margin of vitreous base and extends temporally and nasally. *B*, the posterior flap becomes inverted as tear enlarges.

this produces a buckling effect about 10 mm wide (Fig. 4). However, a broader exoplant may be necessary in myopic eyes. A broader scleral buckle may also be used throughout the limits of the giant tear if the flap appears foreshortened or unusually stiff, because it may be impossible to unfold completely.

Two mattress type scleral sutures are used in each quadrant to secure the exoplant against the sclera and to cause the buckling effect. The anterior scleral bite is made at the ora serrata, and the second bite is made 9.5 to 10 mm posteriorly when a 7 mm exoplant is used (Fig. 5). When a broader buckle is needed, the suture bites are made 3 mm wider than the exoplant material selected. The silicone rubber material is placed around the eye, under the sutures and the rectus muscles before beginning the intravitreal surgery.

A pars plana vitrectomy is then done to create a large fluid-filled space in the vitreous cavity. We prefer divided-system vitrectomy instrumentation (Fig. 6). Any vitreoretinal traction on the retinal flap or other areas of retina posterior to the equator is surgically relieved, and epiretinal membranes causing distortion of folding of the retina are dissected and removed. In eyes with a clear lens and a giant tear of less than 180°, the anterior part of the vitreous gel and the lens are not disturbed. If there is a preexisting visually-significant cataract, or if the retinal tear is greater than 180°, excision of the anterior vitreous gel and a pars plana lensectomy are usually done. In these cases simultaneous fluid-gas exchange is later done with the patient in a prone position to unfold the retinal flap and reattach the retina during surgery.

The edge of retinal flap is grasped with the vitectomy probe or with intraocular forceps and unfolded (Fig. 7). If the flap is mobile and tends to remain unfolded, no special techniques are needed to secure it to the eyewall, and fluid-gas exchange is done as described later. If the flap is quite stiff or foreshortened, or if the tear is 270° or larger, special techniques are used. These included: 1) incarceration of the flap in sclerotomies in the pars plana or the peripheral choroid, and 2) methods for transvitreal suturing of the retinal flap to the eyewall.

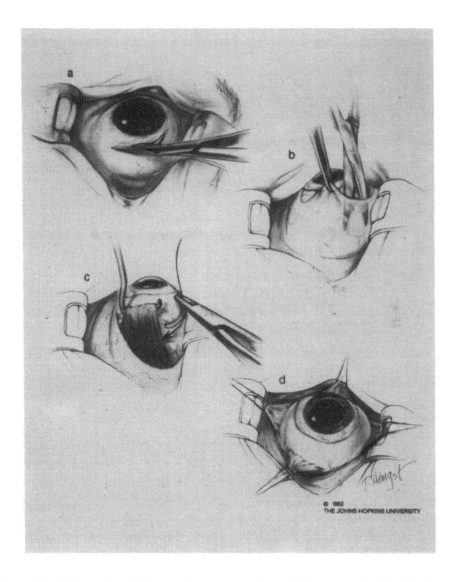

Figure 2. Initial steps in retinal reattachment operation. A 360° conjunctival incision is made 2 mm posterior to the limbus (a) and dissection is done in Tenon's space with blunt scissors (b). Traction sutures are placed beneath each rectus muscle so the eye can be rotated and positioned as necessary during surgery (c and d).

Figure 3. Cryotherapy is applied 360°. The zone of treatment is broader throughout the limits of the giant retinal tear and the anterior applications straddle the ora serrata to treat the elevated anterior edge of the giant tear.

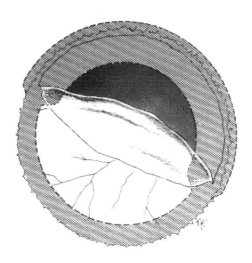

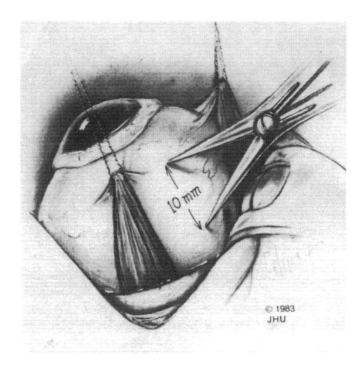

Figure 4. Preparation for scleral buckling. A 10 mm wide buckling effect is planned in most cases extending posteriorly from the ora serrata. Calipers are used to mark the locations for intrascleral suture bites.

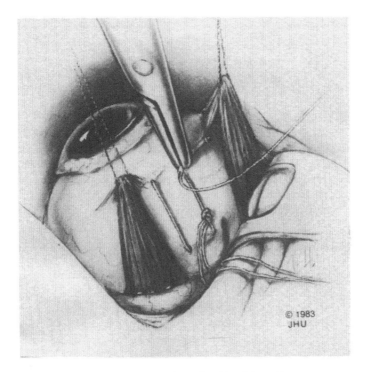

Figure 5. Placement of mattress type sutures for scleral buckling. Two sutures are used in each quadrant. The anterior bite is placed along the line of the rectus muscle insertions which corresponds to the location of the ora serrata.

The edge of the retinal flap can be incarcerated in one or more locations in the pars plana or the peripheral choroid. A pars plana site is chosen if fluid-gas exchange is to be performed in a face-down position because the expanding gas bubble will disengage the retina from the anterior incarceration site. Incarceration sites in the peripheral choroid are preferred if the retinal flap is foreshortened and will not stretch to the pars plana area or if the lens has been preserved and a gas bubble partially filling the vitreous cavity will be used with postoperative rotation of the patient.

The sclerotomy sites used for introduction of the vitrectomy instruments are often used for incarceration of the retinal flap in the pars plana, and the location for the sclerotomy sites may be selected with this latter use in mind. Since the retina will be incarcerated only in the area of the giant tear, there is no danger of damaging the peripheral retina during vitrectomy, and the sclerotomy may be prepared in the posterior part of the pars plana zone rather than at the posterior edge of the pars placita. The number and exact location of the pars plana incisions used to incarcerate the retinal flap depend on the size and location of the giant tear. Usually one incarceration site is planned in each quadrant, and these are evenly spaced so there is about equal distance from the ends of the tear to each incarceration site and between incarceration sites. Sometimes a single incarceration site is used, even if the tear is 180° or larger, when

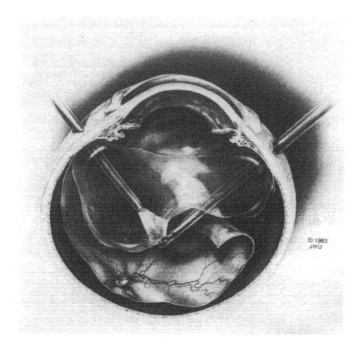

Figure 6. Pars plana vitrectomy is done before unfolding the inverted retinal flap. All of the vitreous gel is removed in aphakic eyes except for the anteroperipheral portion in the region of the vitreous base. .

this results in proper unfolding of the flap so that subsequent fluid-gas exchange is likely to be effective. The edge of torn retina that is judged to correspond to the meridian of sclerotomy is grasped with small forceps and withdrawn into the wound. Intraocular pressure is reduced by lowering the infusion bottle to prevent forceful prolapse of the retina through the scleral incision. As the forceps are withdrawn, the configuration of the retinal flap is monitored to be sure that the tissue is not stretched so severely that posterior tearing of the retina and damage to the optic nerve may occur. If the retina will not stretch to the sclerotomy site, this technique is abandoned and a more posterior sclerotomy is used.

As the intraocular forceps are withdrawn from the wound, the edge of the retina is grasped within the wound margins with small, smooth forceps applied externally, and the intraocular forceps are disengaged. The edge of the retina is then held within the wound as the scleral margins are sutured closed with 7-0 polyglycolic acid suture using a running double figure-of-eight technique (9). This process may be repeated in several locations where necessary to properly unfold the retinal flap (Fig. 8). Secure closure of the sclerotomy wound is necessary to prevent later leakage of fluid or gas during fluid-gas exchange and to prevent further prolapse of retinal tissue. When possible the retinal edge is engaged with a single bite of the suture to secure it in the wound.

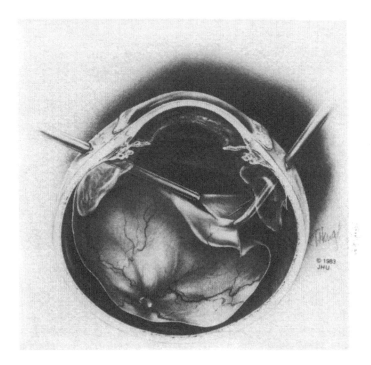

Figure 7. The flap of the giant retinal tear is unfolded after excising the vitreous gel. The torn edge of the retina is grasped with small forceps and unfolded.

The same technique for grasping and incarceration of the retinal flap can be used at locations at or posterior to the ora serrata. Transvitreal suturing techniques can also be used to attach the edge of the retinal flap to the eyewall before fluid-gas exchange (10). Both the retinal incarceration techniques and the retinal suturing methods are done to partially unfold the retinal flap so subsequent fluid-gas exchange is effective in properly unfolding the retinal flap.

In aphakic eyes with tears of greater than 180°, and especially those in which a pars plana incarceration site was used, fluid-gas exchange is performed in a face-down position. Prior to this, each of the sclerotomy incisions, including the infusion cannula site, is permanently closed with sutures.

The gas is injected through a 27 gauge needle, and the eye is rotated so that the bubble floats toward the posterior retina on the side opposite the retinal tear. As the gas is injected, intraocular fluid is displaced out of the eye through a second 27 gauge needle introduced through the limbus into the pupillary space. The fluid-gas exchange is continued until all the intraocular fluid has been replaced by gas (Fig. 9). Then the needle are withdrawn and the patient is returned to a supine posture and the scleral sutures are tightened to elevate the scleral buckle. Small portions of the bubble are aspirated through a 30 gauge needle on a small syringe to soften the globe as the sutures are tied.

Figure 8. Pars plana incarceration results in unfolding of the inverted retinal flap so subsequent use of an intravitreal bubble will position the retina properly against the pigment epithelium.

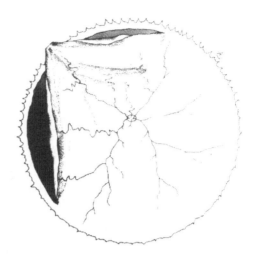

In other eyes, fluid-gas exchange is performed with the patient in a supine position, and 30-50% of the vitreous cavity filled with gas (Fig. 10). In aphakic eyes this is done under direct visualization using the operating microscope and intraocular fiberoptic illumination. In phakic eyes the aid of a biconcave corneal contact lens is needed, or the technique can be done while viewing through an indirect ophthalmoscope. A bubble behind the crystalline lens creates a complicated optical system so that visualization through the operating microscope is not possible with or without a conventional plano-concave contact lens.

When using the supine position, the scleral sutures are usually tightened and tied before the fluid-gas exchange. Thirty to 50% of the vitreous cavity is filled with gas and the sclerotomies are then suture closed. The patient is rotated immediately after surgery so that the bubble unfolds the retinal flap and positions it against the treated pigment epithelium (Fig. 11).

In all cases with giant retinal tears the fundus is examined frequently during the first weeks after surgery. The first week after the bubble absorbs is the most important time, because some portion of the retinal flap may become elevated again causing recurrent detachment with or without complete separation of the flap from the surface of the buckle. We promptly apply photocoagulation to any area of retinal elevation over the buckle. Also, we apply prophylactic photocoagulation to the edge of the retinal tear if it is located near the posterior edge of the buckle or if there is no visible evidence of cryotherapy where the flap is flat on the buckle.

DISCUSSION

Not all eyes with giant retinal tears require vitreous surgery for successful treatment, and many cases can be treated by conventional scleral buckling techniques with or without supplemental injection of gas into the vitreous cavity. Tears without an inverted retinal flap rarely require vitrectomy, and these cases are treated with a low, broad scleral buckle and drainage of subretinal fluid. However, tears with an inverted flap are treated by vitreous surgery to assist in unfolding the flap.

Our early experience using vitreous surgery methods to treat giant retinal tears identified several difficulties and led to refinements in the technique. We now use a broad encircling scleral buckle from the ora serrata to the equator in nearly every case, and

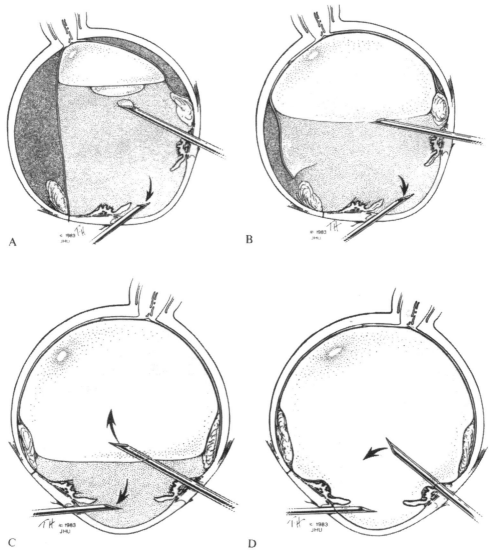

Figure 9. Complete fluid-gas exchange in eye with giant retinal tear treated by pars plana incarceration of retinal flap. *A*, gas is injected through a 27-gauge needle introduced through limbus or pars plana as intraocular fluid is displaced out of the eye through a second needle in the anterior chamber. *B* and *C*, the expanding gas bubble disengages the retinal edge from the pars plana incarceration site as the retina is flattened against the eyewall. *D*, fluid-gas exchange is continued until all intraocular fluid is replaced by gas.

186

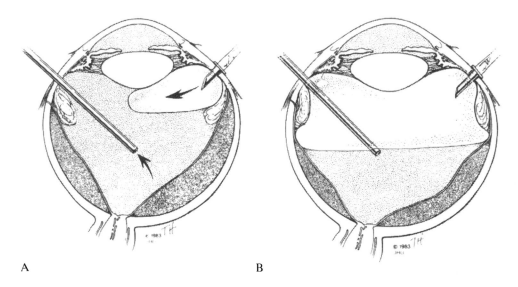

A   B

Figure 10. Fluid-gas exchange performed in supine position to partially fill the vitreous cavity with gas. *A* and *B*, gas is injected through the pars plana infusion cannula as intraocular fluid is displaced out of the eye through a blunt-tipped needle. Visualization is provided by indirect ophthalmoscopy or by operating microscope aided by biconcave corneal contact lens.

we create a broad zone of chorioretinal adhesion on the surface of the buckle by cryotherapy. This virtually eliminates recurrent retinal detachment from unrecognized, iatrogenic or later retinal breaks on the opposite side of the eye or from leakage of subretinal fluid under the anterior flap of the giant tear, around the end of the tear, and across the buckle. The combination of cryotherapy to the anterior flap of the giant tear and intraocular gas will seal the anterior edge, and this prevents leakage of subretinal fluid from that site.

Giant tears as large as 270°, and those with a stiff or contracted flap due to epiretinal membranes or other secondary changes, are difficult to treat by conventional techniques of scleral buckling, vitrectomy and intraocular gas. The intraocular bubble sometimes does not unfold the flap properly, and part of the bubble is occasionally trapped between the flap and the pigment epithelium. The techniques for retinal incarceration or transvitreal suturing are useful in these cases, to be sure the flap is unfolded as fully as possible. The pars plana incarceration technique has the advantage of using the vitrectomy incisions, whereas incarceration sites located more posteriorly or transvitreal suturing are more likely to be associated with permanent fixation of the retinal tear edge.

Although a broad and moderately high scleral buckle is preferred for the reasons mentioned earlier, in some cases no scleral buckle is used. This is done mainly in eyes with a very foreshortened retinal flap in which there is no possibility of unfolding the flap onto a peripheral scleral buckle. Use of an encircling scleral buckle tends to cause further anteroposterior opening of the giant tear. Therefore, in these cases the same methods are used but without the scleral buckle. During the early postoperative time, laser photocoagulation is used to seal the edge of the giant retinal tear in whatever location it has been pressed against the eyewall.

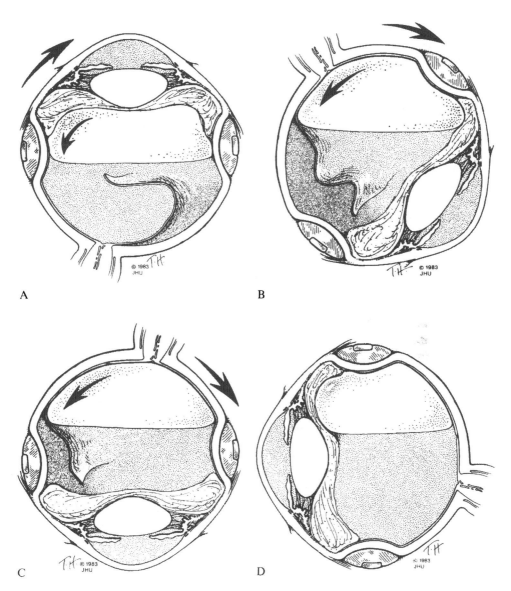

Figure 11. Partial intraocular bubble and postoperative rotation of the patient to unfold flap of giant retinal tear. *A*, bubble filling 30 to 50% of vitreous cavity is used, and patient is rotated so the bubble moves across the retina opposite the location of the retinal tear. *B*, *C* and *D*, the rotation is continued until the intraocular bubble unfolds the retinal flap and positions it against the scleral buckle and the previously treated pigment epithelium.

The sequence of applying cryotherapy and later performing the vitrectomy may be advantageous by removing viable retinal pigment epithelial cells that are liberated into the vitreous cavity during treatment with cryotherapy. After removal of the vitreous gel, we usually lavage the vitreous cavity until all visible cells are removed. Since retinal pigment epithelial cells may contribute to subsequent epiretinal membrane formation and recurrent retinal detachment from proliferative vitreoretinopathy (PVR) (11), removal of most of these cells may lower the incidence of this complication. We have the clinical impression that postoperative PVR is infrequent when these methods are used.

Sterile air is often used as the gas injected into the vitreous cavity when treating giant retinal tears. Air is suitable in most cases because a sufficiently large bubble can be introduced to achieve the mechanical objectives, and the bubble size can be supplemented postoperatively if necessary. However, sulfur hexafluoride (SF_6) mixed with air has the advantage of being absorbed less rapidly because of the lower water solubility of SF_6. This is helpful in cases with giant tears greater than 180° and in cases with tears located inferiorly in which it is difficult to maintain prolonged contact between the flap and the treated pigment epithelium.

The methods described herein represent our current techniques for treating giant retinal tears. They were developed during the course of expanding clinical experience dealing with a variety of complicated situations associated with giant retinal tears. Even so, additional experience will probably enable further refinement of these methods.

REFERENCES

1. Schepens CL, Dobbie JG, McMeele JW (1962): Retinal detachments with giant breaks: Preliminary report. Trans Am Acad Ophthalmol Otolaryngol 66:471-479.
2. Schepens CL, Freeman HM (1967): Current management of giant retinal breaks. Trans Am Acad Ophthalmol Otolaryngol 474-487.
3. Schepens CL (1983): Retinal Detachment and Allied Diseases, Vol. II. Philadelphia: WB Saunders; 520-542.
4. Norton EWD, Aaberg T, Fung W, et al. (1969): Giant retinal tears. I. Clinical management with intravitreal air. Am J Ophthalmol 1011-1021.
5. Freeman HM, Schepens CL, Couvillion GC (1970): Current management of giant retinal breaks. Part II. Trans Am Acad Ophthalmol Otolaryngol 74:59-74.
6. Machemer R, Allen AW (1976): Retinal tears 180° and greater: Management with vitrectomy and intravitreal gas. Arch Ophthalmol 94:1340-1346.
7. Michels RG (1981): Vitreous Surgery. St. Louis, CV Mosby 250-255.
8. Michels RG (1982): Vitreous surgery. In: Manuals Program. San Francisco, Am Acad Ophthalmol 70-72.
9. Michels RG (1981): Vitreous Surgery. St. Louis, CV Mosby, 94.
10. Michels RG, Rice TA, Blankenship G (1983): Surgical techniques for selected giant retinal tears. Retina 139-153.
11. Hilton G, Machemer R, Michels RG, et al. (1983): The Retina Society Terminology Committee: The classification of retinal detachment with proliferative vitreoretinopathy. Ophthalmology 121-125.

Basic and advanced vitreous surgery
G.W. Blankenship, M. Stirpe, M. Gonvers, S. Binder (eds.)
Fidia Research Series, vol. II,
Liviana Press, Padova © 1986

GIANT RETINAL TEAR

M. Gonvers, M.D.

Hôpital Ophtalmologique, Lausanne

There is no doubt that the major characteristic of a giant retinal tear is its rolling over flap, which can only happen if the next three conditions are present:

— the tear must be superior or equal to 180 degrees;
— the vitreous has to be adherent only to the anterior edge of the tear;
— the mid and posterior vitreous must be totally liquified.

On the other hand the situation found in the case of a giant dialysis is totally different and the retinal flap does not have the possibility to roll over, for two specific reasons: first, the vitreous body is adherent to the posterior edge of the tear; secondly, the mid and posterior vitreous is not liquified at all or not as much as in a giant tear.

It is important to make the difference between giant tear and giant dialysis, as the treatment of each condition is totally different. Giant dialysis can be cured with a classical buckle but giant tear must be handled by a vitrectomy technique.

The first logical approach to the treatment of giant tear was described by Machemer et al. (1) and includes these essential steps: a vitrectomy, done to remove the anterior vitreous, followed by radial cuts on the posterior shrunken edge of the retinal tear; then a total filling of the eye with gas, the patient being in a prone position. Finally external coagulation on the retinal tear completed by an encircling buckle.

This technique, however, presents two major disadvantages: first of all, the retinal flap has a great tendency to slip backwards to the posterior pole of the eye. This sliding occurs usually during the operation, when the patient is placed again on his back after filling his whole eye with gas. This sliding can also occur a few days after the operation, when the gas reabsorbs. Secondly, this technique does not prevent the occurrence of proliferative vitreoretinopathy (PVR) which is associated in most cases of giant tear, even if there is no visible proliferation at the time of the operation. This frequent association between giant tear and PVR is due probably to the great bare surface of pigment epithelium which is left uncovered by the retina so that the pigment epithelium cells can widely spread around, in as much that the vitreous is totally liquified.

These two major complications which are very often encountered in the treatment of giant tear made me change my surgical approach to such a disease and instead of using a gas tamponade, I switched over to a temporary tamponade of silicone oil (2). The silicone oil is used exactly in the same way as the gas. It is removed from the eye after six weeks.

The procedure I use starts with a vitrectomy. Usually, the vitreous base is not touched because in the case of giant tear, more than in any other, it is very difficult to cut it with a vitrectomy instrument. Radial cuts are done on the posterior edge of the retinal tear with vitreous scissors. Then, according to the localization of the giant tear, the patient is turned on his right, his left, or is placed face down and a total fluid-silicone exchange is done. Silicone oil is injected at the upper pars plana, on a meridian opposite the giant tear (in a case of a 180° giant tear), while saline is removed at the inferior pars plana, in the area of the giant tear. The silicone bubble when increasing in size unrolls the retinal flap. When the vitreous cavity is filled with silicone, the patient is placed in a normal position and surgery is continued. I should mention at this point that I put an encircling buckle only for giant tears in which one or two of its extremities go down under the horizontal meridian. The reason for doing this will be explained later. The last step of the operation is an extensive xenon photocoagulation done over the whole repositioned retinal flap. Six weeks later the silicone oil is removed from the eye.

What are the advantages of a silicone tamponade over a gas tamponade?
— during the operation the silicone oil prevents posterior sliding of the retinal flap much better than gas;
— the operation is done under excellent visibility and the lens can be left in place which is not possible with the Machemer et al. technique;
— because of the perfect transparency of the silicone oil it is possible at the end of the operation to perform an extensive photocoagulation of the retinal flap without manipulating the eye and this photocoagulation creates immediate strong adherence to the pigment epithelium, which can not be done with external cryopexy;
— in the postoperative course the posterior sliding of the retinal flap is much less frequent, essentially because there is no reabsorption of the silicone oil and the mechanical tamponade of the retina does not decrease, as it does with gas. This positive effect of silicone oil against retinal sliding is much more pronounced in the upper half of the eye than in the lower half:
— silicone oil certainly decreases the danger of PVR. As it is well known, the reapplied retina in a case of a giant tear will always be too short and cannot cover all the pigment epithelium; the pigment epithelium left bare can disseminate a lot of pigment epithelial cells when a gas tamponade is used. With a silicone tamponade this bare epithelium can no longer release its cells. This could be one of the reasons why PVR is less frequent with a silicone tamponade. It is also possible that the silicone tamponade prevents contraction of the invisible preretinal membrane which is already present at the time of surgery. This mechanical property of silicone oil is demonstrated on the animal (3).

Unfortunately silicone oil being lighter than water the tamponade is much more effective for the upper half of the retina than it is for the lower half. A superior giant tear is always perfectly closed by the silicone tamponade and bare pigment epithelium is totally covered. An inferior giant tear is badly tamponaded by the silicone bubble because of the usual accumulation of water in this part of the eye. The only way to tamponade an inferior tear is to put a large encircling buckle which makes the tear come in contact with the silicone bubble. However, the sliding of the posterior flap cannot be properly prevented, and the lower half of the bare pigment epithelium is not covered by the silicone oil which can give rise to a free dissemination of cells.

The specific weight of silicone making it lighter than water, explains why the prognosis of a giant tear is totally different according to the location of the tear. Thus in a statistic of 18 giant tears, the success rate was close to 90% for superior giant tear of 180°, 60% for vertical or inferior giant tear, 35% for 270° giant tear and 3 cases of 360° giant tear were failures. All eyes which had a fully attached retina 6 months or more after silicone removal were considered as successes. Eyes in which silicone oil was not removed were counted as failures even though the macula was attached. In fact, statistical analysis was impossible because of a various degree association of PVR in some cases. However, it is evident that prognosis is excellent for superior giant tear and less good when the giant tear goes below the horizontal meridian. It is hoped that in the future the use of fluorosilicone which is heavier than water will give us a better tamponade of inferior retinal breaks.

REFERENCES

1. Machemer R, Aaberg TM and Norton EWD (1969): Giant retinal tears. II. Experimental production and management with intravitreal air. Trans Amer Ophth Soc 67:394-414.
2. Gonvers M (1983): Temporary use of silicone oil in the treatment of special cases of retinal detachment. Ophthalmologica (Basel) 197:202-209.
3. Gonvers M and Thresher R (1983): Temporary use of silicone oil in the treatment of proliferative vitreoretinopathy. An experimental study with a new animal model. Grafe's Arch Ophthal 221:46-53.

Basic and advanced vitreous surgery
G.W. Blankenship, M. Stirpe, M. Gonvers, S. Binder (eds.)
Fidia Research Series, vol. II,
Liviana Press, Padova © 1986

MANAGEMENT OF GIANT RETINAL TEARS
USING VITRECTOMY AND FLUID/SILICONE-OIL EXCHANGE

P.K. Leaver

Moorfields Eye Hospital, City Road, London EC1V 2PD

During the past 5 years we have been using vitrectomy combined with fluid/silicone-oil exchange in the management of giant retinal tears (GRTs).

Immediate postoperative results were encouraging, complete retinal reattachment with closure of the GRT being achieved in 97% of cases. Review of the same group of patients at 6 months after surgery showed that this success was maintained in 86% of eyes.

We have now reviewed 65 patients with GRTs treated by this method at 18 months after surgery.

PATIENTS AND METHODS

There were 49 males and 16 females, their ages ranging from 4-71 years.

The surgical technique is simple and requires little equipment outside the range of that already used by most vitreous surgeons.

Bimanual closed intraocular microsurgery was performed using common-gauge instrumentation, infusion contact lens and the Zeiss Op Mi VI microscope with X-Y coupling.

All vitreous gel was removed to allow free mobilization of the posterior flap of the GRT. The posterior flap was then unfolded using direct intraocular manipulation with the light-pipe and Charles-flute needle or vitrectomy instrument. Once the flap had been unfolded, silicone-oil of 1000 c/s viscosity was injected via the infusion line which had initially been used for infusion of physiological solution. A compressed-air powered syringe was used to facilitate the injection of silicone oil. The preretinal and subretinal fluid was simultaneously evacuated through a Charles-flute needle as the silicone-oil was injected.

Once the tear had been closed and the retina reattached, cryotherapy was applied to the edge of the posterior flap and throughout 360° A deep, broad circumferential buckle was created inferiorly to support the inferior retina and lower extent of the GRT.

360° prophylactic cryotherapy was applied to the peripheral retina of the fellow eye in the majority of cases.

Surgery was conducted with the patient in the supine position using a standard operating table. Postoperatively the patients were nursed in the face down position for 3 to 4 days. Subsequently they were allowed to mobilize but instructed never to lie in the supine position for extended periods of time.

Silicone-oil was removed from the eye whenever possible after intervals ranging from 5 weeks to 11 months.

RESULTS

Of 65 eyes the retina remained attached after 18 months in 54 (83%). Of the 54 successful cases, 32 (59%) had acuities of 6/60 or better and 14 (26%) had acuities of 6/18 or better. Of the 22 successful cases with acuities of 3/60 or worse, 11 had maculopathy or macular pucker, 7 had cataract, 3 had a combination of cataract and macular disease and one had silicone-oil induced keratopathy and glaucoma.

Of 22 successful cases remaining phakic after 18 months, 5 had oil still in situ while in 17 it had been removed. Only one eye retained a completely clear lens.

In summary, a series of 65 patients with GRTs in whom vitrectomy and fluid/silicone-oil exchange was undertaken is reported.

The surgical method is simple and has been shown to be effective.

Anatomical results at 18 months after surgery indicate a success rate of 83%. Visual results in successful cases range from 6/6 to perception of light only. In 59% visual acuities were found to be 6/60 or better. In the remaining 41% with acuities of 3/60 or worse, the low level of vision was seen to be associated with long term complications attributable equally to the disease process itself and to the late effects of intraocular silicone oil.

Basic and advanced vitreous surgery
G.W. Blankenship, M. Stirpe, M. Gonvers, S. Binder (eds.)
Fidia Research Series, vol. II,
Liviana Press, Padova © 1986

MACULAR HOLE AND RETINAL DETACHMENT

M. Gonvers, M.D.

Hôpital Ophtalmologique, Lausanne

Until recently, the treatment of macular detachment with macular hole was a nightmare for retinal surgeons. Classical treatment included coagulation of the macular hole and buckling of the macula. The surgical procedure was difficult and dangerous and postoperative vision was catastrophic. Most of the time the successfully operated patients complained of seeing much less after the operation than before.

In 1982 a new technique was described (1), in which it was no longer necessary to coagulate the macular hole or to buckle the macula. The operation was very simple since only a straight vitrectomy had to be done, followed by a partial air-fluid exchange. The patient was positioned on his face for 12 hours, just to let the bubble of air close the macular hole while the subretinal fluid reabsorbed by itself.

This technique was based on the following two theoretical ideas: it was thought that in most cases, a macular hole by itself was not able to give rise to a detachment and that vitreous traction was necessary to create a detachment. It was thus imagined that the removal of these tractions should be enough to definitively cure the detachment.

Once the retina reattached, it was decided there was no longer any reason to coagulate the macular hole and destroy the perimacular retina.

Six cases were described in the original paper (1). Their essential characteristics can be summarized as follows:

— myopia ranged from 0 to —19 diopters;
— except for one case which was emmetropic, all the cases had a moderate posterior staphyloma;
— vitreous tractions on the posterior retina were observed in two cases and their presence was presumed in two others.

Up-to-date, two of the six cases redetached, the first one one year after the operation, the second three years later. In these two cases the retina could be reattached only by a new airfluid exchange easily done in the office and since then the retina in both cases has not redetached. It has to be mentioned that an enlargment of the macular hole was documented for these two cases and could be the only explanation for the relapse of detachment.

The follow-up of these two cases is interesting in several ways: it first showed that if a relapse of detachement occurs in an eye which was operated on according to the described technique, it is worth trying a new air tamponade before going in for a more traumatizing technique. It was also learned that vitreous traction does not always play as important a role as it was thought. If these two cases appear to minimize the importance of vitreous traction, a few words have to be said about three other cases which do not belong to this series, and do seem to emphasize the importance of vitreous traction in the pathogenis of detachment with macular hole. These three cases, each with retinal detachment due to a macular hole, had undergone vitrectomy and air tamponade elsewhere; it was assumed by the respective surgeons that in each case the retina was flat the day after the operation but redetached a few days later when the air reabsorbed. When these three referred cases were first examined, it was most interesting to observe that the vitrectomy was very incomplete. These three cases were reoperated and a more complete vitrectomy was performed. Up-to-date these three cases have a totally flat retina.

To make things more complicated, one should mention Miyake's paper (2) in which the author describes a technique to treat detachment with macular hole only with external drainage and air injection, without vitrectomy. This technique was successfully tried by us in one case. Two explanations for the way Dr Miyake's technique could work, can be advanced:
— it is possible that vitreous traction was severed by the air bubble, since the four patients described by Dr Miyake were placed on their face 5 hours a day during a couple of days;
— it is also possible that vitreous tractions separated from the retina, just after the detachment occurred.

In conclusion, on the base of all these observations, the importance of vitreous traction on the occurrence of a detachment with macular hole could vary from one case to another:
— there are cases in which the vitreous is probably very adherent to all or a part of the posterior retina. In these cases vitrectomy is necessary;
— there are certainly other cases in which vitreous traction is very small and can be ruptured just with the help of an air bubble;
— finally, it is possible that in some cases, once the detachment occurs, vitreous traction loses its connection with the retina.

It should be mentioned of course that all these remarks concern eyes in which there is no myopic staphyloma or in which staphyloma is moderate as it is usually the case when myopia does not exceed 15 to 20 diopters. Most retinal detachments with macular holes belong to this category.

However, it is well known that macular hole with retinal detachment can be found in severe myopia, when staphyloma is very marked. In these cases the detachment seems no longer due to vitreous traction but to what should be called an "inverse traction" because the eyewall increases its axial length much more rapidly than the retina. This kind of detachment is much more difficult to treat because usually, vitrectomy alone is uneffective. The following approach can be proposed in these rare cases: a vitrectomy with partial air-fluid exchange and prone positioning should always be the choice procedure. If the retina cannot be permanently reattached, the patient should be reoperated and have a total liquid-silicone exchange, using the macular hole for the internal drainage. Small endo or exolaser coagulations should be placed around the macular hole and the patient asked to sleep on his face for 10 days. After 4 to 6 weeks, if the retina does not detach, silicone oil has to be removed. Another alternative would be to buckle the macula without coagulating it.

In conclusion, the treatment of the majority of retinal detachments with macular hole has been greatly simplified over the last years. However, there are still some rare cases in which major surgery must be considered. The understanding of this type of retinal detachment has been improved but all the problems are not totally solved and discussion is still open.

REFERENCES

1. Gonvers M and Machemer R (1982): A new approach to treating retinal detachment with macular hole. Amer J Ophth 94:468-472.
2. Miyake Y (1984): A simplified method of treating retinal detachment with macular hole. Amer J Ophth 97:243-245.

Basic and advanced vitreous surgery
G.W. Blankenship, M. Stirpe, M. Gonvers, S. Binder (eds.)
Fidia Research Series, vol. II,
Liviana Press, Padova © 1986

TREATMENT OF MYOPIC MACULAR HOLES AND DETACHMENT WITH LIQUID VITREOUS - INTRAVITREAL GAS EXCHANGE

George W. Blankenship, M.D.

The Bascom Palmer Eye Institute
University of Miami School of Medicine, Miami, Florida

Conventional scleral buckling operations for retinal detachments caused by macular holes are very difficult and usually not successful in reattaching the macula and improving vision (1, 2). The more recent advances of pars plana vitrectomy (3) provide a more direct treatment for this condition with improved results. A simple modification of pars plana vitrectomy involving replacement of liquid vitreous with an expanding SF-6 bubble (4) has been used in 4 cases with good anatomical and visual results.

CASE SELECTION

This procedure requires a cooperative patient whose retinal detachment in caused by a macular hole without additional peripheral retinal holes. This type of detachment usually is associated with high myopia, but may also occur following trauma. The formed vitreous must be posteriorly detached without tractional attachments to the macular hole.

This procedure is not recommended for cases in which peripheral retinal holes are present, or where traction remains to the macular area such as may occurr with intraocular proliferative diseases or partial posterior vitreous detachments.

TREATMENT TECHNIQUE

The procedure is performed in the outpatient clinic following a thorough examination, including indirect ophthalmoscopy and fundus contact lens examination, to determine that the posterior vitreous is detached, and to exclude peripheral retinal tears and vitreoretinal attachments to the macula adjacent to the hole. A sterile 5 cc syringe with a 25 gauge 5/8 inch needle is partially filled with 1 cc of filtered 100% SF-6.

After retrobulbar anesthesia has been obtained, a lid speculum is inserted and the patient is positioned in a face down position with the head extended over the end of an examining table.

The surgeon is comfortably positioned beneath the patient's face. The globe is then entered 4 mm peripheral to the limbus in an area that is clearly exposed by inserting the 25 gauge needle through conjunctiva, sclera, pars plana, and formed vitreous, being directed towards the posterior fundus away from the lens and peripheral retina. The tip of the inserted needle can easily be visualized with indirect ophthalmoscopy to insure that the needle tip is clear.

One-fourth cc of SF-6 is then injected into the vitreous cavity and floats superiorly to the posterior fundus further displacing the vitreous towards the dependent anterior portion of the vitreous cavity. Moderate aspiration with the syringe then draws liquid vitreous into the dependent portion of the syringe with the SF-6 remaining in the upper portion of the syringe. The remaining 3/4 cc of SF-6 is injected into the vitreous cavity in 1/4 cc increments with aspiration of 1/4 cc of liquid vitreous between each injection of gas. The needle is then withdrawn from the globe, and the eye is reexamined to exclude elevated intraocular pressure and complications such as lens or retinal damage from the needle, or intraocular bleeding.

A sterile bandage is applied, and the patient returns home with instructions to remain face down for the next 24 hours when a follow-up examination is performed. Laser treatment, if needed, can be applied beneath the intravitreal gas bubble to the edge of the macular hole or in a macular grid pattern. The patient then returns home with instructions to remain face down most of the time for the next few days.

RESULTS

The results are summarized in the accompanying table. Three of the 4 cases had high myopia with posterior staphylomas, and had a long history of decreased vision from myopic macular degeneration with a more recent loss of vision caused by the macular detachment. Patient #2 had a previous pseudophakic retinal detachment which was initially successfully repaired with scleral buckling, but returned 5 weeks after the scleral buckling procedure with a bullous retinal detachment confined to the temporal vascular arcades and an apparent central macular hole without vitreomacular tractional attachments.

The 6 month postoperative visual acuities were improved in each case, but remained reduced because of atrophic macular changes. All of the retinas and maculas were attached 6 months following the procedure. None of the cases developed infections, glaucoma, intraocular bleeding, cataracts, subsequent retinal detachment, or had additional surgery during the 6 months postoperative period.

DISCUSSION

Most retinal detachments associated with an apparent macular hole are caused by peripheral retinal tears (1), and are usually reattached with conventional scleral buckling techniques which close the peripheral retinal hole. Posterior retinal detachments may occur with posterior retinal holes created by traction from contracting proliferative tissues (5), and successful reattachment requires release of the tractional forces. This technique of internal tamponade of the posterior retinal holes by exchanging liquid vitreous with an expanding gas bubble would not be successful in these more typical situations.

Tractional strands of formed vitreous extending from the posteriorly detached vitreous to the macula were not visualized in any of these 4 cases. Presumably, some tractional component existed to produce the retinal detachment and either spontaneously separated from the macula prior to the examination and procedure, or was not visualized at the examination and was released by the expanding gas bubble or during the aspiration of liquid vitreous.

The technique is a simple modification to that described by Gonvers and Machemer (3) with the elimination of vitrectomy instruments since the formed vitreous is not removed. Macular coagulation is probably not necessary as it was not used in their 6 cases, nor in Case 4 of this series. Its use in the first 3 cases was because of apprehension that the detachment would reoccur. The technique is so simple, that it would be easy to repeat and supplement with macular coagulation or with a subsequent pars plana vitrectomy, should the detachment reoccur.

Table

	CASE 1	CASE 2	CASE 3	CASE 4
Age	64	79	77	63
Sex	Female	Male	Female	Female
Eye	Right	Right	Right	Left
Duration Decreased vision				
Total	15 yrs	5 wks	35 yrs	50 yrs
Recent	15 days	5 wks	6 mths	1 week
Ophthalmic problems	High myopia staphyloma	Pseudophakic schleral buckle	High myopia staphyloma amblyopia	High myopia staphyloma
Visual acuities				
Preop	6/200	6/200	4/200	3/200
6 months postop	20/200	20/200	6/200	20/100
Laser treatment following gas injections	Yes	Yes	Yes	No
Macula and retina 6 months postop	Attach	Attach	Attach	Attach

REFERENCES

1. Aaberg TM (1970): Macular Holes. a review, Surv Ophthalmol, 15:139-162.
2. Kloti R (1974): Silver clip for central retinal detachment with macular hole. Mod Prob Ophthalmol, 12:330-336.
3. Gonvers M, Machemer R (1982): A new approach to treating retinal detachment with macular hole. Am J Ophthalmol, 94:468-72.
4. Norton EWD (1973): Intraocular gas in the management of selected retinal detachments. Trans Am Acad Ophthalmol Otolaryngol, 77:Op-85-98.
5. Blankenship GW (1983): Posterior retinal holes secondary to diabetic retinopathy. Arch Ophthalmol, 101:885-887.

Basic and advanced vitreous surgery
G.W. Blankenship, M. Stirpe, M. Gonvers, S. Binder (eds.)
Fidia Research Series, vol. II,
Liviana Press, Padova © 1986

RETINAL DETACHMENT WITH MACULAR HOLE

Mario Stirpe and Carlo Villani

Fondazione Oftalmologica 'G.B. Bietti', Piazza Sassari, 5, Roma.

According to the observations of Machemer, "attraction forces" created by a continuous absorption of fluid by the pigmented epithelium keep the retina attached to the underlying planes. Following this observation, Machemer and Gonvers showed that a relaxing of any vitreo-retinal traction by vitrectomy makes possible the reattachment of a detached retina with macular hole. By relaxing traction on the retina, posterior scleral buckles and cryo or laser treatment can be avoided. Without scar adhesions, however, any tangential traction on the retina, even if it is not near the macular hole, can cause a new subretinal infiltration of fluid through the re-opened central hole.

Many surgeons still continue to treat the macular hole after vitrectomy. Most frequently used are laser treatments applied around the macular hole.

CLINICAL OBSERVATIONS AND TECHNIQUES

In five eyes with elevated myopia and a macular hole with retinal detachment not exceeding the paramacular vascular arcades, we noted that a complete reattachment of the central retina was possible by performing laser treatment external to the vascular arcades. Evidently a scar adhesion of the retina at the right point succeeded in overcoming the tractional forces of the vitreous on the retina (Figs. 1,2,3).

In one eye, however, in which the vitreo-retinal contraction continued, the retina, notwithstanding treatment, became completely detached, and many small holes appeared on the treated area. All this showed us that the removal of posterior vitreal traction is the best treatment, and also that treatment on the paramacular vascular arcades can keep the central retina attached, even if a posterior stapyloma is present. In order to avoid the possibility of a redetached retina, at the end of the vitrectomy and after absorption of subretinal fluid, we performed four or five endocryocoagulations around the paramacular vascular arcades (Fig. 4).

This treatment in one eye showed that the central retina can remain attached after an equatorial proliferation with peripheral and post-equatorial retinal detachment (Fig. 5).

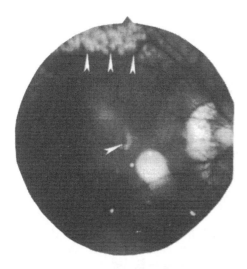

Figure 1. Photocoagulative treatments (see arrows) around posterior retina detachment with macular hole (see arrow).

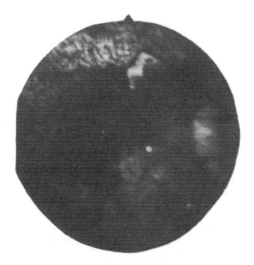

Figure 2. Preretinal hemorrhage after detachment of tractional vitreous.

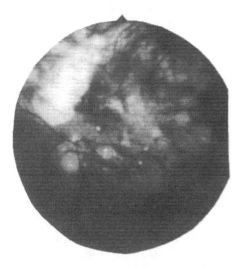

Figure 3. Adhesion of the central retina.

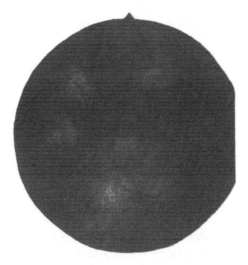

Figure 4. Endocryocoagulations after vitrectomy in retinal detachment with macular hole.

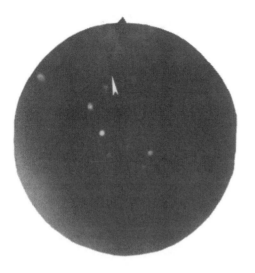

Figure 5. The central retina remains attached (see arrow) notwithstanding a peripheral and post-equatorial retinal detachment after equatorial proliferation.

CONCLUSIONS

The cryo treatment as described above does not limit the possibility of central functional recovery.

Endocryocoagulation, as compared with photocoagulation has the advantage that it can be performed at the same time as the vitrectomy, even if the retina is not completely adherent.

The beginning of cicatrization, that occurs before the complete reabsorption of the air introduced for internal tamponade, protects against the possibility of a precocious redetachment of the central retina.

Basic and advanced vitreous surgery
G.W. Blankenship, M. Stirpe, M. Gonvers, S. Binder (eds.)
Fidia Research Series, vol. II,
Liviana Press, Padova © 1986

VITRECTOMY FLUID-GAS EXCHANGE
IN THE TREATMENT OF MACULAR HOLE

R. Tittarelli, S. Benedetti, P.K. Leaver*

University Eye Clinic, Ancona; *Moorfields Eye Hospital, City Road,
London EC1V 2PD

In the past retinal detachment (R.D.) by macular hole (M.H.) always presented considerable problems both from the surgical point of view and functional recovery. Many surgeons studied the results of the use of several techniques in order to solve these problems, but much too often these attempts were unsuccessful, as they presented a great number of intraoperative and postoperative complications, which were quite difficult to manage (1-5,7-22). Later on with the advent of vitrectomy, the pathogenesis of retinal detachment seemed to be connected with vitreous traction; when this concept was accepted it was quite easy to think of managing R.D. by M.H. with vitrectomy and internal tamponade (Gonvers, Machemer, Tittarelli-Benedetti).

For a better understanding of the success of this method we must consider the peculiar anatomo-pathologic characteristics of the macular area. For example, a decreasing corion-capillary cellularity involved with aging processes, and an increase of PAS-positivity between Bruch lamina and choriocapillaries which can signify an increase in mucopolisaccarides. Furthermore, we have to consider a weak cohesion between pigmented epithelium and photoreceptors because in this area we find only cone receptors, and finally most of these patients are high myopes and therefore affected by atrophic areas of the choriocapillaries.

Several factors can assume a great importance in order to understand the reasons of failures with conventional surgery techniques. In particular: the optic nerve proximity to the macular area, the extreme vascularization, the difficulties in approaching this area, and sometimes the scleral thinning. For this reason the complications with conventional techniques are due, most of the time, to unintentional subretinal fluid drainage, choroidal hemorrage, vitreous hemorrage and scleral rupture in suturing.

There are some cases in which the R.D. by M.H. can be associated with trauma, retinal degeneration, intraocular inflammation, vascular insufficency and so on. But most of all, the preoperative biomicroscopic examination is not quite the same as the one performed during the operation. In fact the vitreous situation can be summarised in posterior vitreous detachment (PVD), total PVD with lacuna and epiretinal membrane, partial PVD with many connections with the internal limiting membrane. These different situations can explain the success, of a very simple procedure, such as injecting air in the cases of total PVD and contraction, but the failure of this procedure when there are remnants of traction or invisible epiretinal membrane over the macula.

Among our cases during 1982, we selected two patients for vitrectomy; in one case we unintentionally drained externally and injected SF^6 (Sulfur hexafluoride gas); in the other patient it was sufficient to drain subretinal fluid externally and inject gas to flatten the retina. These two patients were high myopes but it was impossible to visualize biomicroscopically any retinal membrane or vitreous strands.

The success of using internal tamponade suggested that probably some of the residual vitreous strand could be broken, and for better control of this procedure we decided to introduce vitrectomy. After some months of this experience we found the paper presented by Gonvers and Machemer on the same subject and this encouraged us to continue with this procedure.

Our conclusions were also due to the experience of the vitreo-retinal group of Moorfield's Eye Hospital in London.

About the surgery technique, we perform a pars plana vitrectomy and gas-fluid exchange. Most of the time a lensectomy is also performed because of the beneficial effects on the optics of a high myopic eye, and better intraoperative viewing of the fundus. Furthermore, in high myopes we perform an equatorial cryo of 360° and a cirling band to prevent redetachment. It is unnecessary to treat the macular area with any sort of retinopexy to prevent any further damage to fotoreceptors and because the internal tamponade seems to be effective in restoring the pigment epithelium pumping mechanism.

About the results, four patients were followed at Moorefield's Eye Hospital in London and three cases were operated in the Eye Clinic of Ancona with the maximum follow-up being 24 months.

We had only one redetachment after six months which was successfully treated by epimacular membrane peeling and fluid gas exchange.

REFERENCES

1. Aaberg TM, Blair CV and Gass J D M (1970): Macular holes. Am J Ophthal, 69:555.
2. Arruga H (1946): Chirurgia ocular. Salvat Edit, Barcellona
3. Bagolini B and Peduzzi M (1979): Implant de silicone armé dans le tratement chirurgical du décollement de la rétine avec tou maculaire, F.F.O., 161-163.
4. Bangerter A (1940): Operations methode zym Verschluss von Netzhautlochern am hinteren Augenpol in besonderen von Mculalochern. Ophthal, 100:351-354.
5. Cattaneo D (1956): Fori maculari e distacco di retina. Boll. Ocular 35: 1029.
6. Gonvers M, Machemer R (1982): A new approach to treating retinal detachment with macular hole. Am J Ophthal, 94:468.
7. Guist G (1933): Die ablatio-operation mit Aetzkali und ihr weiterer Ausban, Kli Mbl Augenheilk, 90, 71.
8. Haut J, Lecoq PJ, Cley C, Limon S and Moschos M (1972): Traitement par époge en silicone

elastique localisée et cryotherapie des décollements de rétine par trou maculaire, Arch. Ophtal, Paris, 32- 8-9, 541-548.

9. Haut J (1980): Traitement chirurgical des decollements de rétine avec trou maculaire par la technique de la vitrectomie associé a la injection de silicone-liquid, J Fr Ophtal, vol. 3-2, 115-118.

10. Kloti R (1974): Silver clip for central retinal detachment with macular hole, Mod Probl Ophthal Basel 12, 330-336.

11. Leaver PK (1975): Macular hole and retinal detachment. Trans Ophthal Soc U.K. 95, pp. 145-147.'

12. Linder K (1932): Ueber eine neue Operations-methode fur Netzhaitabhebungen bei Netzhautadefekten am hinteren Augenpol, Graefes Arch J Ophthal, 128, 654.

13. Mamoli L (1937): Un cas de décollement de la rétine avec trou de la macula. Tentative de thérapeutique transbulbaire. Ann Oculist, Paris 174, 309.

14. Margherio RR and Schepens CL (1972): Macular breaks. I Diagnosis etiology and observations. Am J Ophthal, 74, 219.

15. Margherio RR and Schepens CL (1972): Macular breaks II Managements, Am J Ophthal, 74, 233-240.

16. Meyer-Schwickerath G (1959): Indications and limitations of light-coagulations of the retina. Trans Am Acad Ophthal, Otolaring 63, 725.

17. Pannarale MR (1963): Techniques du traitement de décollements avec déchirurespostérieures Comm.to colloque deu Club Gonin Amers foort 29 Avril 3 Mai 1963 (Mod Probl Ophtal, vol. 4).

18. Pannarale MR (1966): Techniques de traitement du décollement avec déchirures trés postérieures. Bibl. Ophtal, 70, 239.

19. Paufique L and Bonnet M (1966): Traitement du décollement de la rétine avec déchirure vraie de la macula par la technique de la "poche sclérale". Bull Soc Opht de France, 9, 863-866.

20. Paufique L and Bonnet M (1968): Traitement du décollement de la rétine avec déchirure vraie de la macula par la technique de la "poche sclérale". Ann Ocul, Paris, 201, 290-303.

21. Rosengreen B (1960): Indentation of the sclera by means of a silver ball in the surgical treatment of retinal detachment. Acta Ophthal (Kbh) 38,109-114.

22. Theodossiadis G (1982): Traitement du décollement de la rétine consécutif à un trou maculaire et sans aiilication d'aucune forme d'énergie. J Fr Ophtal 5, 6-7, 427-431.

23. Tittarelli R, Benedetti S, Valazzi CM (1982): Considerazioni sul trattamento chirurgico del distacco di retina da foro maculare, atti del LXII congresso della Società Italiana d'Oftalmologia (Roma, 3-5 dicembre 1982). Ed Pluri-Grafica Sicula, Messina, 187-191.

Basic and advanced vitreous surgery
G.W. Blankenship, M. Stirpe, M. Gonvers, S. Binder (eds.)
Fidia Research Series, vol. II,
Liviana Press, Padova © 1986

COMPLICATIONS OF RETINAL DETACHMENT

John Scott

14 Bowers Croft, Cambridge CB1, 4RP, England

Many retina surgeons refer to two groups of retinal detachment, simple and complicated, distinguishing between the two perhaps by whether they are successful at the first operation! An agreed definition of a complicated case has not been found although by general usage where vitreous pathology becomes clinically obvious the term 'complicated' is often employed. Many authors in discussing the concept of complication of retinal detachment, concentrate on the vitreous with the understanding that some form of proliferation occurs involving retinal pigment epithelium and perhaps macrophages from other sources. Little attention has been paid to the possibility that other intraocular tissues may be affected by the detached retina itself. That other tissues might be affected by the disease itself is of paramount importance in considering the complications of surgery and it is this idea that I should like to suggest to you in this presentation. In the limited time available I should like to concentrate primarily on the lens, for cataract has long been a recognised and common complication of many intraocular diseases.

The close relationship between the retina and lens begins in embryonic life where lens induction is dependent upon the presence of the optic vesicle which later differentiates to form the retina and pigment epithelium; without the optic vesicle no proliferation occurs within the ectoderm to form the lens placode. After formation of the infant lens proliferation of lens epithelium proceeds at an extraordinarily slow rate and indeed does so only to keep up with lens fibre formation. Disturbance of the rate or character of lens epithelium differentiation results in cataract of various kinds familiar to us all. Little is known of the factors which control lens epithelial behaviour, although much has been discovered about the factors controlling lens transparency and it has perhaps been an obsession with the belief that cataract is primarily a disorder of protein metabolism in mature lens fibres that has taken interest away from other aspects of epithelial behaviour which may be much more influential in cataract formation. Little has been written on the relationship between retinal detachment and cataract, a fact emphasised by the statements in Duke-Elder that "Long standing retinal detachment is often followed by cataract of a secondary variety''. That this is only partly true I will hope to show you.

My interest in cataract after retinal detachment was aroused some years ago, by the observation that when lens opacities following retinal reattachment using liquid silicone were operated, by extracapsular methods, the anterior capsule was extremely tough and could only be incised with difficulty. Histology of the anterior capsule showed fibroblastic metaplasia of the anterior epithelium. This was an extraordinary finding, for the idea that an epithelium of ectodermal origin could change into fibroblasts was unknown to pathologists working in other areas of the body. However, there was no doubt that the source of the fibroblasts was in the lens itself and not from extraneous cellular invasion.

Extreme opacification of the posterior capsule after extracapsular extraction led us to develop intracapsular techniques of cataract following treatment of proliferative vitreoretinopathy with liquid silicone, and whole lenses became available for histological study. These lenses were removed from one to several years after successful retinal reattachment surgery and showed characteristic changes. The anterior epithelium was often multilayered, and showed cystic swelling of the cytoplasm. The anterior epithelium extended posteriorly to line the posterior capsule where aberrant lens fibres formed in the shape of balloon cells which rapidly disintergrated. The equatorial bow completely disappeared and new lens fibres therefore failed to form, and in the anterior epithelium ectopic fibre-forming foci were often seen. Sometimes, but, not in all lenses. fibroblastic metaplasia was seen in both anterior and in migrated posterior epithelium.

Many will draw the natural conclusion that the cataract which I have described is a direct result of the use of liquid silicone, and I would have agreed with you until four years ago. At that time I began to look at blind detached eyes untreated with silicone which had suffered retinal detachment some years before and noticed that many eyes were affected by cataract of the kind which we had seen after the use of liquid silicone. Only the eyes which had persistent retinal detachment unaffected by proliferative vitreoretinopathy had clear lenses.

An interesting case was treated some years ago where bilateral giant tears occurred within two weeks of each other. One eye was successfully treated using liquid silicone and the other was considered untreatable. Fifteen months later both lenses became opaque within one month of each other. Thus one eye with silicone and a flat retina and the other untreated with a detached retina developed cataract at the same time.

There are two further aspects of cataract following retinal detachment which are of interest: first, the speed with which the lens becomes opaque which is often very rapid indeed together with the sudden maturation and swelling of the lens; and second, the constant interval between retinal detachment and the development of a mature cataract which in the case of giant tears is around sixteen months. In P.V.R. the interval may be much greater due to the less massive loss of new lens fibres formation in these cases. These various aspects of cataract have led us to use the term ''retinogenic'' and to believe that they are the result of the effect of retinal detachment on lens epithelial proliferation and not the influence of liquid silicone on the theoretical passage of metabolic substrates across the back of the lens.

An obvious comment would be that what I have described is no different to any other so-called secondary cataract, and with regard to the actual occurrence of epithelial migration this is certainly true. However, it is the scale of migration which is so characteristic of retinogenic cataract, together with the development of epithelial metaplasia and the cessation of new lens fibre formation. The latter phenomenon is probably the cause of the acute swelling of the lens where massive loss of control of transparency results from aging of most, if not all, recent metabolically active lens fibres at the same time. Constant replacement of lens fibres is necessary for continuing lens transparency and in retinogenic cataract this does not occur. The possibility that the cataract may be due to chronic uveitis is reduced by the examination of the histology of iris taken at iridectomy during the cataract surgery. In 50 consecutive cases only one specimen showed any evidence of inflammatory cells and this case had been complicated by acute glaucoma secondary to acute lens swelling. The loss of fibre production in retinogenic cataract results from disturbance of the epithelium at the epithelial equatorial bow where epithelial cells migrate and proliferate posteriorly and this effect occurs very early after giant tear formation or the development of proliferative complications of retinal detachment, so that it is unlikely that even if you believe that silicone causes these problems its removal will affect the likelihood of subsequent development of cataract. Once the equatorial bow has dispperead it cannot reform so that cataract is inevitable.

So it would appear that cataract following complicated retinal detachment is yet another example of the massive proliferative response of ocular tissue to severe retinal disease.

There is one other proliferative response which I should like to discuss and that is in the angle of the anterior chamber. Eyes long blind with retinal detachment show a unique change in the angle, and this is creeping peripheral anterior synechia formation. This curious problem begins in the trabecular meshwork and extends centrally producing progressive shallowing of the anterior chamber. Again this may be an example of metaplasia, for the endothelium of the trabeculum and cornea appears to proliferate and develop fibroblastic activity. Concentration resulting in progressive closure of the anterior chamber angle. These cells may originate from the posterior segment, but, clinical evidence makes this unlikely. Trabeculectomy preparations showed only very few macrophages and intracellular silicone adhesions were not seen. Glaucoma does follow successful reattachment of retinas affected by massive vitreoretinal proliferation and in these cases a closed zipped up angle is usually found. It is very likely that proliferative changes in the angle account for these pressure rises, and only unsuccessful cases will enjoy the comfort of a normal or low intraocular pressure, where persistent retinal detachment accounts for high outflow of aqueous.

Finally it will not have escaped your notice that one or two reports have crept into the popular literature where eyes long blind from unsuccessful silicone surgery for complicated retinal detachment have been described at length and the pathology of these long blind eyes have been attributed to the use of liquid silicone. I would ask you to consider the possibility that perhaps an eye blind for years with retinal detachment might show pathology due to reasons other than the use of liquid silicone among which will be widespread proliferative disease resulting from the effects of the retinal detachment itself. We might broaden the definition of complicated retinal detachment to include complications involving tissues other than the retina itself: in the lens, the cornea and in the trabecular endothelium, and probably in the other ocular tissues as well, so that consideration of the possible complications of the disease must be compared with the direct effects of the operation itself.

Basic and advanced vitreous surgery
G.W. Blankenship, M. Stirpe, M. Gonvers, S. Binder (eds.)
Fidia Research Series, vol. II,
Liviana Press, Padova © 1986

PROLIFERATIVE VITREORETINOPATHY AND SURGICAL APPROACH

M. Gonvers, M.D.

Hôpital Ophtalmologique, Lausanne

In 1979 a new technique for the treatment of detachment with advanced proliferative vitreoretinopathy (PVR) was developed (1). An extensive preretinal peeling, a six weeks tamponade with silicone oil and a panphotocoagulation were the three major characteristics of the original technique which was used from 1979 to mid-1983. The surgical procedure was done in four steps:

1. During a first operation a pars plana vitrectomy was performed, completed by preretinal peeling. A high encircling buckle was placed around the eye and the operation ended with a partial gas-fluid exchange. The patient was then positioned on his face for one night.

2. The day following, when the retina was totally reattached, the vitreous cavity was totally filled with silicone oil, the patient being placed on his right or left side with the help of a rotating operating table. The operation was completed by heavy xenon coagulations placed on the buckle.

3. Panretinal laser photocoagulation was done a few days later.

4. Six weeks later silicone oil was removed.

The advantages of the technique were as follows:
— first of all, the success rate was fairly good, around 65%;
— in spite of the multiple operations, the technique was not traumatising for the eye as each operation was of short duration;
— the operative danger was reduced to a minima.

However, the disadvantages were also numerous:
— the technique was time-consuming for the surgeon as well as for the patient;
— the first two major operations, usually done under general anesthesia, were performed in less than a 48 hour interval;
— a rotating operating table was necessary for the injection of silicone;

— after the first operation the patient had to be put on his face for 12 hours;

— the visibility of the fundus when performing the second operation was not always very good, because fibrin and blood could accumulate on the posterior side of the lens or on the corneal endothelium after the prone positioning, and photocoagulation was not always possible after the injection of silicone oil.

In mid 1983 the technique was simplified and reduced to one major operation and one minor operation, the principle of the technique being the same.

The major operation done under general anesthesia starts with a vitrectomy and peeling procedure. The Sutherland intraocular forceps are used as the choice instrument for membrane peeling. Then a high encircling buckle is put around the eye and internal drainage is performed. Subretinal fluid is aspirated through any preexisting posterior retinal hole, but in most cases an iatrogenic hole has to be made in the posterior retina with the help of a newly designed instrument which is called a retinal perforator (2). This instrument, when introduced into the eye, can aspirate at the outer part of its tip, a small area of retina which is immobilized and stretched before it is punched out by a needle. The needle is pushed forward by a spring located in the handle of the instrument, and set off when a trigger is activated. Then a total fluid-silicone exchange is started. Subretinal fluid is first aspirated through the needle of the retinal perforator while silicone is injected. Fluid-silicone exchange is finished with a tapered needle, the retinal perforator just providing illumination. When the vitreous cavity is filled with silicone oil and the retina totally attached, extensive xenon photocoagulation is performed.

The minor operation consists in removing the silicone: it is done six weeks later, under local anesthesia. This operation is very easy since the sclerotomy is reopened, and silicone oil expelled from the eye by an infusion of Ringer's solution.

The advantages of the new technique over the old one are evident:

— the surgical problems are solved practically in one operation;

— the technique is less time-consuming for the surgeon and the patient;

— only one general anesthesia is necessary;

— the whole operation is done under excellent conditions of visibility, the media remaining crystal clear from the beginning to the end of the operation;

— there is no need of a rotating operating table;

— the patient does not have to be placed in a prone position as in the case when a gas tamponade is used;

— the technique can also be used in aphakic cases.

This technique, however, is not without its disadvantages:

— the major surgical procedure is difficult, more dangerous, and usually lasts more than three hours;

— the internal drainage can sometimes be complicated by retinal bleeding;

— the filling of silicone oil is not as total as it was with the old technique, as the vitreous base, which cannot be totally removed during the vitrectomy, does not have time to collapse and dehydrate. Consequently, the inferior meniscus of water which is always present under the bubble of silicone oil, is larger than in the first technique, and inferior tamponade not as good. For this reason a higher inferior buckle is necessary.

In conclusion this simplified technique, which has conserved the major principles of the original technique and given the same success rate, saves a lot of time for both surgeon and patient, with a minimum of increase in surgical risks.

REFERENCES

1. Gonvers M (1982): Temporary use of intraocular silicone oil in the treatment of detachment with massive periretinal proliferation. Preliminary report. Ophthalmologica (Basel) 184:210-218.
2. Gonvers M (1984): Retinal perforator for internal drainage. Amer J Ophth 97:786-797.

Basic and advanced vitreous surgery
G.W. Blankenship, M. Stirpe, M. Gonvers, S. Binder (eds.)
Fidia Research Series, vol. II,
Liviana Press, Padova © 1986

VALIDITY OF SCLERAL SURGERY FOR THE TREATMENT OF VITREO-RETINAL TRACTIONS AND PROLIFERATIONS

Mario R. Pannarale

Clinica Oculistica I, Università 'La Sapienza' Roma

Scleral indentation techniques can be used not only to close retinal breaks but also to reduce vitreo-retinal tractions and retractions. To a certain extent proper applications of scleral indentations can sometimes avoid or at least restrict the use of vitreous surgery.

However, vitreous surgery is mandatory when relevant vitreo-retinal tractions or retractions are present: it can be used, when retinal detachment is present, before or simultaneously with scleral surgery.

Scleral indentation techniques can reduce circumscribed tractions or retractions or extensive tractions. Size and height of scleral indentations should be selected in accordance with tractions or areas of vitreo-retinal retractions.

Scleral undermining is necessary, if the sclera is thick to reduce tractions or vitreo-retinal retractions. Therefore lamellar scleral resections of variable shape (trap-door, pouch, tunnel, etc.) should be performed.

The size of these resections will be selected in accordance with the extension of vitreo-retinal tractions and retractions. The height of scleral indentation will be adequate to the extension of the traction using a material, such as silicon rubbe, that can mould to the shape of indentation.

In other words, scleral buckles will be made to reduce circumscribed traction or retraction by means of moulded silicon rubber, cut off from a block of "soft" Dow Corning Co. Silastic (Fig. 1), and, if necessary, by scleral undermining.

Scleral sutures placed on buckles should exert as much indentation as required. Therefore scleral sutures, in case of intrascleral buckle made by trap-door, pouch or tunnel scleral resection, should be placed on the external scleral flaps, as shown in Fig. 2, and the more the sutures are tightened the more the implant is pushed towards the center of the globe. When an episcleral buckle has to be used upon thin or already altered sclera, sutures should be sufficiently closed and inserted into resistant sclera to obtain an adequate indentation. In these cases, when silicon sponge is preferred, sutures should be very close indeed so as to avoid exterior herniation of the sponge (Fig. 3).

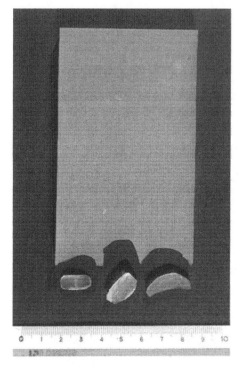

Figure 1. Moulded silicon rubber, cut from a block of "soft" Dow Corning Co. Silastic.

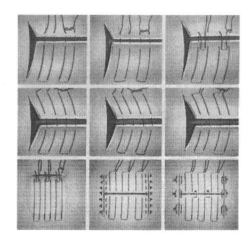

Figure 2. In case of an intrascleral buckel, scleral sutures should be placed in the external scleral flaps, and the more the sutures are tightened the more the implant is pushed towards the center of the globe.

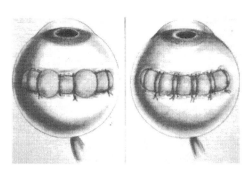

Figure 3. In case of an episcleral buckle, especially when silicon sponge is prefered, sutures should be very close so as to avoid exterior herniation of the buckle.

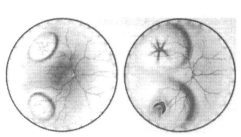

Figure 4. See text.

Numerous and various cases of vitreo-retinal tractions and retractions could be met in vitreo-retinal surgery.

Some examples of simple clinical features will now be discussed for better understanding.

A case of retinal detachment is shown in the drawing of Fig. 4, with a superior-temporal break and a star-shaped fold in the inferior temporal quadrant. In this case, besides break buckle, a sclero-choroidal buckle of the star-shaped fold will be necessary, together with cryotreatments at its level, so as to fix retina to choroid.

A case of retinal detachment (Fig. 5) with an inferior temporal break and vitreo-retinal traction in the temporal quadrants: even in this case, besides break buckle, a scleral indentation of the vitreo-retinal traction will be performed together with cryo-treatment.

In tractional retinal detachment, which is a frequent complication of proliferative diabetic retinopathy, scleral indentation of major tractional or retractional areas will be useful even after vitrectomy, to favour also vitreo-retinal adhesion by the means of cryo. In the drawing of Fig. 6 tractional areas from vitreo-retinal proliferation are shown; scleral indentation will be made at their level (both full thickness and with undermining) together with cryoapplications and subretinal fluid drainage.

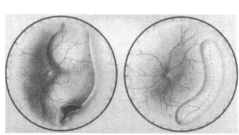

Figure 5. See text.

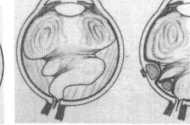

Figure 6. See text.

The treatment of extensive vitreo-retinal tractions will be the same as for the circumscribed ones. Scleral indentations will be large according to the larger extension of tractions and retractions, by means of larger buckles, or fully circular (circling bands).

Actually the application of proper scleral indentations to tractions and retractions can solve those cases which on preoperative examination exibit a definite indication for vitrectomy techniques.

Vitrectomy could be planned sometimes after scleral surgery and internal tamponage have been performed.

A preoperative drawing or map should be prepared with indication of vitreo-retinal tractions and areas of vitreo-retinal retractions. These could be identified as lying along a globe circumference, or irregularly placed at various levels. In the first case a circling indentation (band) would simultaneously reduce all tractions whereas in the second the circling band would reduce as many tractions as possible, and other apposite buckles would reduce tractions elsewhere.

A circling band should be placed along the globe equator or anteriorly or posteriorly. It could be parallel to the equator or oblique (Fig. 7). It is not infrequent in retinal detachment surgery to have to cope with more or less circumferential pre-equatorial tractions, even with involvement of pars ciliaris retinae. These tractions usually correspond to the vitreous base and seldom could be removed by vitrectomy because it would have to be performed in the far periphery, with serious danger to the peripheral retina and zonule structures. In these cases with extensive pre equatorial tractions, a circling element anterior to the equator would be sufficient, and if that is the case, by internal tamponage with air or gas that could detach anterior vitreous bands from retina.

Similar surgical criteria would be employed in some cases of traumatic retinal detachment following globe perforations, with proliferation at the vitreous base and traction on peripheral retina.

Moreover a post-equatorial circling element can damage vortex veins. The compression of their venous trunk or their "caput medusae" can cause choroidal detachment or ocular hypertension, especially when two veins are involved. Choroidal detachment could occur at the time of surgery, altering the validity of scleral indentations, or in the postoperative period. Ocular hypertension can cause central artery occlusion with irreparable functional loss.

To avoid the critical points of vortex veins it will be useful to avoid their compression moving circling bands anteriorly or posteriorly, or cutting appropriate "holes" inside the buckles to make room for the vein.

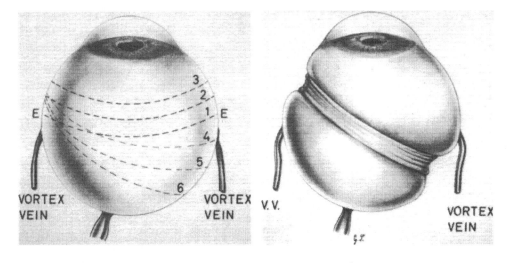

Figure 7. A circling band should be placed along the globe equator or anteriorly or posteriourly, and parallel to the equator or oblique.

Figure 8. When an oblique circling band has to be used, it should run posterior to emergence of one or more vortex veins, to avoid the compression of their venous trunk or their "caput meduse".

When an oblique circling band has to be used, it should run posterior to one or more vortex veins (Fig. 8): but no more than two, to safeguard posterior choroidal reflux. Very oblique circling bands could be employed when a regular series of peripheral tractions (in one or two quadrants) and posterior tractions (in the other one or two) could be connected by a regular circumferencial indentation line.

Oblique circling bands could be even selected to raise a posterior buckle, beside anterior ones, to reduce a major traction (Fig. 9).

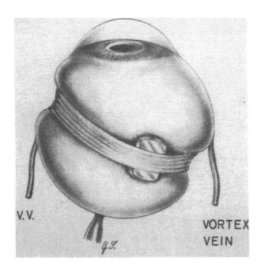

V.V.

VORTEX
VEIN

Figure 9. See text.

Before vitrectomy gained universal acceptance, and precisely between 1960 and 1970, I often used these surgical techniques of scleral indentation to reduce vitreo-retinal tractions in the management of tractional retinal detachment of proliferative diabetic retinopathy. In fact when posterior tractions or retractions were present I used scleral indentations with buckles associated with an oblique circling band (Fig. 6). Even today I sometimes use this technique, together with vitrectomy.

Width and height of circling elements used in the reduction of vitreo-retinal tractions and retractions should be chosen with regard to them, giving priority to materials appropriate for width and elasticity.

Vitreo-retinal tractions, with circumferential and narrow band extension, could be also reduced by circular bands with very narrow indentation surface (such as encircling threads). But their narrow indentations will seldom be sufficient and therefore silicon rubber circling bands should be preferred. These ones, selected with various widths, can produce a progressive indentation effect due to their elasticity.

To increase indentation surface the surgeon could use the well known additional silicon implants articulated with silastic band as proposed by the Boston School.

Scleral surgery according to the above mentioned criteria works in the reduction of mild tractions and retractions. In other cases vitreous surgey is needed with its various techniques such as vitrectomy, and other internal tamponade techniques.

Basic and advanced vitreous surgery
G.W. Blankenship, M. Stirpe, M. Gonvers, S. Binder (eds.)
Fidia Research Series, vol. II,
Liviana Press, Padova © 1986

SUBRETINAL PROLIFERATION

Mario Stirpe

Fondazione Oftalmologica 'G.B. Bietti', Piazza Sassari, 5, Roma

Complications connected with retinal detachment either before or, more frequently, after surgery, have been variously defined according to the way in which different authors have interpreted the pathological process (MVR, MPR, MPP). In order to arrive at a uniform terminology, this condition has finally been called RD with PVR. The definition MPP, however, which is in keeping with histological findings, still remains the most synthethic and complete definition of this pathology.

Until it became possible to treat preretinal proliferations, little attention was paid to subretinal ones. Both are part of the same pathological pattern, although either may occur as the sole objective manifestation. Subretinal proliferation may assume a variety of morphologic aspects: strands, single or multiple, sometimes of dendritic structure or as concentric rings around the optic nerve, inverted stellar folds, and/or plaques, sometimes extensive (Fig. 1). A condition necessary for the development of subretinal membranes is retinal detachment, and since their development is a slower process than that of preretinal membranes, the retina must remain detached for a certain length of time. While in fact early surgery for retinal detachment does not appear to influence the development of preretinal proliferation, it certainly does influence the possibility of subretinal proliferation.

From the histological point of view, subretinal membranes, like preretinal ones, originate from glial elements and pigmented cells, but their possibility for extension is much more limited because of the lack of a framework like the vitreous. Any congestion of the uveal membrane during surgery which is accompanied by an increase in cellular elements and fibrin in the subretinal space may bring about the extension of preexisting subretinal membranes. If a gap in the overlying retina opens a line of communication between the subretinal proliferation and the vitreous chamber, proliferation may extend towards the interior, thus giving rise to a pattern that can be called "shirt-button" proliferation (Fig. 2).

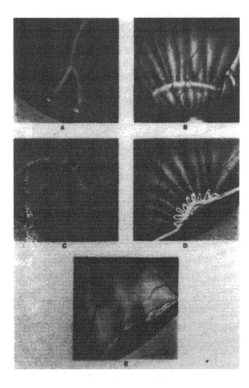

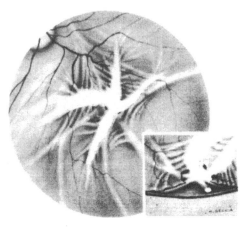

Figure 2. "Shirt-button" proliferation

Figure 1. Subretinal proliferations:
a) strands
b) dendritic form
c) concentric ring around the optic disc
d) inverted stellar fold
e) plaque form

Subretinal membranes in the shape of strands are more frequently found in young subjects. In a study of children under 8 years old, these were present in 21 out of 93 eyes, and in practically every case of retinal detachment of more than 3 months' standing. However, in only three cases did the presence of these membranes interfere with the success of a normal operation for retinal detachment. Among these 93 cases, a more complete pattern of MPP was found in only three cases; two, of traumatic origin, had plaques of subretinal proliferation.

The fact that children have less tendency to develop preretinal rather than subretinal membranes is probably accounted for by the persistent adherence of the vitreous to the retina even after retinal detachment.

SURGERY

In a paper published in AJO in 1980, R. Machemer described for the first time the surgical technique for the resection of strand-shaped subretinal membranes which were responsible for the lifting of the retina. This is the most frequent type, and surgery yields good results. Strand-shaped subretinal membranes are often not connected with the retina, even if they require surgery, but stretch from one meridian to the other, thus lifting the retina just as a sheet is suspended from a clothes-line. Once resected, these membranes retract, and the retina can again settle down (Fig. 3). The surgical technique is fairly simple: after the vitreous has been removed, a small opening is created

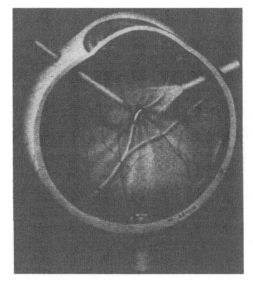 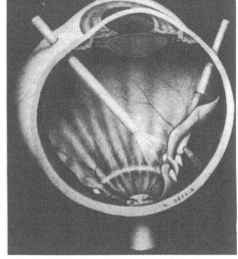

Figure 3. Resection of cord-like (in strands) subretinal membranes.

Figure 4. Resection of ring-like subretinal proliferation.

in the peripheral retina through which a pair of bent scissors with short blades is introduced (MPC scissors are the ideal instrument); these are used to hook and resect the membranes. The optic fibers in front of the retina provide satisfactory illumination during the cutting (Fig. 4). After this operation is completed, slight pressure should be applied to the retina in order to make sure that there is no further obstacle to its settling down. Short membrane segments may sometimes be connected to the overlying retina. The points of attachment can easily be identified because they are marked by pigment at the level of the corresponding retinal surface.

Inverted star folds can be treated by a scleral buckle if they are distant from the center. On the contrary, extensive plaque-shaped proliferations can be removed only by wide openings in the peripheral retina (Fig. 5). In the case of extensive plaque-shaped proliferation, it is important to consider, before surgery, the possibility of functional recovery, since this type of proliferation is likely to deprive the overlying retina of any possibility of nutritional exchange. In two very young subjects with retinal detachment and in whom vitrectomy could be avoided, we were able to demonstrate that short and repeated transcleral freezing at any one point led to the breaking of subretinal proliferative strands (Fig. 6). Freezing through the vitreous chamber at a point of the retina corresponding to the subretinal membrane brought about retinal contraction where the freezing had been applied (Fig. 7). A later operation showed that the damage caused to the retina by freezing had contributed to the extension of subretinal proliferation towards the interior (Fig. 8).

In the absence of vitreous detachment, the possibilities for epiretinal proliferation are likely to be limited. In order to avoid surgical approach through the vitreous chamber, we have recently used YAG laser in cooperation with B. Lumbroso for the cutting of subretinal proliferative strands. Results have been satisfactory and have shown that this

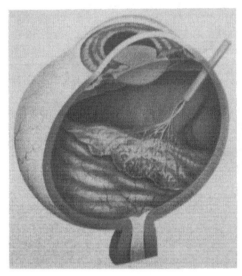

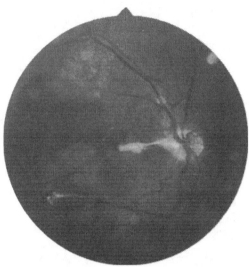

Figure 5. Removal of extensive subretinal pro-liferation (dendritic form or plaque form).

Figure 6. Breaking of a subretinal strand by means of transcleral cryopexy.

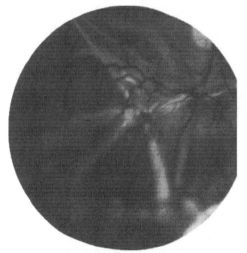

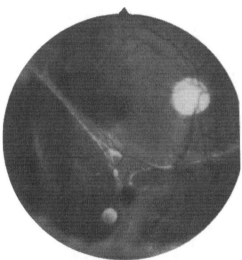

Figure 7. Epiretinal proliferation after internal freezing of retinal strands ("shirt-button" extension).

Figure 8. Distension of the retina after removing epiretinal proliferation and cutting subretinal strands.

instrument can also be used in retinal surgery. Once strand-shaped membranes have been resected, the retina settles down and the retinal holes opened by YAG laser can be closed by laser photocoagulation.

At present, we are studying the action of YAG laser on eyes with silicone oil. If silicone oil does not become emulsified during YAG laser application, YAG laser could be used for the resection of subretinal membranes found after vitrectomy while silicone oil used as an internal tamponade is still inside.

Basic and advanced vitreous surgery
G.W. Blankenship, M. Stirpe, M. Gonvers, S. Binder (eds.)
Fidia Research Series, vol. II,
Liviana Press, Padova © 1986

THE USE OF SILICONE OIL FOLLOWING FAILED VITRECTOMY FOR RETINAL DETACHMENT WITH ADVANCED PROLIFERATIVE VITREORETINOPATHY

Brooks W. McCuen II, Maurice B. Landers III, Robert Machemer

Duke University Eye Center, Box 3802, Durham, North Carolina

Recent reports suggest that sophisticated vitreous surgical methods allow increasing success in reattaching retinas with advanced proliferative vitreoretinopathy. By utilizing such techniques as broad scleral buckling, intra and postoperative fluid-gas exchange, and endolaser photocoagulation some surgeons now claim over 75% success in these cases. Nevertheless, a significant number of eyes still fail despite these measures (1,2). Encouraged by the work of Scott, Gonvers, Zivojnovic and others, we at Duke University have approached these failures over the past 3 years by reoperation with silicone oil (3-5). This report briefly reviews our techniques, results, and complications in these difficult cases.

SURGICAL TECHNIQUE

Eyes with recurrent retinal detachment after vitrectomy for PVR are reoperated with repeat vitrectomy and membrane peeling. Particular attention is paid to the removal of vitreous and epiretinal membranes anteriorly. If adequate release of anterior traction cannot be achieved, or if dense subretinal proliferation is present then the retina is diathermized and a relaxing retinotomy is performed with the vitreous cutter or microscissors.

Scleral buckle revision, if judged necessary, is then performed followed by fluid-gas exchange with internal drainage of subretinal fluid. A posterior drainage retinotomy is created if necessary to allow complete retinal reattachement. A gas-silicone oil exchange is then performed by injection of silicone oil through the infusion cannula while venting gas anteriorly. Transvitreal cryopexy to the retinotomy sites is achieved through the silicone oil. In many cases either complete or peripheral panretinal endo-argon photocoagulation was administered also through the oil, while in other cases postoperative slit-lamp photocoagulation was employed.

RESULTS

Between August 1981 and March 1984 we employed silicone oil injection in 44 eyes all of which had previously failed vitrectomy and membrane peeling for retinal detachment with proliferative vitreoretinopathy. Excluded from this series were retinal detachments associated with giant retinal tears, penetrating ocular trauma, and proliferative diabetic retinopathy. All eyes had a minimal follow-up of 6 months and no eye was lost to follow-up. 86% of eyes had proliferative vitreoretinopathy in the "D" category of the grading system proposed by the Retina Society (6) (Table 1).

Table 1 . *Results of silicone oil injection after failed vitrectomy for retinal detachment with advanced proliferative vitreoretinopathy*

PVR GRADE	EYES (%)	EYES ANATOMICALLY REATTACHED (%)	EYES REATTACHED WITH VA $\geqslant$ 5/200 (%)
C1	0 (0)	0 (0)	0 (0)
C2	4 (9)	4 (100)	3 (75)
C3	3 (7)	2 (67)	2 (67)
D1	14 (32)	10 (71)	5 (36)
D2	16 (36)	8 (50)	3 (19)
D3	7 (16)	4 (57)	3 (43)
	44 (100)	28 (64)	16 (36)

An average of 3.31 previous vitreoretinal procedures had been performed on these eyes before reoperation with silicone oil, and 30% of the patients had no useful vision in their fellow eye.

An eye was considered an anatomic success only if the retina was 100% reattached posterior to the encircling buckle with 6 months follow-up. Utilizing this criterion we were able to achieve anatomic success in 64% of operated eyes. We found that there was a statistically significant correlation with improved success rate in those eyes that received either intraoperative or postoperative peripheral scatter laser photocoagulation and in those eyes in which there was a broad scleral buckle present at the end of the procedure. We found that in those cases where retinal reattachment was achieved, 57% of the eyes had a visual acuity of 5/200 or better.

Despite these encouraging results, complications associated with silicone oil injection were both frequent and severe. Recurrent retinal detachment posterior to the encircling buckle occurred at some point in the postoperative course in 52% of these eyes. Repeated vitrectomy procedures after silicone oil injection were performed in 10 cases with ultimate retinal reattachment achieved in 7 of the 10. Ultimately, however, 36% of the eyes in this series had some subretinal fluid present posterior to the buckle at the end of follow-up.

Corneal decompensation was also a major problem occurring in 34% of the eyes in this series. In 4 eyes with successfully reattached retinas, penetrating keratoplasty has re-established ambulatory visual function.

In our series visual loss due to postoperative glaucoma was unusual. Much more common was the occurrence of postoperative hypotony, although this did not appear to affect the final visual outcome.

In an effort to minimize the postoperative complications due to silicone oil, it is our goal to remove the oil after sustained retinal reattachment has been achieved for 3-6 months. We have removed the silicone in 69% of the eyes in this series that were both anatomic and visual successes. No eye in our series in which the silicone oil has been removed has redetached so far.

CONCLUSIONS

We feel that retinal detachement complicated by advanced proliferative vitreoretinopathy is better treated by conventional vitreous surgical techniques rather than by primary silicone oil injection. When sophisticated vitrectomy and membrane peeling techniques, including broad scleral buckling, peripheral intra- or postoperative scatter laser photocoagulation, and postoperative augmentation fluid-gas exchange have failed to achieve sustained retinal reattachment, however, our results suggest that reoperation with silicone oil injection may allow successful anatomic and visual results in a significant percentage of these otherwise very poor prognosis cases.

It is to be emphasized that when the physician and the patient embark on a course involving silicone oil injection that both must be prepared for multiple further surgical interventions with the eventual goals of complete anatomic reattachment and the ultimate removal of the oil kept clearly in mind.

ACKNOWLEDGMENTS

This study was supported by National Eye Institute Grant EY 02903 and the Helena Rubinstein Foundation.

REFERENCES

1. Sternberg P Jr, Machemer R: Results of conventional vitreous surgery for proliferative vitreoretinopathy. Am J Ophthalmol. Accepted for publication.
2. Jalkh AE, Avila MP, Schepens CL, et al (1984): Surgical treatments of proliferative vitreoretinopathy. Arch Ophthalmol; 102:1135-39.
3. Scott JD (1975): The treatment of massive vitreous retraction by the separation of preretinal membranes using liquid silicone. Mod Probl Ophthalmol; 15:285-90.

232

4. Zivojnovic R, Mertens DAE, Peperkamp E (1982): Das flussige silikon in der amotiochirurgie (II) Bericht uber 280 falleweiter entwicklung der technik. Klin Mbl Augenheilk; 181:444-52.
5. Gonvers M (1982): Temporary use of silicone oil in the treatment of detachment with massive periretinal proliferation. Ophthalmologica; 184:210-18.
6. The Retina Society Terminology Committee. The classification of retinal detachment with proliferative vitreoretinopathy. Ophthalmology; 90:121-5.

Basic and advanced vitreous surgery
G.W. Blankenship, M. Stirpe, M. Gonvers, S. Binder (eds.)
Fidia Research Series, vol. II,
Liviana Press, Padova © 1986

BEHAVIOUR OF RETINAL PROLIFERATION AFTER SILICONE OIL INJECTION

Mario Stirpe

Fondazione Oftalmologica 'G.B. Bietti', Piazza Sassari, 5, Roma

Silicone oil is injected into the vitreous chamber at the end of surgery for retinal detachment with PVR if the condition is severe enough to convince the surgeon that success is not sufficiently guaranteed. The purpose of the injection of silicone oil into the vitreous chamber is to maintain a tamponade for a prolonged period of time. As a matter of fact, silicone oil cannot inhibit the proliferative process but it is apt to condition its progress in some way.

CLINICAL OBSERVATIONS AND METHODS

In order to avoid immediate removal of actively proliferating fibroblasts in case of very recent proliferation occurring after retinal detachment, we have used the following method.

The membranes are carefully detached from the back, and silicone oil is injected underneath. After this procedure, the proliferative process appears to continue only at the level of the pre-equatorial and equatorial areas along the plane created by the still undeveloped membranes on the anterior portion of the silicone oil meniscus. The areas at the back of the oil bubble and peripherally where a portion of vitreous of almost normal appearance remains are spared. When the membranes and silicone oil are subsequently removed, a greater success seems possible (Figs. 1,2,3,4). The contraction of the pre-equatorial membranes may cause peripheral tears or dialyses of the retina in rare cases (Fig. 5). There is no risk of silicone oil infiltrating beneath the retina. This is due to the presence of cicatricial barrage at the level of the encircling buckle, and because the roof formed by the membranes contains the oil posteriorly. Tears are, at any rate, closed before removing the silicone oil.

The most common procedure is to introduce silicone oil into the vitreous chamber

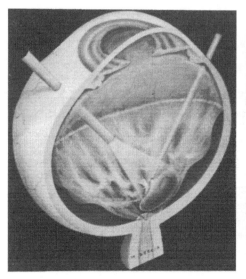

Figure 1. The membranes are elevated from the posterior retina and silicone oil is injected underneath.

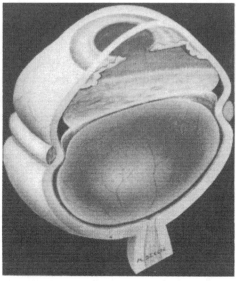

Figure 2. Proliferation continues on the anterior portion of the silicone oil meniscus.

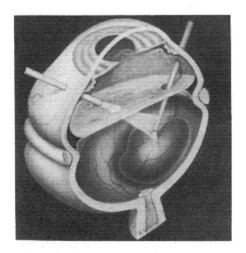

Figure 3. Removal of silicone oil by cannula through the plane of the membranes.

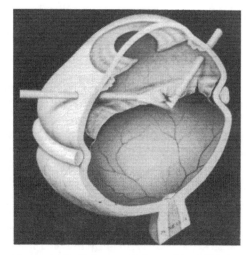

Figure 4. Radial cuts of the residual fibrous ring after removing the plane of the membranes.

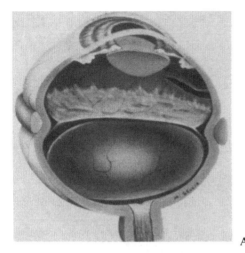

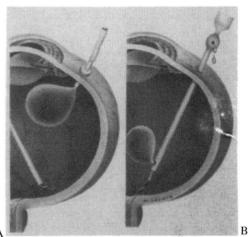

A

B

Figure 5. Dialysis of the retina due to a contraction of pre-equatorial membranes.

Figure 6. Fluid/silicone oil exchange: (a) silicone oil is introduced through the infusion cannula; (b) silicone oil is introduced by means of a special two-way needle connected to a pneumatic syringe.

after having removed vitreous and membranes. This can be done by directly exchanging the fluid with silicone oil (Fig. 6), or by first exchanging the fluid with air, and immediately afterwards, air with silicone oil (Figs. 7a,7b). In these cases, the vitreous chamber can be filled completely or partly with silicone oil. If the vitreous chamber is filled only partially and proliferative activity is still present, membrane formation is mostly observed in the pre-equatorial, equatorial and post-equatorial areas of the lower quadrants.

If the vitreous chamber is filled completely with silicone oil, recurrent proliferation in the lower quadrants appears to be more limited. However, there is the possibility of a more serious complication related to peripheral proliferation. In 7 eyes treated with silicone oil injection, we found that between 30 days and 2 months afterwards, pigmented elements appeared in subconjunctival tissue at the pars plana level around the points where vitrectomy instruments had been introduced during surgery. The pigmented areas tended to spread during the subsequent weeks. In 3 of these cases, we removed the silicone oil. Up to that time, the retina had been perfectly adherent, but within a week of extracting the silicone oil, severe retinal proliferation had developed in all three cases; the uselessness of further intervention was obvious. In the remaining 4 cases, the oil was not removed, and after a period of 5 to 8 months, the pigmented area became attenuated and even completely disappeared. When the silicone oil was finally removed, the retina stayed adherent. However, all these eyes were markedly hypotonic, and one of them developed a progressive condition of subatrophy.

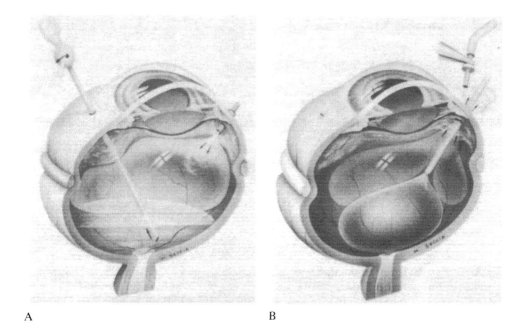

A   B

Figure 7. (a) Fluid/air and (b) air/silicone oil exchange.

We removed the subconjunctival tissue containing the pigmented elements. The histological slides were examined by Machemer, who found a large number of macrophages. The origin of these (from pigmented epithelium or from ciliary body) is still uncertain.

COMMENT

The presence of silicone oil in the vitreous chamber does not prevent membrane proliferation. However, this proliferation occurs more readily in spaces left free of silicone oil, particularly if vitreous residues are present. If we look at the surface of the silicone oil introduced into the vitreous chamber after severe MPP, we see in some cases numerous pigmented elements on the oil meniscus. This may mean that if proliferation continues, many cellular elements distribute themselves over the silicone oil meniscus just as they spread over the external surface of the vitreous. Since silicone oil is not a biological medium, they cannot develop. If the membranes are removed by the previously described method, and silicone oil is injected underneath, proliferation continues at the pre-equatorial and equatorial level along the framework to which the membranes previously adhered, which has been shifted but not removed (Fig. 8). The most peripheral portion of the retina is usually not involved in the proliferative process. The posterior portion may be involved in the circumscribed proliferation. If after vitrectomy the silicone oil does not fill the vitreous chamber completely, proliferation occurs mainly in the lower portions of the retina, exactly as is the case when vitrectomy is not followed by silicone oil injection (Fig. 9).

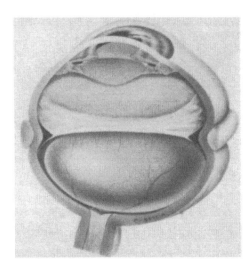

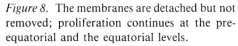

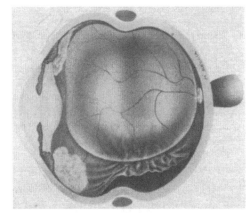

Figure 8. The membranes are detached but not removed; proliferation continues at the pre-equatorial and the equatorial levels.

Figure 9. The membranes are completely removed and silicone oil partially fills the vitreous chamber; proliferation can continue on the inferior quadrants of the retina.

There appear to be three reasons for this:
1) Silicone oil floats upwards, thus leaving the lower surface of the retina free.
2) Cellular elements are likely to deposit at the bottom, probably due to gravity.
3) These are the areas where after massive proliferation it is more difficult to remove all residues of vitreal cortex.

If the vitreous chamber is completely filled with silicone oil, many cellular elements appear to migrate towards the region of the ora serrata where the residual vitreous tissue offers a more favorable medium. It is certainly here that membrane proliferation occurs which then extends towards the posterior surface of the lens (Fig. 10). One of the most serious detrimental effects of this type of proliferation probably occurs at the level of the ciliary body and becomes manifest through the marked decrease of aqueous humor production.

At first, we believed this to be the consequence of a toxic condition of the ciliary body caused by the presence of silicone oil. Proof to the contrary came from the finding that this complication never occurred when silicone oil was used for reasons other than massive proliferation (giant tears with retinal eversion, choroid angiomata with secondary RD, recurrent hemorrhage after vitrectomy, etc.).

238

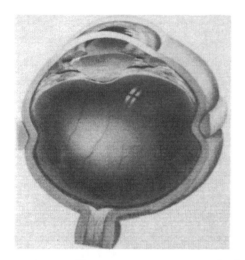

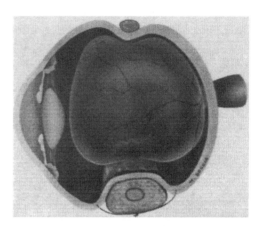

Figure 10. The membranes are completely removed and the silicone oil completely fills the vitreous chamber; proliferation can occur at the peripheral level.

Figure 11. Membranes which recur posteriorly can be removed even with the presence of silicone oil.

Silicone oil may influence the development of membranes in one site rather than another, depending on the amount and the way in which it has been introduced into the vitreous chamber. In keeping with these clinical findings, in the presence of RD with PVR, we prefer to fill the vitreous chamber only partly with silicone oil and to condition the patient to an adequate positioning.

All recurrent membranes may still be removed even with the presence of silicone oil (Fig. 11) except those developing at the extreme periphery of the retina.

Basic and advanced vitreous surgery
G.W. Blankenship, M. Stirpe, M. Gonvers, S. Binder (eds.)
Fidia Research Series, vol. II,
Liviana Press, Padova © 1986

SURGICAL TREATMENT OF MACULAR PUCKER

Ronald G. Michels

The Vitreoretinal Service, Department of Ophthalmology,
Johns Hopkins University School of Medicine, Baltimore, Maryland.

Nonvascularized cellular membranes growing on the inner retinal surface (epiretinal membranes, ERM's) occur in a number of clinical conditions including: 1) idiopathic membranes in patients of all ages, but especially during the latter decades of life, 2) following otherwise-successful retinal reattachment surgery, and 3) as a secondary change associated with blunt or penetrating ocular injuries, intraocular inflammation, vitreous hemorrhage, non-proliferative retinal vascular disorders and following ocular surgery. These epiretinal membranes may cause differing amounts of visual loss due to the abnormal tissue covering and/or distorting the macular area (macular pucker) and sometimes causing vascular leakage and intraretinal edema.

SURGICAL TECHNIQUE

Pars plana vitrectomy methods can be used to remove these abnormal membranes. The surgery is performed using divided-system vitrectomy instrumentation with an infusion cannula, a fiberoptic light probe and a vitrectomy instrument introduced through separate pars plana incisions. Usually a posterior vitreous detachment is present, and the posterior two-thirds of the vitreous gel is excised. All significant intravitreal opacities are removed, and the posterior vitreous surface is separated from the underlying retina and excised if a pre-existing posterior vitreous detachment is not present. Care is taken to avoid damage to the lens or trauma to chorioretinal tissue elevated on a previous scleral buckle if the macular pucker occurred after previous retinal surgery.

The epiretinal membrane covering or distorting the macula is engaged with a hooked needle or special vitreoretinal pick, and it is gently separated from the inner retinal surface (Fig. 1). Care is taken to avoid excessive traction on the retina, and various manipulations are made to aid in separating this tissue. These manipulations include: 1) side-to-side movement with the vitreoretinal pick to break delicate adhesions between the membrane and the underlying retina, 2) use of special intraocular forceps to grasp the partially separated membrane and 3) use of the vitrectomy instrument or intraocular scissors to divide the membrane at points of firm attachment to the retina.

The membrane can sometimes be separated effectively using only a vitreoretinal pick. However, use of forceps to assist in grasping the membrane after a portion has been separated minimizes fragmentation of the abnormal tissue. It is often necessary to engage the membrane sequentially from various directions. The abnormal tissue is removed from the eye using the cutting-aspiration port of the vitrectomy instrument or with special intraocular forceps.

We have used these techniques to remove epiretinal membranes affecting the macula in various clinical conditions including: 1) following otherwise-successful retinal re-

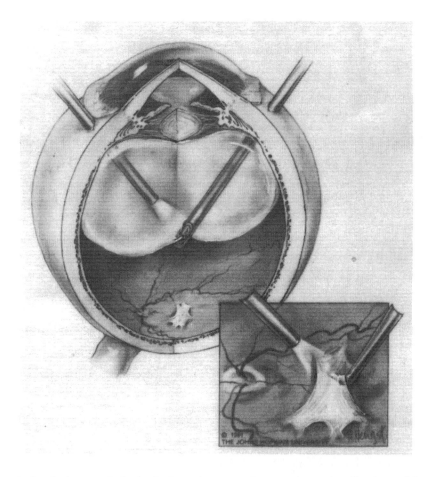

Figure 1. Surgical removal of epiretinal membrane causing macular pucker. Portions of detached posterior vitreous gel are excised first. The epiretinal membrane is then dissected from the inner retinal surface with a vitreoretinal pick (inset).

attachment surgery (Fig. 2), 2) membranes occurring after blunt ocular injuries, 3) following photocoagulation of peripheral retinal lesions (Fig. 3), 4) after longstanding vitreous hemorrhage, 5) after intraocular inflammation (Figs. 4, 5), and 6) idiopathic membranes in young patients (Fig. 6) and elderly patients (Fig. 7).

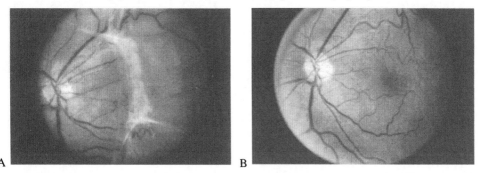

A   B

Figure 2. *A*, Preoperative appearence of prominent macular pucker after retinal reattachment surgery. *B*, Appearance after removal of abnormal epiretinal tissue.

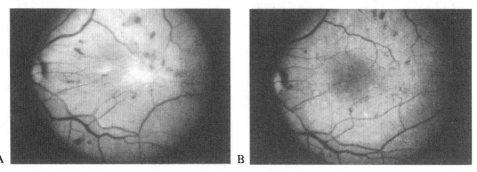

A   B

Figure 3. *A*, White epiretinal membrane occurring after scatter retinal photocoagulation for proliferative diabetic retinopathy. *B*, Postoperative appearance after removal of abnormal epiretinal membrane.

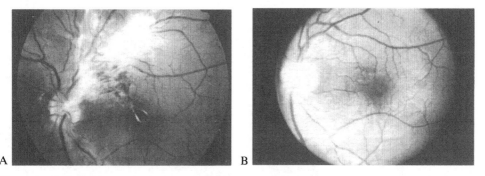

A   B

Figure 4. *A*, Prominent epiretinal membrane along superotemporal arcade causing traction on macular area after resolution of idiopathic vitritis. *B*, Postoperative appearance after removal of epiretinal membrane.

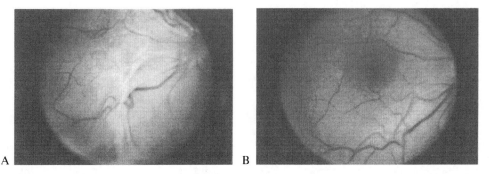

Figure 5. *A*, Preoperative appearance of thick membrane covering posterior pole associated with uniocular uveitis. *B*, Postoperative appearance after removal of thick epiretinal membrane.

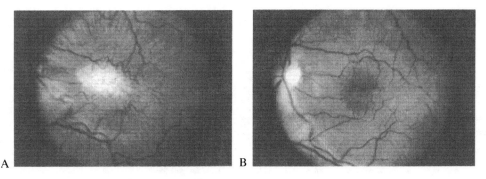

Figure 6. *A*, Prominent idiopathic macular pucker in young patient. *B*, Postoperative appearance after removal of thick epiretinal membrane.

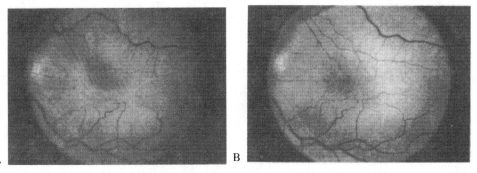

Figure 7. *A*, Preoperative appearance of thin epiretinal membrane in elderly patient. *B*, Postoperative appearance after removal of thin epiretinal membrane.

RESULTS AND COMPLICATIONS

We recently reviewed the records of 130 consecutive cases of epiretinal membranes associated with various conditions and removed by vitreous surgery (1). This series includes 72 male and 58 female patients with an age range from nine to 77 years and a median age of 60 years.

In this series the epiretinal membrane occurred after otherwise-successful surgery for rhegmatogenous retinal detachment in 78 eyes (60%). The membrane was idiopathic in 28 eyes (22%). It was associated with other ocular disorders in 20 eyes (15%). Four additional cases (3%) involved eyes that were also normal in other respects but these patients were relatively young (12, 17, 34 and 35 years of age, respectively). The latter four cases were classified as being possibly developmental although documented membrane growth in two eyes suggested that they may have been of an acquired type.

Portions of the abnormal epiretinal tissue were successfully removed in 128 of the 130 cases. In one eye no epiretinal membrane could be found even though a prominent retinal fold was present in the posterior pole.

The postoperative visual acuity improved at least two lines on the Snellen chart in 108 eyes (83%), (Table 1). The final visual acuity ranged from 20/20 to 20/400 (Table 2). Most of the 20 eyes with final visual acuities of 20/200 or 20/400 had severe pre-existing macular damage.

Intraoperative complications occurred in some patients. Retinal breaks anterior to the equator were found intraoperatively in six eyes (5%) and these were treated by cryotherapy and intraocular air injection with or without a localized scleral buckle. No posterior retinal breaks occurred in this series. A small amount of bleeding from the inner retinal surface occurred in most eyes as the membrane was removed. This was usually limited to small, petechial hemorrhages on the inner retinal surface. In no eye was persistent bleeding a problem.

Postoperative complications included sterile (culture negative) endophthalmitis in one case and infective (culture proven, Staphylococcus epidermidis) endophthalmitis in a second case. Both of these eyes obtained a successful result with postoperative visions of 20/25 and 20/100 respectively. Other, more frequent, postoperative complications included rhegmatogenous retinal detachment in eight eyes. In five cases the detachment occurred within four weeks after the vitrectomy and may have been due to peripheral retinal breaks that occurred during the vitrectomy operation but were not recognized. In the other three eyes retinal detachment occurred more than two months after the vitrectomy due to new retinal breaks in areas that had been thoroughly examined before and where no retinal break was seen previously. In each case the retina was successfully reattached with additional scleral buckling operations.

Progressive lens opacities occurred postoperatively in 31 (34%) of the 90 phakic eyes during the follow-up period. These were usually nuclear sclerotic lens changes. Three eyes underwent cataract extraction during the follow-up interval.

Postoperative recurrence of epiretinal membranes was infrequent. In four case (3%) a sizable amount of epiretinal membrane recurred. In several other cases postoperative photographs taken at six-month intervals showed an increased sheen of the internal limiting membrane suggesting the presence of a thin ERM. However, in no case in this series did an epiretinal membrane occur to the extent present preoperatively, and in no case did a recurrent membrane significantly reduce the visual acuity below the best postoperative level.

Table 1. *Change in vision after vitrectomy*

	Vision improved	Vision same
Retinal detachment (78)	64 (82%)	14 (19%)
Idiopathic (28)	23 (82%)	5 (18%)
Other disorders (20)	19 (95%)	1 (5%)
Developmental (4)	2 (50%)	2 (50%)
Total Eyes (130)	108 (83%)	22 (17%)

Table 2. *Final vision after vitrectomy*

Final vision	Detachment	Idiopathic	Other	Dev.	Total
20/20	2	2	1	—	5 (4%)
20/25 - 20/40	16	13	11	1	41 (31.5%)
20/50 - 20/100	48	8	7	1	64 (49%)
20/200	9	4	—	2	15 (11.5%)
20/400	3	1	1	—	5 (4%)
	78	28	20	4	130

DISCUSSION

We now use vitreous surgery to treat selected cases with epiretinal membranes causing macular pucker and significant visual loss to a level of 20/80 or worse (2-6). Patients usually appreciate both an improvement in visual acuity and also a reduction in distortion (metamorphopsia). However, vision rarely returns to a normal level and some subjective distortion often persists as well.

There are wide variations in the physical characteristics of epiretinal membranes. Thick membranes are usually the easiest to remove although membranes of various sizes and consistency can be successfully treated. The presence or absence of a partially elevated edge of the membrane, noted preoperatively, is not a factor in case selection. The majority of cases in our series did not have a partially elevated edge and yet the membrane could be readily engaged and removed (4, 7).

The occurrence of small petechial hemorrhages on the inner retinal surface when the membrane is removed suggests a firm adherence between the membrane and the basal lamina of the retina. Indeed, ultrastructure study of epiretinal membranes removed by vitreous surgery shows large amounts of internal limiting membrane adherent to the abnormal tissue in most cases (6, 8, 9). This indicates that once an epiretinal membrane is removed from an area of retina, no further dissection should be done in that region even though the retinal surface may still appear abnormal. Postoperatively the wrinkled and distorted retina develops a more normal location and appearance in one to four weeks.

In some cases linear white zones in the inner retinal layers are noted preoperatively (4). This white appearance remains after removing the epiretinal membrane, and it then disappears during the first 48 to 72 hours after surgery. The white intraretinal changes are usually present near the peripheral margin of the membrane and probably represent a zone of obstructed retrograde axoplasmic flow. This may account, in part, for the damaging effect that epiretinal membranes have on visual function in some eyes.

Although no posterior retinal breaks occurred in our series, important intraoperative and postoperative complications were encountered, and this possibility must be considered in any eye being evaluated for possible removal of an epiretinal membrane. Progressive postoperative lens opacification is of special significance since it occurred in 31 (34%) of 90 phakic eyes in this series. These lens changes occurred despite absence of apparent mechanical damage from the vitrectomy instrument and despite use of less than 100 cc of an enriched physiologic irrigating solution. We do not know whether these lens changes are the result of vitreous surgery alone or if they are associated with the underlying ocular disorder or previous surgical procedures. Further analysis of cases with idiopathic membranes is planned to determine the incidence and severity of postoperative nuclear sclerotic lens changes directly attributable to vitreous surgery. In a separate study of diabetic eyes undergoing vitrectomy, a statistically-significant correlation was shown between postoperative nuclear sclerotic lens changes and older patient age (10).

In summary, vitreous surgery now provides an effective means to remove epiretinal membranes causing macular pucker in various clinical situations and to achieve partial visual improvement in severely affected eyes. Because the final postoperative vision often ranges between 20/25 to 20/100, patients with preopertive vision of 20/100 or less are usually selected for surgery. The operation can be performed in eyes with better vision, but surgery is usually not advised in cases with vision better than 20/60. Serious intraoperative and postoperative complications are infrequent, and they can usually be treated effectively. The incidence of clinically-significant recurrent epiretinal membrane is low. Of special concern is the risk of later nuclear sclerotic lens change.

REFERENCES

1. Michels RG: Vitrectomy for macular pucker. Ophthalmology (in press).
2. Machemer R (1978): The surgical removal of epiretinal macular membranes (macular puckers) (in German). Klin Monatsbl Augenheilkd; 173:36-42.
3. Michels RG and Gilbert DH (1979): Surgical management of macular pucker after retinal reattachment surgery. Am J Ophthalmol; 88:925-929.
4. Michels RG (1981): Vitreous surgery for macular pucker. Am J Ophthalmol; 92:628-639.
5. Charles S (1981): Epimacular proliferation, in Schachet WS (ed): Vitreous Microsurgery, Baltimore, Williams & Wilkins Co, Chapter 8, pp 131-133.
6. Michels RG (1982): A clinical and histopathological study of epiretinal membranes affecting the macula and removed by vitreous surgery. Trans Am Ophthalmol Soc; 80:580-656.

7. Michels RG (1981): Vitreous Surgery. St. Louis, CV Mosby Co, pp 357-362.

8. Kampik A, Kenyon KR, Michels RG, Green WR and de la Cruz ZC (1981): Epiretinal and vitreous membranes. A comparative study of 56 cases. Arch Ophthalmol. 99:1445-1454.

9. Lindsey PS, Michels RG, Luckenbach N, Green WR (1983): Ultrastructure of epiretinal membrane causing retinal starfold. Ophthalmology; 90:578-583.

10. Novak MA, Rice TA, Michels RG and Auer C: The lens after diabetic vitrectomy. Ophthalmology (in press).

Basic and advanced vitreous surgery
G.W. Blankenship, M. Stirpe, M. Gonvers, S. Binder (eds.)
Fidia Research Series, vol. II,
Liviana Press, Padova © 1986

PREOPERATIVE IRIS ANGIOGRAPHY:
A PROGNOSTIC TOOL FOR DIABETIC PATIENTS

Robert Machemèr

Duke University, Dept. of Ophthalmology, Durham, North Carolina
(Reported by Severino Fruscella)

Iris neovascularization is one of the most severe ocular complications occuring after vitrectomy in diabetic patients. This complication can be predicted by performing preoperative iris fluorescein angiography.

A study of iris fluorescein angiograms of patients undergoing vitrectomy and effected by proliferative diabetic retinopathy was carried out. The first important finding was that most of the patients, though with no biomicroscopy evidence of rubeosis iridis, showed rather intense fluorescein leakage.

The findings showed a statistically significant correlation between the severity of preoperative fluorescein leakage and the development of rubeosis iridis 6 months after the operation.

The more extensive the diffusion of the contrast medium in preoperative fluorescein agiograms, the higher the degree of post-operative iris neovascularization.

We conclude that iris fluorescein angiography is a valuable tool to predict the possible development of rubeosis iridis; intra or early postoperative photocoagulation therapy should be recommended for high risk patients. There is evidence that pan-retinal photocoagulation causes a partial decrease or the complete regression of iris neovascularization.

Basic and advanced vitreous surgery
G.W. Blankenship, M. Stirpe, M. Gonvers, S. Binder (eds.)
Fidia Research Series, vol. II,
Liviana Press, Padova © 1986

PROGNOSTIC VALUES OF PREOPERATIVE FINDINGS FOR DIABETIC VITRECTOMY

George W. Blankenship, M.D.

The Bascom Palmer Eye Institute, University of Miami School of Medicine
Miami, Florida

Recommending vitrectomy, like any surgical procedure, requires that the probable results of the vitrectomy are better than other forms of treatment or the natural course of the disease. To better predict the results of vitrectomy for diabetic retinopathy complications, various previtrectomy findings were compared with the 6 month visual results.

MATERIALS AND METHODS

One thousand, two hundred and twenty-three diabetic vitrectomy cases performed by the full time faculty of the Bascom Palmer Eye Institute were reviewed with 1,056 (86%) having 6 month follow-up examinations, 47 (4%) patients having died, 19 (2%) eyes having been enucleated, 59 (5%) cases being excluded because of subsequent vitrectomy operations, and the remaining 42 (3%) cases being lost to follow-up.

The best corrected preoperative and 6 month postoperative visual acuities were grouped into broad categories: 1) reading vision, 6/5 to 6/12 (20/15 to 20/40); 2) decreased visual acuity but not legal blindness, 6/15 to 6/60 (20/50 to 20/200); 3) ambulating visual acuity, 6/90 to 1/60 (20/300 to finger counting); 4) minimal visual function, (hand movements to light perception); and 5) no light perception. Since small changes in acuity at such poor levels are difficult to interpret, a successful 6 month visual result required improvement by at least one category. The influence of preoperative findings was evaluated by subdividing each finding and comparing each with the 6 month visual result.

Information regarding the patients' general characteristics, past ophthalmic and medical histories, best corrected visual functions, and ophthalmic findings with slit lamp microscopy, gonioscopy, fundus contact lens, and indirect ophthalmoscopy was recorded at the preoperative and 6 month follow-up examinations. Data regarding the operative procedures, complications, and findings were also recorded. All of the information was computerized.

Occasionally, the follow-up data were incomplete due to inadequacies of examinations performed elsewhere, or more often, because opacities in the optical media made visualization of more posterior structures impossible.

The influence of operative complications was so great that it precluded the evaluation of other influencing factors. Therefore, when evaluating factors other than operative complications, the 281 cases in which complications occurred were excluded and the remaining 775 cases were analyzed.

RESULTS

The patient's age, sex, known duration of diabetes, and treatment for control of diabetes did not have a significant influence on the 6 month visual results. Likewise, the visual results were not significantly influenced by the eye involved, presence of cataract, or a history of previous vitrectomy.

Table 1 shows the 6 month visual success rate with the incidence of operative complications. When complications did not occur, 54% of the cases had substantially improved visual acuities compared with only 26% when iatrogenic retinal tears developed.

The duration of decreased vision which existed at the time of vitrectomy was not important in the cases having vitrectomy for dense, non-clearing vitreous hemorrhages, but was very important for those having traction detachments involving the macula. A successful result was obtained in 75% of the vitreous hemorrhage cases when the loss of vision had been 2 months or less compared with 69% when the loss of vision had been present for longer than a year (Table 2) for the vitreous hemorrhage cases.

Table 1. *Diabetic vitrectomy success rate*

OPERATIVE COMPLICATIONS		
NONE	775 cases	54%
HOLE	218	26%
BLEEDING	40	38%
BOTH	23	22%

Table 2. *Diabetic vitrectomy success rate for vitreous hemorrhage (394 cases)*

DURATION OF PREOP VISUAL ACUITY (MONTHS)		
0-2	48 cases	75%
3-6	110	70%
7-12	99	71%
13 +	137	69%

The success rates compared to the duration of decreased vision for traction detachments involving the macula are shown in Table 3 with a significantly smaller incidence of successful results when vitrectomy was delayed.

Eyes with preoperative iris neovascularization did much poorer than eyes without iris neovascularization, especially when the peripheral iris and angle were involved (Table 4).

The visual results obtained in vitreous hemorrhage cases with attached maculas are much better than those cases where the macula is detached either with or without vitreous hemorrhage as shown in Table 5.

The extent of neovascularization in the diabetic proliferative tissue was also found to correlate with the visual results (Table 6). A much higher incidence of successful results was obtained when proliferative retinopathy was not found during the vitrectomy, compared with only a 14% incidence of successful visual results obtained with the 21 cases in which very extensive neovascularization was present.

Table 3. *Diabetic vitrectomy success rate for macular detachments (183 cases)*

DURATION OF PREOP VISUAL ACUITY (MONTHS)		
0-2	62 cases	42%
3-6	60	32%
7-12	30	23%
13+	31	20%

Table 4. *Diabetic vitrectomy success rate*

PREOP IRIS NEOVASCULARIZATION		
NONE	653 cases	55%
PUPIL	75	42%
PERIPHERAL	47	32%

Table 5. *Diabetic vitrectomy success rate*

PREOP MACULAR STATUS		
ATTACHED	496 cases	66%
DETACHED	279	32%

Table 6. *Diabetic vitrectomy success rate*

NEOVASCULAR COMPONENT		
NONE	32 cases	69%
ATROPHIC	416	56%
SOME	306	49%
FLORID	21	14%

DISCUSSION

The unfortunately high incidence of operative complications is characteristic of diabetic vitrectomy, especially when the earlier cases are included. The poor results associated with cases having complications was due to both the frequent inability to repair the complications and obtain good anatomical results, and the retinas prone to complications were usually atrophic and unable to provide good visual function even if the vitrectomy was anatomically successful. The exclusion of cases with operative complications accounts for the higher incidence of successful visual results and the smaller number of cases analyzed than in other previous reports of vitrectomy results.

The advantages and disadvantages of performing diabetic vitrectomy for vitreous hemorrhage shortly after the onset of hemorrhage and loss of vision, compared with deferring vitrectomy until a later time, will hopefully be answered by the Diabetic Retinopathy Vitrectomy Study (1), but the retrospective analysis of cases in this report does not indicate a strong preference in the timing of vitrectomy for diabetic vitreous hemorrhage. However, vitrectomy should be performed relatively quickly following detachment of the macula, as has been previously reported (2, 3).

The higher incidence of postoperative iris neovascularization and neovascular glaucoma with subsequent blindness is obviously much higher in eyes with preoperative iris neovascularization (4). Although many of the eyes with preoperative iris neovascularization also had neovascular glaucoma, 32% had a successful visual result 6 months following vitrectomy and most were associated with regression of the iris neovascularization (5).

The poor visual results associated with extensive neovascular proliferation has been previously described (3, 6) with most of the eyes having extensive postoperative inflammation, vitreous cavity flare, subsequent iris neovascularization and glaucoma, and rapid deterioration to phthisis and blindness.

REFERENCES

1. Kupfer C (1976):The diabetic retinopathy vitrectomy study. Am J Ophthalmol, 81:687-90.
2. Aaberg TM (1981): Pars plana vitrectomy for diabetic traction retinal detachment. Ophthalmology, 88:639-42.

3. Hutton WL, Bernstein I, Fuller D (1980): Diabetic traction retinal detachment; factors influencing final visual acuity. Ophthalmology, 87:1071-7.
4. Blankenship G (1980): Preoperative iris rubeosis and diabetic vitrectomy results. Ophthalmology, 87:176-82.
5. Scuderi JJ, Blumenkranz MS, Blankenship G (1982): Regression of diabetic rubeosis irides following successful surgical reattachment of the retina by vitrectomy. Retina, 2:193-196.
6. Machemer R, Blankenship G (1981): Vitrectomy for proliferative diabetic retinopathy associated with vitreous hemorrhage. Ophthalmology, 88:643-6.

Basic and advanced vitreous surgery
G.W. Blankenship, M. Stirpe, M. Gonvers, S. Binder (eds.)
Fidia Research Series, vol. II,
Liviana Press, Padova © 1986

LENS INFLUENCE ON IRIS NEOVASCULARIZATION AND GLAUCOMA

George W. Blankenship, M.D.

The Bascom Palmer Eye Institute
University of Miami School of Medicine, Miami, Florida

Iris neovascularization and neovascular glaucoma following pars plana vitrectomy for diabetic retinopathy have been major complications during the early postoperative course. A retrospective analysis of diabetic vitrectomy cases, and a prospective randomized study find a direct relationship between postvitrectomy aphakia and the development of iris neovascularization and secondary glaucoma.

MATERIALS AND METHODS

One thousand, one hundred sixty-one consecutive diabetic vitrectomy cases performed at the Bascom Palmer Eye Institute by the full time faculty were reviewed with 980 (84%) having 6 month follow-up examinations, 46 (4%) patients having died, 19 (2%) eyes having been enucleated, 51 (4%) being excluded for having subsequent vitrectomy operations, and the remaining 65 (6%) being lost to follow-up. The 980 cases with 6 month follow-up were subdivided into 331 (34%) which retained clear lenses at the end of the vitrectomy procedure, 543 (55%) which had lensectomy combined with the vitrectomy, and the remaining 106 (11%) cases having had previous cataract surgery before the vitrectomy.

In a separate prospective study a randomized decision was made to remove or retain clear lenses of informed consenting patients undergoing pars plana vitrectomy for diabetic retinopathy complications. Six month follow-up information for eyes without previtrectomy iris neovascularization was available for 20 eyes randomly assigned to having lens removal combined with vitrectomy, and 23 randomly assigned to lens retention.

Information regarding the patients' general characteristics, past ophthalmic and medical histories, best corrected visual functions, and ophthalmic findings with slit lamp microscopy, gonioscopy, fundus contact lenses, and indirect ophthalmoscopy was recorded at the preoperative and 6 month follow-up examinations. Data regarding the operative procedures, complications, and findings were also recorded. All of the information was computerized.

Occasionally the follow-up data were incomplete because of inadequacies of examinations performed elsewhere or, more often, because of the inability to visualize structures located posterior to opacities in the optic axis.

RETROSPECTIVE RESULTS

Preoperatively, there was a substantially higher incidence of peripheral iris neovascularization in those cases having previous cataract surgery than in the other two groups (Table 1). During the 6 months following vitrectomy, several eyes, especially in the aphakic groups, had further deterioration with corneal opacification which obscured the iris at the 6 month examination. In all probability these eyes also had extensive peripheral iris neovascular involvement. Table 2 shows the incidence and geographic distribution of postoperative iris neovascularization in the 3 groups with most of the phakic eyes without iris neovascularization, but the majority of aphakic eyes having iris neovascularization with an essentially equal involvement of those having lensectomy during vitrectomy and those having previous cataract surgery before vitrectomy.

About 1/2 of the eyes with peripheral iris neovascularization developed neovascular glaucoma (Table 3) with a much higher and essentially identical incidence in the 2 groups of aphakic eyes.

Table 1. *Lens status and diabetic vitrectomy iris neovascularization preop*

	Phakic (331)	Lensectomy (543)	Preop aphakic (106)
NONE	92%	83%	74%
PUPIL	7%	11%	4%
PERIPHERAL	1%	6%	22%

Table 2. *Lens status and diabetic vitrectomy iris neovascularization postop*

	Phakic (331)	Lensectomy (543)	Preop aphakic (106)
NONE	72%	48%	47%
PUPIL	10%	7%	3%
PERIPHERAL	16%	38%	41%
CAN'T EXAMINE	2%	7%	9%

Table 3. *Lens status and diabetic vitrectomy incidence of neovascular glaucoma*

PHAKIC (331 cases)	7%
LENSECTOMY (543 cases)	25%
PREOP APHAKIC (106 cases)	22%

PROSPECTIVE RANDOMIZED RESULTS

Cases with preoperative iris neovascularization, lens opacities, or previous lens removal were excluded from the group of cases being reported. Six months following vitrectomy the 20 eyes randomly assigned to having lensectomy with vitrectomy had a 50% incidence of peripheral iris neovascularization, compared with only 17% of the 23 eyes randomly assigned to the lens retention group (Table 4).

The majority of eyes in each group had intraocular pressures within an acceptable range 6 months following vitrectomy (Table 5), but during the 6 month follow-up period, neovascular glaucoma had occurred in 35% of the aphakic eyes and in only 13% of the phakic eyes.

Table 4. *Lens status and diabetic vitrectomy 6 months post vitrectomy iris neovascularization (exclude pre-vit. iris neovascularization)*

	Aphakic (20)	Phakic (23)
NONE	40%	65%
PUPIL	5%	9%
PERIPHERAL	50%	17%
CAN'T EXAMINE	5%	9%

Table 5. *Lens influence and diabetic vitrectomy 6 months post vitrectomy I.O.P. (exclude pre-vit. iris neovascularization)*

	Aphakic (20)	Phakic (23)
00-05 mm Hg	20%	26%
06-30	55%	74%
31 +	25%	0%
(NEOVASC. GLAU)	35%	13%

DISCUSSION

The development of iris neovascularization and secondary neovascular glaucoma following diabetic vitrectomy has been previously correlated with postoperative retinal detachment (1, 2). A substantial number of cases in this report may have had retinal detachments following vitrectomy, which were obscured by anterior segment and vitreous opacities, and probably contributed to the high incidence of iris neovascularization and glaucoma.

The retained lens provides a protective barrier between the anterior and posterior segments (3). This barrier effects results in the lower incidence of iris neovascularization and neovascular glaucoma (4, 5, 6). The higher incidence of iris neovascularization before vitrectomy in the preoperative aphakic eyes is also related to the loss of this protective barrier effect of the lens. While the barrier effect is beneficial in reducing the incidence of iris neovascularization and glaucoma, it definitely decreases the clearing rate of subsequent vitreous cavity hemorrhage (5), for which vitreous cavity washout or air fluid exchange procedures might be required.

More recently, the incidence of iris neovascularization was also found to be lower in eyes whith previtrectomy panretinal photocoagulation (6). A previous review of Miami vitrectomy cases (7) had failed to appreciate this beneficial effect.

Iris neovascularization and neovascular glaucoma will continue to occur after vitrectomy for diabetic retinopathy complications, but can be minimized by previtrectomy panretinal photocoagulation, retention of clear lenses, and reattachment of postvitrectomy retinal detachments.

REFERENCES

1. Michels RG (1978): Vitrectomy for complications of diabetic retinopathy. Arch Ophthalmol, 96:237-246.
2. Aaberg TM, Van Horn DL (1978): Late complications of pars plana vitreous surgery. Ophthalmology, 85:126-140.
3. Michels RG (1976): Vitreoretinal and anterior segment surgery through the pars plana. Part I. Ann Ophthalmol, 8:1353-1381.
4. Blankenship G, Cortez R, Machemer R (1979): The lens and pars plana vitrectomy for diabetic retinopathy complications. Arch Ophthalmol, 97:1263-1267.
5. Blankenship GW (1980): The lens influence on diabetic vitrectomy results, report of a prospective randomized study. Arch Ophthalmol, 98:2196-2198.
6. Rice TA, Michels RG, Maquir MG, Rice EF (1983): The effect of lensectomy on the incidence of iris neovascularization and neovascular glaucoma after vitrectomy for diabetic retinopathy. Am J Ophthalmol, 95:1-11.
7. Goodard R, Blankenship G (1980): Panretinal photocoagulation influence on vitrectomy results for complications of diabetic retinopathy. Ophthalmol, 87:183-188.

Basic and advanced vitreous surgery
G.W. Blankenship, M. Stirpe, M. Gonvers, S. Binder (eds.)
Fidia Research Series, vol. II,
Liviana Press, Padova © 1986

DIABETIC TRACTION DETACHMENT

M. Gonvers, M.D.

Hôpital Ophtalmologique, Lausanne

Diabetic traction detachment can be encountered in two different situations: associated with vitreous hemorrhage when the detachment is diagnosed only by B-Scan or with a clear vitreous when the detachment can be seen ophthalmoscopically.

When diabetic traction detachment occurs in addition to vitreous hemorrhage, it is an indication for immediate vitrectomy, in so far as there is a reasonable chance of visual recovering (that is, the loss of vision must not be too long-dated, the optic nerve and the retina still retaining some visual function). Wherever the detachment is located, a vitrectomy must be performed because the associated vitreous hemorrhage is an aggravating factor in the detachment and indicates most of the time that diabetic retinopathy is active.

When there is no vitreous hemorrhage, the decision for surgery will rely on the localization of the detachment. Only detachments which include the macula and date no more than a few months will be operated on for the following two reasons: first, because operative risks are justified by the loss of central vision, secondly because a recently detached macula has a chance of recovering its function. On the other hand, extramacular localized detachments should usually not be touched because their spontaneous evolution is slow and does not justify the operative risk of a vitrectomy. In fact, Charles showed that in one year, only 10% of extramacular detachments progressed to the macula.

Total retinal detachment with or without vitreous hemorrhage can be submitted to vitreous surgery if, however, the following conditions are fulfilled:

— loss of vision does not date more than 1-2 years;
— the retina must be sufficiently vascularized;
— the retina must not be atrophic, that is, ophthalmoscopically transparent;
— the optic nerve must not be pale;
— the condition of the anterior segment must be acceptable.

The surgical technique in diabetic traction detachment includes two steps. The first one aims to cut over 360° the posterior face of the vitreous body which is usually stretched between the periphery of the eye and the posterior proliferans. This is a very important step which must be perfectly mastered by the beginning surgeon before he goes any further. The second step is epiretinal surgery which aims to cut off all tangential tractions at the retinal surface. This surgery is reserved to the experienced surgeon. These tractions can be removed by the different techniques which sometimes may be combined: the first is segmentation, the second delamination.

The aim of segmentation is to divide the epiretinal proliferans into small islands of tissue which are left in place, each island corresponding to a vascular unit. This technique, which was described in detail by Aaberg, has the advantage of not being dangerous but does not allow good hemostasis because of the difficulty to coagulate vessels which bleed under an island of proliferans. This technique which is used less and less has, however, some indications:

— when it is mandatory to minimize operative risks as in the case of an only eye with good preoperative vision;
— when the proliferans is very fibrous and adherent to the retina, and cannot be peeled off;
— when the proliferans is not very vascularized;
— when there is a shallow detachment with minor tractions.

In fact, in most cases, delamination is the choice technique. It allows total removal of the epiretinal proliferation from the retinal surface. One way to perform this type of surgery is to grasp the edge of the proliferans with the vitreous instrument and cut all the connections between the retina and the proliferans with vitreous scissors.

The delamination technique has a good indication in the case of disc proliferans and peripapillary traction detachment with nasal traction of the macula (which can be detached or not detached).

Delamination is also a good technique when the proliferans is very vascularized. When a posterior retinal hole is located in an area of traction detachment, delamination alone can totally flatten the retina, a condition necessary to close the hole: in such cases, as it will be pointed out later, delamination is often associated with a temporary tamponnade of silicone oil. The association of delamination and silicone is also used in tough cases with total traction detachment.

Even if delamination is much more dangerous than segmentation it does present a lot of advantages:

— hemostasis is much easier because the feeder vessels of the proliferans which originate from the retinal vessels can be easily coagulated right at the surface of the retina;
— the risk of rebleeding is 50% less with delamination than it is with segmentation;
— reapplication of the retina is more fully achieved when tractions are totally removed. This fact must be kept in mind when the macula is detached, when endophotocoagulation is considered and in the case of posterior retinal hole;
— at long term it is possible that a perfect reapplication of the retina decreases the risks of rubeosis.

As mentioned before, silicone oil is used in a few cases of diabetic retinal detachment, as a temporary tamponade, in addition to delamination. Clinical experience shows that silicone oil has some very interesting properties in diabetic retinopathy:

— silicone oil gives fantastic hemostasis, probably because of its surface tension effects at the level of the retina;

— silicone oil is the best tamponade for a huge posterior retinal tear;

— in any situation and at any time silicone oil allows a perfect control of the situation of the fundus so that additional photocoagulation or any other surgery can be done if necessary;

— silicone oil acts against rubeosis iridis and this fact has now become clinical evidence.

These properties are used in the following situations:

— in very tough cases which usually include total traction detachment;

— in huge iatrogenic or natural posterior tear;

— in traction detachment combined with unclear rhegmatogenous detachment;

— in cases with major risks of neovascular glaucoma, especially when endophotocoagulation cannot be performed during the vitrectomy;

— in cases which repeatedly rebleed and where corneal decompensation does not allow any other treatment; silicone oil is then injected as a blind procedure.

In conclusion, the prognosis of diabetic traction detachment has been greatly improved by the association of vitrectomy with segmentation or delamination of proliferans, completed sometimes by a temporary tamponade of silicone oil.

Basic and advanced vitreous surgery
G.W. Blankenship, M. Stirpe, M. Gonvers, S. Binder (eds.)
Fidia Research Series, vol. II,
Liviana Press, Padova © 1986

VITREOUS SURGERY FOR PROLIFERATIVE DIABETIC RETINOPATHY

Ronald G. Michels, M.D.

The Vitreoretinal Service, Wilmer Ophthalmological Institute,
Johns Hopkins University School of Medicine, Baltimore, Maryland

Proliferative diabetic retinopathy can cause visual loss by various mechanisms including complications from neovascular and fibrovascular tissue growth causing vitreous hemorrhage, detachment or distortion of the retina, and/or traction on the optic nerve. Extraretinal complications of proliferative diabetic retinopathy often cause severe visual loss, and these complications can now be successfully treated by vitreous surgery in the majority of cases. The principles and techniques of surgery, as well as the visual results and lasting structural effects, depend on the unique pathophysiology of the extraretinal proliferative process.

PATHOGENESIS OF PROLIFERATIVE DIABETIC RETINOPATHY

Exact features of proliferative diabetic retinopathy vary widely, but the disorder is characterized by neovascular, and later, fibrovascular proliferative tissue extending from the retina into the vitreous cavity. This often begins as neovascularization on the optic nervehead and in other locations such as along the temporal vascular arcades and in the midperiphery adjacent to areas of capillary nonperfusion. The etiology of the neovascular process is not known, but it is presumed to be caused by angiogenic substance(s) produced by hypoxic retinal tissue.

Growth of extraretinal neovascular and fibrovascular tissue is quite dependent on the posterior vitreous surface. Neovascularization originating on the optic nervehead occasionally invades the adjacent vitreous gel, but proliferative tissue beginning elsewhere grows almost exclusively along the posterior vitreous surface. This proliferation often causes changes in the vitreous gel, resulting in partial posterior vitreous detachment with separation of the cortical vitreous from the retina. The vitreous remains attached to the anterior retina at the vitreous base and at each area of posterior fibrovascular proliferation.

The mechanism causing separation of the posterior vitreous surface is uncertain, although it is probably due to contraction of fibrovascular tissue growing along its surface. After separating from the retina the vitreous often develops a funnel-shaped configuration, and it extends between the vitreous base anteriorly and the areas of fibrovascular proliferation posteriorly. The taut posterior vitreous surface then causes anteroposterior traction on the areas of vitreoretinal attachment.

Further fibrovascular tissue growth may then occur along the posterior vitreous surface. Often the more peripheral margins of the abnormal tissue are elevated and the more posterior margins lie flat along the plane of the inner retina following the contour of the trampoline-like posterior vitreous surface where it bridges between one area of retina and another. When little or no posterior vitreous detachment occurs, the proliferative tissue grows along the plane of the inner retinal surface, and it may develop widespread adhesions to the retina.

Fibrovascular tissue growth and secondary changes in the vitreous gel can cause further complications. These include: 1) hemorrhage into the vitreous gel and/or into the preretinal space behind the separated cortical vitreous, 2) traction retinal detachment, 3) traction on the optic nervehead, and 4) retinal breaks with or without rhegmatogenous detachment. Fibrovascular tissue growing along the inner retinal surface can also contract, causing tangential traction on the retina and resulting in visual loss from distortion or displacement of the macular or the peripapillary retina.

The posterior vitreous surface, therefore, is of great importance in the pathogenesis of extraretinal features of proliferative diabetic retinopathy and its secondary complications (1-6). This is readily confirmed by observing the natural course of eyes with these progressive features and studying the structural relations encountered during preoperative evaluation and vitreous surgery. The objectives of vitreous surgery and the long-term effects of vitrectomy are, in turn, determined by this fundamental structural pathophysiology.

SURGICAL OBJECTIVES AND TECHNIQUES

The purpose of vitreous surgery is twofold: to reverse pre-existing blinding complications of the proliferative retinopathy, and to alter the later course of this often-progressive disease by removing the posterior vitreous surface on which abnormal fibrovascular tissue mainly grows. Therefore, the general surgical objectives are to: 1) remove any visually-significant intravitreal opacities, 2) excise the posterior vitreous surface, and 3) remove and/or segment portions of preretinal (elevated) and epiretinal (flat) fibrovascular tissue. Excision of the posterior vitreous surface serves to relieve pre-existing anteroposterior and tangential traction on areas of vitreoretinal attachment, and it removes the "scaffold" necessary for further growth of elevated fibrovascular tissue. These basic surgical objectives are the same in all such eyes, although the indications for surgery and the features of the vitreoretinal anatomy vary widely from case to case, and therefore different techniques may be needed.

We prefer divided-system vitrectomy instrumentation, such as the O'Malley Ocutome system, because of the small size of each instrument and because the bimanual method and the ease of substituting instruments one for another facilitate a wide range of ancillary techniques (Figs. 1 and 2). Lens removal is performed when cataract changes are severe enough to interfere with safe performance of the operation or to significant-

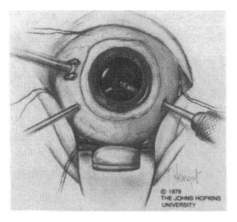

Figure 1. Divided system instrumentation for pars plana vitrectomy using O'Malley Ocutome System. Separate scleral incisions are made for introduction of: (1) infusion cannula, sutured to the sclera, (2) vitrectomy cutting probe, and (3) fiber-optic illuminator. (Courtesy of The Johns Hopkins University).

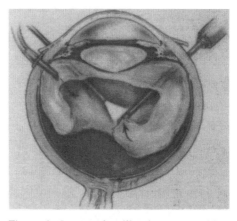

Figure 2. Intraocular illuminator provides reflex-free illumination as opaque vitreous gel is cut and removed via vitrectomy cutting probe. Separate infusion cannula replaces intraocular volume loss as opaque tissue is removed. (Courtesy of the Johns Hopkins University).

ly reduce the postoperative vision. Otherwise, lens removal is avoided so as to preserve a more physiologic optical system and to reduce the risk of postoperative rubeosis iridis (7, 8). A cataractous lens is usually removed through the pars plana incision using an ultrasonic needle and the vitrectomy probe (Fig. 3) (9). If the cataract is of extremely

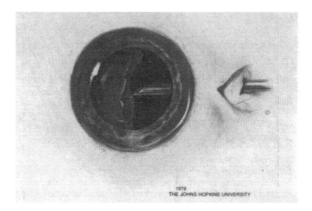

Figure 3. Pars plana approach for removal of cataractous lens in conjunction with vitrectomy. Ultrasonic needle is used to emulsify and remove the firm, opaque lens nucleus. Remaining cortical material and lens capsule are then excised with vitrectomy probe. (Courtesy of The Johns Hopkins University).

hard consistency, it is removed through the limbus using an intracapsular technique.

The vitreous gel is then excised with the vitrectomy probe (Fig. 4). In phakic eyes the anterior vitreous gel is preserved unless it is opaque. The posterior vitreous surface

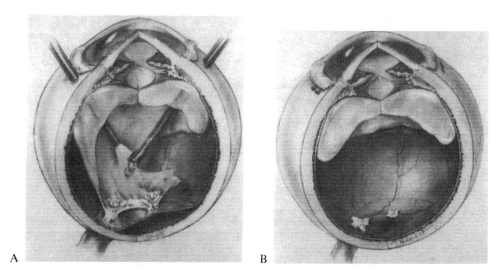

A   B

Figure 4. Excision of vitreous gel in diabetic eye with posterior traction retinal detachment. *A*, The central vitreous gel is excised, and the posterior vitreous surface is then cut to relieve traction between the vitreous base anteriorly and zones of fibrovascular proliferation posteriorly. *B*, Release of anteroposterior vitreous traction and cutting of fibrovascular tissue into separate islands permits traction retinal detachment to settle. (Courtesy of The Johns Hopkins University).

is incised with the vitrectomy probe in a midperipheral location where there is a safe distance between the vitreous and the underlying retina, and any unclotted blood in the preretinal space is removed. Additional portions of the posterior vitreous surface are then excised in a circumferential direction until the entire cone-shaped vitreous surface has been divided, thereby relieving all anteroposterior traction.

The cortical vitreous further posterior is then excised. The techniques required to do this vary, depending on the specific vitreoretinal anatomy. If the vitreous is separated from the retina except at attachments to one or more stalks of elevated fibrovascular tissue, then all of the vitreous and most of the fibrovascular tissue is readily excised, leaving only portions of the fibrovascular stalks where they grow out of the retina. These remaining portions are treated with bipolar diathermy (10).

Often sizable portions of the posterior vitreous surface have not separated from the retina, and fibrovascular tissue has grown along the vitreous surface, extending between those places where the proliferation originated. This results in sheets of epiretinal tissue that have a curvilinear or geographic configuration. Commonly this proliferation occurs around the optic nervehead and along the temporal vascular arcades, and it may encircle the macula. The posterior vitreous surface over the macula may be separated from the retina like a trampoline, or it may remain adherent to the underlying retina.

The posterior part of the cortical vitreous is first excised between zones of fibrovascular proliferation using the vitrectomy probe or vitreoretinal scissors (11). Remaining edges of the posterior vitreous surface involved with fibrovascular tissue may be treated with bipolar diathermy. Other portions of the posterior vitreous surface, with or without fibrovascular proliferation, are then separated from the retina using a vitreoretinal pic when this can be done safely. The objective is to divide the posterior zone of cortical vitreous and fibrovascular tissue into separate islands in order to minimize traction on the underlying and adjacent retina (Fig. 5).

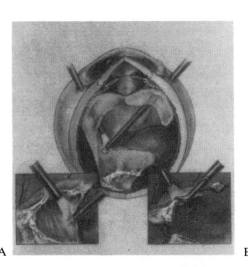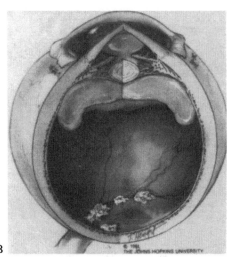

A   B

Figure 5. Vitrectomy for complicated diabetic retinopathy with widespread epiretinal fibrovascular tissue growth. *A*, Vitreous opacities are removed and anteroposterior traction relieved by excising the posterior vitreous gel, including the posterior vitreous surface. Cortical vitreous extending across the posterior pole is then cut with the vitrectomy probe (left inset). Fibrovascular tissue is cut into various separate islands using vitreoretinal scissors (right insert). *B*, Release of vitreous traction and segmentation of fibrovascular tissue results in improved vision and stable posterior-segment relations. Residual islands of fibrovascular tissue remain *in situ*. (Courtesy of The Johns Hopkins University).

When sizable portions of epiretinal tissue can be separated from the retina, this tissue is excised with the vitrectomy probe. Scissors are used to transect localized tissue bridges after identifying a cleavage plana between the abnormal tissue and the underlying retina. Therefore, the posterior vitreous surface, including portions involved by fibrovascular tissue growth, is removed except at places of firm attachment to the retina, which often correspond to the origins of neovascular proliferation.

The extent to which this objective of removing the posterior vitreous surface and epiretinal tissue can be safely achieved varies greatly, depending on the complexity of the vitreoretinal anatomy. However, even in difficult cases, the posterior vitreous surface can usually be removed even though the amount of proliferation is great and the process is longstanding.

Any bleeding is stopped before completing the operation, and bipolar diathermy

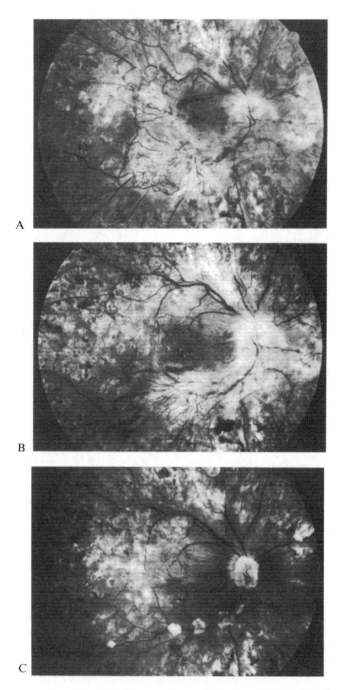

Figure 6. Vitrectomy for progressive fibrovascular proliferation. *A*, Epiretinal fibrovascular tissue surrounds the optic nerve and is growing along the inferotemporal arcade despite extensive scatter retinal photocoagulation. *B*, Two months later fibrovascular tissue covers the macular area. This tissue is growing on the posterior vitreous surface that is not separated from inner retina.

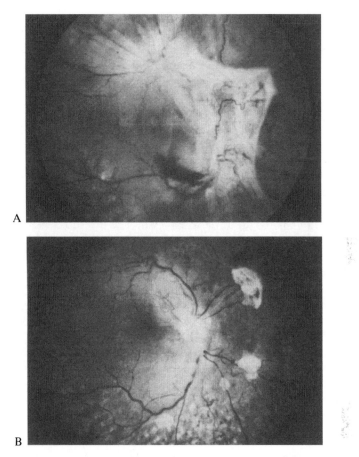

Figure 7. Vitrectomy for progressive fibrovascular proliferation. *A*, Fibrovascular tissue covers the optic nerve and peripapillary retina causing progressive distortion and detachment of the underlying retina and macula. *B*, Appearance six weeks after vitrectomy. Most of the abnormal tissue was removed and the peripapillary retina has become reattached.

is often used to treat the cut edges of fibrovascular tissue. Any retinal breaks are also treated, and subretinal fluid can be evacuated through suitable posterior breaks to flatten the retina and position the edges of each tear near the pigment epithelium (12, 13). Any retinal breaks are then treated by transscleral cryotherapy or by transvitreal cryotherapy (14) or photocoagulation (15). An air bubble is placed inthe vitreous cavity to provide temporary internal tamponade of the retinal break(s) (12, 13). A scleral buckle is also used beneath each retinal break if there is persistent traction from remaining vitreous or tangential traction from adjacent areas of residual fibrovascular tissue.

Figure 6. (continued) C, Appearance one month after pars plana vitrectomy. The abnormal fibrovascular tissue was removed except for several islands remaining on the optic nerve and along the inferotemporal arcade where firm attachments to the underlying retinal vessels were encountered.

RESULTS

We operated on 596 consecutive eyes with severe visual loss from complications of proliferative diabetic retinopathy. This group includes 253 females and 266 males, with ages ranging from 20 to 80 years and with a median age of 48 years. The right eye was operated on in 294 patients and the left eye in 302 patients. In 77 patients both eyes were operated on at different times.

Follow-up information at least six months after surgery was available on 579 patients. The average interval of follow-up was 19 months. Two patients died during the interval between three months and six months after the operation. These two eyes are included in the statistical analysis, with the visual acuities and physical findings as noted at least three months after the operation.

A successful result with visual acuity of 5/200 or better and stable anatomic findings was achieved in 384 (66%) of these 579 eyes. The threshold visual level of 5/200 was selected as a measure of success because with this amount of vision a patient can usually ambulate unaided, using only one eye. A successful result was obtained in 189 (76%) of 248 eyes with preoperative vitreous hemorrhage but without previous retinal detachment involving the macula A successful result was obtained in 116 (59%) of 195 eyes with tractional retinal detachment involving the macula preoperatively. A successful result was obtained in 60 (54%) of 111 eyes with a preoperative combined traction and rhegatogenous retinal detachment.

The postoperative visual acuity in these 579 eyes in given in Table 1. The final levels of vision in most cases depended on the amount of pre-existing intraretinal vascular damage and residual effects from retinal detachment or distortion of the macula due to fibrovascular tissue. Our data are similar to the experience of others (16-21) in treating diabetic patients (Tables 2, 3).

Table 1. *Final visual results after vitrectomy (579 eyes)*

Final V.A.	Hemorrhage only	Traction R.D.	Rhegmato- genous R.D.	Other	Total
20/20	10	3	2	1	16 (3%)
20/25-20/50	63	12	13	4	92 (16%)
20/60-20/100	42	25	12	8	87 (15%)
20/200	42	39	12	2	95 (16%)
20/300	12	10	7	2	31 (5%)
20/400	8	16	5	0	29 (5%)
5/200-9/200	12	11	9	2	34 (6%)
1/200-4/200	6	4	5	1	16 (3%)
HM*	12	13	9	1	36 (6%)
LP*	25	25	14	0	64 (11%)
NLP*	16	36	23	4	79 (14%)
	248	195	111	25	579 (100%)

* HM = Hand motions; LP = Light perception; NLP = no light perception

Table 2. *Results of vitrectomy in simple diabetic vitreous hemorrhage*

Authors	No. eyes	V.A. improved*	V.A. unchanged	V.A. worse
Machemer et al[17]	414	242 (59%)	84 (21%)	87 (20%)
Blankenship[15]	299	182 (61%)	66 (22%)	50 (17%)
Peyman et al[14]	109	72 (66%)	29 (27%)	8 (7%)
Michels and Rice	248	189 (76%)	59 (24%)	

* V.A., visual acuity

Table 3. *Results of vitrectomy in simple diabetic traction detachment*

Authors	No. eyes	V.A. improved*	V.A. unchanged	V.A. worse
Blankenship[15]	168	42 (26%)	62 (37%)	63 (37%)
Tolentino et al[16]	82	50 (61%)	13 (16%)	19 (23%)
Aaberg[18]	125	90 (72%)	35 (28%)	21 (17%)
Charles[19]	341	228 (67%)	113 (33%)	
Michels and Rice	195	116 (59%)	79 (41%)	

* V.A., visual acuity

DISCUSSION

Vitreous surgery provides important new capabilities to deal with certain blinding complications of proliferative diabetic retinopathy, and the majority of these eyes can now be successfully treated. The objectives of surgery are based on the pathophysiologic changes causing visual loss; and these objectives consist of removal of intraocular opacities and/or excision of portions of vitreous gel together with the posterior vitreous surface, which is usually involved to some extent by fibrovascular tissue growth. Excising the posterior vitreous surface has the effect of relieving anteroposterior traction between the vitreous base and the posterior retina, and of relieving tangential or transverse traction between one area of posterior retina and another. By separating and/or segmenting selected epiretinal membranes, the effects of traction on the retina are further reduced, traction retinal detachment can settle postoperatively, and retinal breaks can be conveniently treated by ancillary methods. The effectiveness of the operation depends on the extent to which these objectives can be achieved. A successful result with improved vision is achieved in 50 to 75% of eyes. The level of postoperative vision depends on the amount of permanent retinal damage from the proliferative tissue, the extent of intraretinal vascular abnormalities, and any effects from hemosiderosis.

A successfully completed vitrectomy also has an important beneficial effect on the further course of the posterior segment condition. Elevated extraretinal fibrovascular proliferation does not occur when the scaffold of the posterior vitreous surface has been removed. Postoperatively, neovascularization growing along the inner retinal surface only rarely occurs (22). Therefore, the incidence of further vitreous hemorrhage is probably reduced, as is also the possibility of additional structural damage involving the retina. These features corroborate the previous clinical observation that progressive proliferative retinopathy does not occur in eyes with a posterior vitreous detachment. This suggests that the posterior vitreous surface is an obligatory scaffold for extraretinal tissue growth and is an important part of the pathophysiologic process causing visual loss (1, 2, 22).

The observation that removal of the posterior vitreous surface usually stops extraretinal fibrovascular proliferation also raises questions regarding the optimum time for surgical intervention, and the combination of vitreous surgery with retinal photocoagulation. Many operative failures are due to advanced structural changes that cannot be reversed, and earlier surgery might sometimes be more effective. On the other hand, the risks of intraoperative bleeding and postoperative rubeoisis iridis are higher when vitreous surgery is done while there is active fibrovascular proliferation in the posterior segment. Therefore, scatter retinal photocoagulation is our preferred initial treatment for eyes with early proliferative retinopathy, because it controls the neovascular process and prevents blindness in most eyes and because it is associated with only a small risk of serious complications (23-25).

When photocoagulation cannot be safely done or when severe visual loss occurs despite its use, vitreous surgery permits partial restoration of vision in most cases. Vitrectomy is now recommended for treatment of nonclearing vitreous hemorrhage of at least six months duration, and prompt surgery is considered in eyes with recent macular traction detachment, complicated combined traction and rhegmatogenous detachment, and other eyes with visual loss due to distortion of the macula or traction on the optic nerve. Although the risks of vitreous surgery are substantial, eyes with a successful result have a much improved long-term prognosis, because the operation directly alters the pathophysiologic process that is causing blinding complications (22, 26).

REFERENCES

1. Davis MD (1965): Vitreous contraction in proliferative diabetic retinopathy. Arch Ophthalmol 74:741-751.
2. Michels RG (1978): Vitrectomy for complications of diabetic retinopathy. Arch Ophthal. 96:237-246.
3. Machemer R (1978): Pathogenesis of proliferative neovascular retinopathies and the role of vitrectomy: A hypothesis. Int Ophthalmol 1:1-3.
4. Michels RG (1981): Indications and results, In: Vitreous Surgery. St. Louis: The C.V. Mosby Co., pp. 21-227.
5. Foos RY, Kreiger AE, Porsythe AB and Zakka KA (1980): Posterior vitreous detachment in diabetic subjects. Ophthalmology 87:122-128.
6. Takahashi M, Trempe CL, Maguire K, and McMeel JW (1981): Vitreoretinal relationship in diabetic retinopathy. Arch Ophthalmol 99:241-245.
7. Blankenship G, Cortez R and Machemer R (1979): The lens and pars plana vitrectomy for diabetic retinopathy complications. Arch Ophthalmol 97:1263-1267.

8. Rice TA, Michels RG, Maguire MG and Rice EF (1983): The effect of lensectomy on the incidence of iris neovascularization and neovascular glaucoma after vitrectomy for diabetic retinopathy. Am J Ophthalmol 95:1-11.

9. Benson WE, Blankenship GW and Machemer R (1977): Pars plana lens removal with vitrectomy. Am J Ophthalmol 84:150-152.

10. Charles S, White J, Dennis C and Eichenbaum D (1976): Bimanual, bipolar intraocular diathermy. Am J Ophthalmol 81:101-102.

11. Meredith TA, Kaplan HJ and Aaberg TM (1980): Pars plana vitrectomy techniques for relief of epiretinal traction by membrane segmentation. Am J Ophthalmol 89:408-413.

12. Charles S (1977): Fluid-gas exchange in the vitreous cavity. Ocutome Newsletter 2(2):1.

13. Michels RG (1981): Surgical objectives and techniques, In: Vitreous Surgery, St. Louis: The C.V. Mosby Co., pp. 176-192.

14. Machemer R and Aaberg TM (1979): Posterior segment indications, In: Vitrectomy (ed 2). New York. Grune & Stratton, pp. 120-123.

15. Charles S: Vitreous Microsurgery. Baltimore: Williams and Wilkins Co. (in press).

16. Peyman GA, Huamonte FU, Goldberg MF et al (1978): Four hundred consecutive pars plana vitrectomies with the Vitrophage. Arch Ophthalmol 96:45-50.

17. Blankenship G (1979): Pars plana vitrectomy for diabetic retinopathy: A report of eight years's experience. Mod Prob Ophthalmol 20:376-386.

18. Tolentino FI, Freeman HM and Tolentino FL (1980): Closed Vitrectomy in the management of diabetic traction retinal detachment. Ophthalmology 87:1078-1089.

19. Machemer R and Blankenship G (1981): Vitrectomy for proliferative retinopathy associated with vitreous hemorrhage. Ophthalmology 88:643-646.

20. Aaberg TM (1981): Pars plana vitrectomy for diabetic traction retinal detachment. Ophthalmology 88:639-642.

21. Charles S (1980): Vitrectomy for retinal detachement. Trans Ophthalmol Soc UK 100:542-549.

22. Rice TA and Michels RG (1980): Long-term anatomic and functional results of vitrectomy for diabetic retinopathy. Am J Ophthalmol 90:297-303.

23. The Diabetic Retinopathy Study Research Group (1976): Preliminary report of effects of photocoagulation therapy. Am J Ophthalmol 81:383-396.

24. The Diabetic Retinopathy Study Research Group (1978): Photocoagulation treatment of proliferative diabetic retinopathy: The second report of diabetic retinopathy study findings. Ophthalmology 85:82-106.

25. The Diabetic Retinopathy Study Research Group (1979): Four risk factors for severe visual loss in diabetic retinopathy. Arch Ophthalmol 97:654-655.

26. Blankenship G (1981): Stability of pars plana vitrectomy results for diabetic retinopathy complications. Arch Ophthalmol 99:1009-1012.

Basic and advanced vitreous surgery
G.W. Blankenship, M. Stirpe, M. Gonvers, S. Binder (eds.)
Fidia Research Series, vol. II,
Liviana Press, Padova © 1986

REMOVAL OF FIBROVASCULAR DIABETIC MEMBRANES

Mario Stirpe and Bernardo Billi

Fondazione Oftamologica 'G.B. Bietti', Piazza Sassari, 5, Roma

The biggest problem in the surgery of advanced proliferative diabetic retinopathy with tractional retinal detachment concerns the removal of the fibrovascular membranes at the apex of the vitreal cone that exerts traction on the retina. These membranes can at times be very limited; this happens when there has been a precocious posterior vitreous detachment. In this case, after the vitreal cone has been removed and the point of the adhesion between the vitreous cortex and the membrane is cut, the retina returns to a flattened position. Sometimes, however, the epiretinal proliferations are very extensive and very closely attached to the underlying retina. This happens in cases in which there has been no posterior vitreous detachment or when such a posterior vitreous detachment has occured later and to a more limited degree (1,2). In these cases, the epicenter of the proliferation is usually in the optic disc or between the paramacular vascular arcades. In the latter cases, fibrovascular proliferations can extend bridge-like between the two arcades or remain attached to the central part of the retina (1,2,3). In these areas, if the detachment is not too old, the retina is sufficiently resistent. A new adhesion of the retina can be obtained by dividing the epiretinal tissues into small islands corresponding to the original fibrovascular stem (segmentation technique), (1,2,4,5), or by removing the epiretinal tissues completely.

This can be done by carefully elevating the epiretinal tissues and cutting with vitreal, angle-shaped micro-scissors that cut horizontally all the connections between epiretinal proliferations and the underlying retina (delamination technique) (3).

The segmentation technique has the advantage of reducing the risk of the operation by shortening the duration of the surgery, but there is the possibility of further retinal detachment due to tangential traction or further bleeding because of incomplete closure of new vessels.

The delamination technique, because it permits the complete removal of the epiretinal membranes, has the advantage that it offers a more stable retinal adhesion,

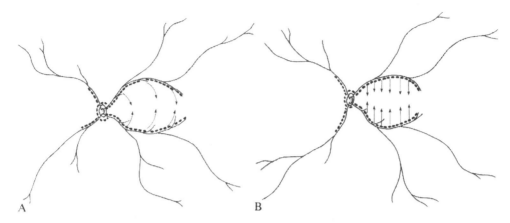

Figure 1. Fibrovascular membranes frequently originate at the optic disc and at the paramacular vascular arcades, and can extend either bridge-like between the two arcades (a) or along the central retina (b).

lessens the risk of further bleeding, and allows precocious post-operative photocoagulation, but it has all the general risks of protracted surgery.

Fibrovascular proliferations can be present also in superior temporal and nasal, and inferior nasal post-equatorial regions. This happens in cases of long-standing diabetic

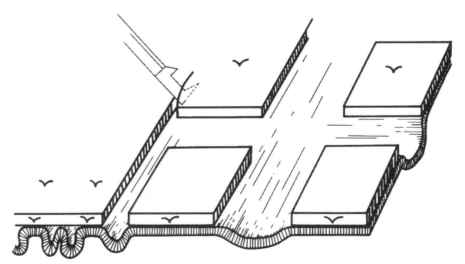

Figure 2. Segmentation technique.

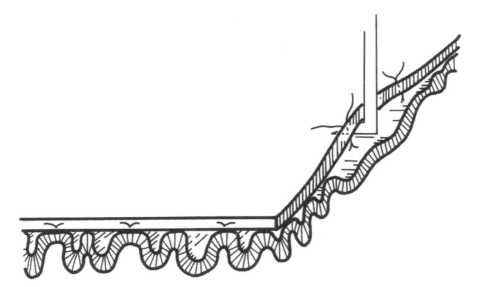

Figure 3. Delamination technique.

fibrovascular proliferations. In these cases the retinal detachment frequently occurs initially in these regions. The membranes are of particularly fibrous consistency and strongly attached to the retina; the underlying retina is extremely fragile.

When this condition is present in the nasal region, a segmentation of the mem-

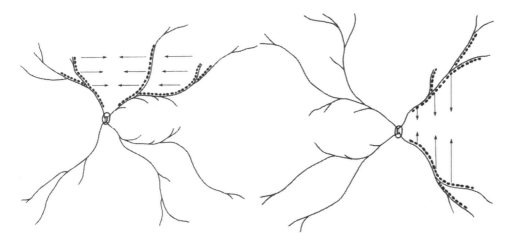

Figure 4. Fibrovascular proliferations can be present also in superior temporal and nasal, and inferior nasal post-equatorial regions.

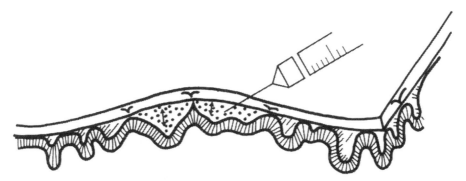

Figure 5. Fibrovascular membranes can be elevated by introducing a viscoelastic substance between the retina and the epiretinal membranes.

branes with the scleral buckle is sufficient to release any traction on the optic nerve head and on the macular area. When the proliferation is in the post-equatorial area of the superior quadrant, on the contrary, total removal of the membranes or a more complete segmentation of them is necessary because the membranes are directly connected to the temporal superior vascular arcades and exert traction on the macular area.

It is frequently difficult to remove fibrovascular membranes that are closely connected to the retina; the underlying retina is very fragile and the areas adjacent to the elevated retina are frequently anchored to the underlying planes by the scars of previous photocoagulative treatments. Also, very little traction can cause a retinal break in the underlying area or at the level of the border between the elevated retina and the photocoagulative scars.

A good method for elevating epiretinal membranes is to push the retina towards the posterior plane while the membranes are pushed in an anterior direction. This can be done by introducing a viscoelastic substance between the retina and the epiretinal membranes.

For this surgical procedure we use a pneumatic syringe controlled by a foot-switch connected to a needle for lymphatic vessels and bent at the apex at a right angle (6).

When a sufficiently large portion of the membrane has been detached, the connections between the retina and the membrane are cut.

The substance used for the detachment of membranes is IAL (sodium hyaluronate; P.M. between 500,000 and 730,000; intrinsic viscosity 10-13 dl/g, produced by Fidia Pharmaceutics).

REFERENCES

1. Machemer R, Aaberg TM (1979): Posterior segment indications. In: Vitrectomy (2 ed) New York, Grune & Stratton, pp. 71-75.
2. Michels RG (1981): Indications and results. In: Vitreous Surgery, St Louis, C V Mosby Co, pp. 21-227.

3. Charles S (1981): Proliferative Diabetic Retinopathy. In: Vitreous Microsurgery, Baltimore, Williams & Wilkins, pp. 107-118.
4. Blankenship G (1979): Pars plana vitrectomy for diabetic retinopathy: A report of eight years experience, Mod Prob Ophthalmol, 20:376-386.
5. Meredith TA, Koplan HJ, Aaberg TM (1980): Pars plana vitrectomy techniques for relief of epiretinal traction by membrane segmentation, Am J Ophthalmol, 89:408-413.
6. Stirpe M: Pneumatic Syringe Used in the Surgery of Fibrovascular Membranes, Amer J Ophth, in press.

Basic and advanced vitreous surgery
G.W. Blankenship, M. Stirpe, M. Gonvers, S. Binder (eds.)
Fidia Research Series, vol. II,
Liviana Press, Padova © 1986

ARGON LASER ENDOPHOTOCOAGULATION

Maurice B. Landers III

Department of Ophthalmology, Duke University Medical Center,
Durham, North Carolina, U.S.A.

Argon laser photocoagulation has been demonstrated to be useful in the treatment of diabetic retinopathy, retinal breaks and rubeosis iridis. Many individuals who undergo vitreous surgery can benefit from photocoagulation at that time to treat retinal breaks or proliferative diabetic retinopathy. It is possible that such photocoagulation may prevent neovascular glaucoma in some cases.

The first successful surgical endophotocoagulation system was designed by Charles. He used the O'Malley xenon arc portable photocoagulator attached to a specially designed fiber optics probe (1). The use of this endophotocoagulator provided the ability to precisely localize treatment to specific lesions, to treat posterior retinal breaks at the time of vitreous surgery, and to avoid the problem of having to carry out photocoagulation through the hazy ocular media in the immediate post-operative period. However, this photocoagulation system, using a xenon light source, had several short-comings. Excessive heat was generated within the optical system and damaged the fiber optics probe. It was difficult to routinely use the probe in an air-filled eye. Finally, the white light produced a wide angle of beam divergence at the probe tip requiring the probe to be held near the retina for good photocoagulation treatment. In some places this resulted in retinal damage from the probe tip itself.

Nevertheless, the advantages of endophotocoagulation were clear. An endophotocoagulation system permitted pan-retinal photocoagulation at the time of vitrectomy, rather than at some future time. A well-controlled system permitted photocoagulation burns involving only the outer portions of the retina including the retinal pigment epithelium. Thus selected burns could be made which did not involve the overlying nerve fiber unlike endodiathermy treatment.

With the above characteristics in mind, an argon laser intraocular photocoagulation system was designed and tested in the laboratory. This system was subsequently used in a series of patients (2). This argon laser endophotocoagulation system used a standard argon laser connected to a 12 foot long, sterilizable fiber optics cable with a 20 gauge metallic probe tip. The fiber optics cable was of a very low light-loss variety so that an insignificant amount of the laser power was lost in passing through the cable.

The water-cooled argon laser produces a beam of 1.5 mm in diameter and a beam divergence of approximately 0.65 millirad. With the 20 gauge probe inside the eye and the 50 micron fiber optic filament in the center of the probe, a spot size of approximately 3 mm is produced when the end of the fiber optic probe is 1 cm away from a flat target and a 300 micron spot when the probe is 1 mm from the target. The fiber optics probe can be held as far as several millimeters from the retina and still produce a retinal burn. This has increased the safety factor of endophotocoagulation considerably.

The system was initially tested in experimental animals. The retina of the monkey was treated with an exposure time of 0.2 seconds and varying spot sizes. As the tip was removed from proximity to the retina, the spot grew in size. The system allows rapid photocoagulation with laser lesions being delivered at a rate of 2 per second easily.

The argon laser endophotocoagulation lesions in the experimental animal were examined by light microscopy and compared with lesions made in a similar part of the retina of the same animal using the standard clinical argon laser photocoagulation system with a beam passing through the cornea and lens to reach the retina. The histologic appearance of the two types of laser photocoagulation burns was noted to be identical. The clinical appearance of the laser photocoagulation burns, both in the experimental animal and in the human patients, was identical in the post-operative period for standard external clinical photocoagulation treatment and endophotocoagulation.

Visualization of the retina in clinical argon laser endophotocoagulation can be carried out in both phakic and aphakic fluid-filled eyes using the standard infusion operating contact lens. Visualization of the retina in a completely gas-filled aphakic eye can be achieved without an operating contract lens by using the operating microscope alone. In the phakic eye filled with gas, visualization of the retina requires a special high minus contact lens of approximately 93 diopteres on the surface of the cornea (3).

Endophotocoagulation of the far peripheral retina is aided by the use of a prism-shaped corneal contact lens. Using this rotating contact lens and alternating the endophotocoagulation probe in different ports of a multiport vitrectomy system, it is possible to carry out extensive endophotocoagulation involving essentially the entire mid-peripheral and peripheral retina.

SUMMARY

An argon laser endophotocoagulation system has been developed which allows rapid, precise, accurate photocoagulation to be carried out at the time of vitreous surgery. This can be done safely with the probe being a significant distance from the retina if necessary. Photocoagulation can be carried out in fluid-filled or air-filled eyes without damage to the equipment. With the use of supplemental contact lenses, complete pan-retinal photocoagulation can be carried out rapidly during the time of vitreous surgerey in both fluid-filled and air-filled eyes, whether phakic or aphakic.

REFERENCES

1. Charles S (1981): Endophotocoagulation, William and Wilkins, Baltimore, Md, pp. 82-96.
2. Landers MB, Trese MT, Stefansson E and Bessler M (1982): Ophthalmology 89 (7):785-788.
3. Landers MB, Stefansson E and Wolbarsht MT (1981): American Journal of Ophthalmology, 91: 611-614.
4. Tolentino F, Freeman H and Schepens C (1972): Observation and Illumination System for Closed Vitreous Surgery. In: Freeman HM, Hirose F and Schpens C (eds.): Vitreous Surgery and Advances in Fundus Diagnosis and Treatment. Appleton-Century Crofts, New York, p. 139.

Basic and advanced vitreous surgery
G.W. Blankenship, M. Stirpe, M. Gonvers, S. Binder (eds.)
Fidia Research Series, vol. II,
Liviana Press, Padova © 1986

CATARACT WITH RUBEOSIS IRIDIS: ITS TREATMENT

Severino Fruscella, Piero Lischetti, Mario Stirpe

Fondazione Oftalmologica 'G.B. Bietti', Piazza Sassari, 5,Roma

Rubeosis iridis, with or without ocular hypertension, is a frequent complication in vascular diseases of the retina.

The hypoxia of ocular tissues that results from serious vascular diseases of the retina is the most frequently accepted cause of this complication.

Photocoagulative treatments of the retina performed in order to ablate non-perfused tissue and to improve perfusion of the remaining retina can lead in many cases to a lessening of the rubeosis.

When a significant cataract is present, however, posterior photocoagulative treatment is not possible. Direct photocoagulation of vessel neoformation in the iris is not beneficial because the neovascularization recurs quickly.

On the other hand, extraction of the cataract, when new vessels are present in the iris, leads to recurring anterior hemorrhages.

The use of intraocular, bimanual, bipolar diathermy on eyes that may still have some visual function allows the closing of the new vessels of the iris at the time of surgery, the removal of a large section of the iris, and the extraction of the cataract (Fig. 1).

In order to prevent bleeding during the resection of the iris and the extraction of the cataract, the new vessels must be cauterized around the entire pupillary border, along the meridians of 2:00 and 10:00 o'clock, and along the base of the iris between these two meridians (Fig. 2).

This is done in order to avoid traction on the pupillary border, and so that the incision follows the points of the previous cauterization (Fig. 3).

The closing of the vessels of the pupillary border must be done with the anterior chamber closed.

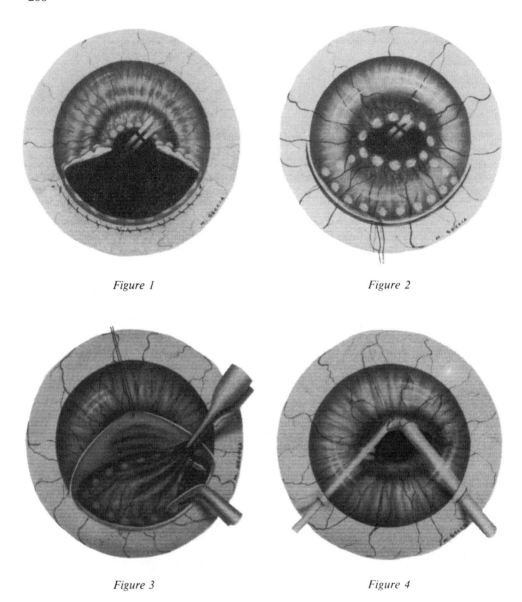

Figure 1   *Figure 2*

Figure 3   *Figure 4*

TECHNIQUES

Two electrodes are introduced, one of which is a needle that injects fluid continuously in order to avoid any possibility of contact with the corneal endothelium (Fig. 4).

The passage of the current between the two electrodes permits complete closure of the newly formed vessels (Fig. 5).

Cauterization of the vessels at the base of the iris is performed with the anterior chamber open (Fig. 6).

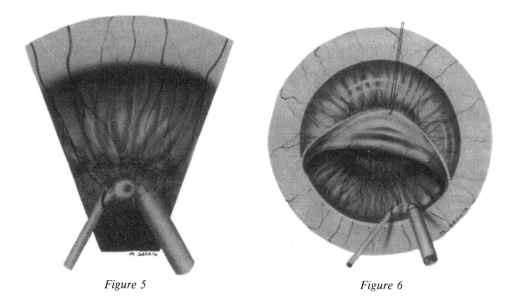

Figure 5   Figure 6

It has been noted that cauterization of the iris can cause lesions on the anterior capsule of the underlying lens. The extraction of the cataract is therefore performed according to the extracapsular technique. It is preferable to extract the nucleus by means of a hook or cryo because expression of the nucleus can cause bleeding. A vitrectomy can be performed after this procedure, if there is significant blood in the vitreous or a traction retinal detachment.

Basic and advanced vitreous surgery
G.W. Blankenship, M. Stirpe, M. Gonvers, S. Binder (eds.)
Fidia Research Series, vol. II,
Liviana Press, Padova © 1986

LONG TERM DIABETIC RETINOPATHY VITRECTOMY RESULTS: 10 YEARS FOLLOW-UP

George W. Blankenship and Robert Machemer, M.D.

The Bascom Palmer Eye Institute
University of Miami School of Medicine, Miami, Florida
and
Duke University Eye Center
Duke University School of Medicine, Durham, North Carolina

Since the development of pars plana vitrectomy (1) this procedure has become the standard from of treatment for dense non-clearing vitreous hemorrhages, and traction retinal detachments involving the macula caused by diabetic retinopathy. This report concerns the visual and anatomical results 10 years following vitrectomy for diabetic retinopathy.

MATERIALS AND METHODS

Between 1970 and 1973, 202 pars plana vitrectomies for complications of diabetic retinopathy were performed by the full time faculty of the Bascom Palmer Eye Institute. Many of these procedures involved patients with severe diabetic medical problems, and unfortunately there was a substantial mortality rate with 101 (50%) of the patients having died within 10 years of the vitrectomy. Some eyes became phthisical and painful and 14 (8%) were enucleated; 15 (7%) cases were lost to follow-up. The remaining 72 (35%) patients were available for 10 year follow-up examinations and are the subject of this report.

Information regarding the patients, and findings of their eye examinations preoperatively, 6 months, 2 years, 5 years, and 10 years following vitrectomy were recorded and computerized.

RESULTS

The main indication for vitrectomy for this series was dense nonclearing vitreous hemorrhage which involved 52 (72%) of the 72 cases, with 16 (22%) having traction detachments involving the macula, and the remaining 4 (6%) having both vitreous hemor-rhage and macular detachments.

During the 10 years following vitrectomy most of the cases did not require additional surgery, but within 6 months of vitrectomy, 8 (11%) had scleral buckles, 4 (5%) had glaucoma operations, and 1 (1%) had photocoagulation. Between 6 months and 5 years of the vitrectomy an additional 3 (4%) had scleral buckles, 1 (1%) had glaucoma surgery, 3 (4%) had cataract extractions, 3 (4%) had vitreous cavity washouts for recurrent hemorrhage, and 1 (1%) had photocoagulation. Two (3%) additional eyes had cataract surgery between the 5 and 10 year follow-up examinations.

The levels of visual acuity at the preoperative, 6 month, 5 year, and 10 year follow-up examinations are shown in Table 1. The visual results comparing the preoperative and 10 year follow-up examinations are shown in Figure 1 with 42% of the eyes maintaining 6/60 or better visual acuity.

Table 1. *Diabetic vitrectomy visual acuities (72 cases)*

	Prep op	6 mths	5 year	10 year
6/6 - 6/12	3%	7%	13%	14%
6/15 - 6/60	7%	49%	37%	28%
6/90 - 1/60	23%	18%	13%	11%
H.M. - L.P.	67%	21%	11%	17%
N.L.P.		5%	26%	30%

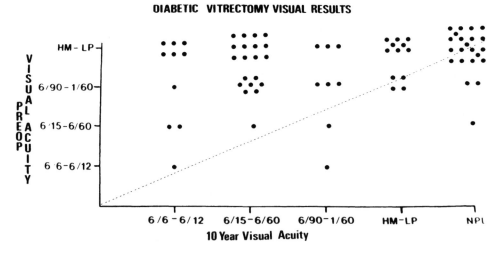

Figure 1. Scattergram showing the preoperative visual acuities and the 10 year visual acuities for each of the 72 eyes. Each dot represents one eye. Dots above the diagonal line had improved visual acuities, dots below the diagonal line had worse final visual acuities, and dots on the diagonal line had unchanged visual acuities.

After the 6 month follow-up examination, the visual acuities were fairly stable with 9 (13%) of the 72 cases having further improvement in vision, 29 (40%) maintaining the same level of acuity, but 38 (47%) having poorer vision at 10 years (Figure 2). Most of the cases with improved vision at 10 years compared to 6 months had gradual clearing of residual vitreous cavity blood or cataract surgery following the 6 month examination. The unsuccessful cases with dramatic loss of vision between the two examinations usually had only hand movements or light perception acuity at 6 months and subsequently became blind and phthisical. An obvious cause for more subtle loss of vision following the 6 month examination was usually not apparent but was probably related to increased retinal and disc ischemia from occlusive vascular problems.

Most of the cases did not develop iris neovascularization during the 10 year follow-up period, but this did involve the pupil of 3 (4%) cases, and the peripheral iris and angle of an additional 16 (27%) cases. Lens removal was a frequent component of the procedures due to preexisting lens opacities and to improve the clearing rate of recurrent vitreous hemorrhage. Iris neovascularization occurred much more frequently in the aphakic eyes and usually developed within the first 6 months after vitrectomy.

Most of the cases (64%) did not have glaucoma at any of the follow-up examinations, but 11 developed neovascular glaucoma as a complication of the iris and angle neovascularization, usually occurring within 6 months of the vitrectomy and involving aphakic eyes as shown in Table 2. The eyes with iris neovascularization and glaucoma subsequently became phthisical and blind, usually following the 2 or 5 year follow-up

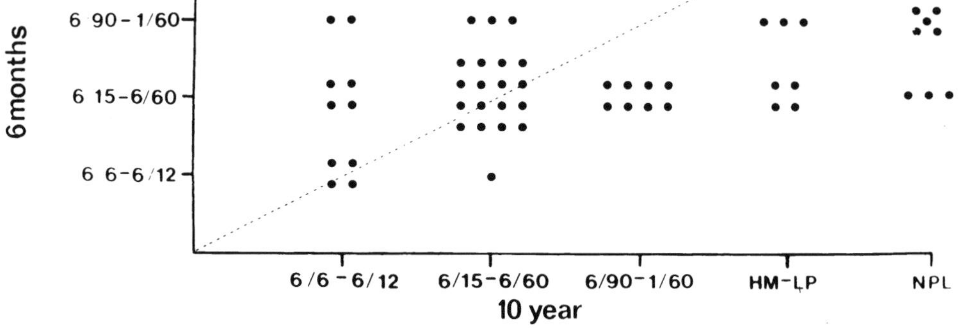

Figure 2. Scattergram showing the 6 month postvitrectomy visual acuities, and the 10 year postvitrectomy visual acuities for each of the 72 eyes. Each dot represents one eye. Dots above the diagonal line had improved visual acuities, dots below the diagonal line had worse visual acuities, and dots on the diagonal line had unchanged visual acuities.

Table 2. *Diabetic vitrectomy glaucoma (72 cases)*

	Neovascular glaucoma	Open angle glaucoma
ONSET FOLLOWING VITRECTOMY		
0-6 months	9	4
6m-2 years	2	4
5-10 years		8
LENS STATUS		
Phakic	1	1
Aphakic	10	15

examinations. An additional 16 eyes developed open angle glaucoma which tended to occur during the later follow-up period, was usually medically controlled, and again almost exclusively involved aphakic eyes.

At the end of vitrectomy 20 eyes were phakic with 5 (25%) remaining clear at the 10 year follow-up examination, an additional 5 had lenses removed during the 10 years, and the remaining 10 developed cataracts usually in conjunction with more serious problems such as neovascular glaucoma and retinal detachment which would prevent visual improvement with cataract surgery.

Most of the eyes with extensive iris neovascularization underwent phthisis with opacification of the cornea and anterior segment obscuring the posterior segment structures in many cases. The large majority of vitreous cavities remained clear as shown in Table 3, and 83% of the vitreous cavities that were clear at 6 months continued to be clear at 10 years; 1 (3%) became opaque, and the remaining 8 (14%) were obscured by corneal and anterior segment opacities.

The retinas usually remained attached as shown in Table 4, but unfortunately anterior segment opacities obscured the retinas in a large number of the cases at 5 and 10 years following vitrectomy.

None of the 72 cases were observed to have any recurrent neovascular proliferation of the discs or retinas during the 10 year follow-up period.

Table 3. *Diabetic vitrectomy vitreous cavity (72 cases)*

	Pre op	6 mths	5 year	10 year
CLEAR	22%	81%	71%	67%
OPAQUE	78%	7%	1%	3%
OBSCURED		12%	28%	30%

Table 4. *Diabetic vitrectomy retinal status (72 cases)*

	Pre op	6 mths	5 year	10 year
ATTACHED	47%	63%	64%	64%
PERIMACULAR DETACHMENT	25%	8%	6%	1%
MACULAR DETACHMENT	18%	4%		1%
TOTAL DETACHMENT	10%	7%	1%	1%
OBSCURED		18%	29%	33%

DISCUSSION

The vitrectomy procedures in this series were performed during the start of pars plana vitreous surgery, during a time of rapidly changing instrumentation and techniques (1, 2). Various aspects of these cases have been previously reported such as a general description of the cases (3), the surgical complications (4), and the 5 year findings (5). This series is quite similar to the initially successful cases reported by Rice and Michels (6) with most of the complications occurring within the first 6 months of surgery, and good stability of the visual results during the follow-up period.

Improvements in vision following the 6 month examination was usually due to further clearing of vitreous cavity hemorrhages and in a few cases from cataract extraction. Loss of vision when severe was related to further deterioration of unsuccessful cases which subsequently became phthisical and blind. When there was only a mild deterioration of vision an obvious cause was usually not apparent and presumably was caused by gradual progressing ischemia and atrophy by the vasoocclusive component of diabetes.

The rapid developement of iris neovascularization and neovascular glaucoma in association with aphakia has been previously reported (7, 8), but the more gradual development of open angle glaucoma in aphakic eyes in less known. This late development of glaucoma stresses the importance of regular follow-up examinations, and hopefully these cases will continue to be medically controlled.

The successful clearing of the vitreous cavities and reattachments of the retinas, and the stability of these successful anatomical results without additional neovascular proliferation occurring, again documents the tremendous contribution of pars plana vitreous surgery in regaining good visual function for patients previously blinded by diabetic retinopathy.

REFERENCES

1. Machemer R (1972): A new concept for vitreous surgery. 2. Surgical technique and complications. Am J Ophthalmol, 74:1022-3.
2. Parel JM, Machemer R, Aumayr W (1974): A new concept for vitreous surgery. 4. Improvements in instrumentation and illumination. Am J Ophthalmol, 77:6-12.
3. Mandelcorn MS, Blankenship G, Machemer R (1976): Pars plana vitrectomy for the management of severe diabetic retinopathy. Am J Ophthalmol, 81:561-70.
4. Faulborn J, Conway BP, Machemer R (1978): Surgical complications of pars plana vitreous surgery. Ophthalmol, 85:116-25.
5. Blankenship GW (1981): Stability of pars plana vitrectomy results for diabetic retinopathy complications; a comparison of five-year and six-month postvitrectomy findings. Arch Ophthalmol, 99:1099-1012.
6. Rice TA, Michels RG (1980): Long-term anatomic and functional results of vitrectomy for diabetic retinopathy. Am J Ophthalmol, 90:297-303.
7. Blankenship GW (1980): The lens influence on diabetic vitrectomy results; report of a prospective randomized study. Arch Ophthalmol, 98:2196-2198.
8. Rice TA, Michels RG, Maquire MG, Rice EF (1983): The effect of lensectomy on the incidence of iris neovascularization and neovascular glaucoma after vitrectomy for diabetic retinopathy. Am J Ophthalmol, 95:1-11.

Basic and advanced vitreous surgery
G.W. Blankenship, M. Stirpe, M. Gonvers, S. Binder (eds.)
Fidia Research Series, vol. II,
Liviana Press, Padova © 1986

MANAGEMENT OF POSTVITRECTOMY DIABETIC VITREOUS HEMORRHAGE

George W. Blankenship, M.D.

The Bascom Palmer Eye Institute
University of Miami School of Medicine, Miami, Florida

Following diabetic vitrectomy the vitreous cavity can become hazy and opaque with blood. The postvitrectomy vitreous cavity blood can originate from dispersion of residual previtrectomy blood released by the peripheral formed vitreous skirt, or from additional bleeding following vitrectomy from various sources such as residual fundus neovascularization, pars plana entry sites, and iris neovascularization. In most cases an obvious source of this blood cannot be identified.

Vitreous cavity blood following vitrectomy not only interferes with visual function but also prevents adequate fundus examination and laser treatment, if indicated. Good visual and anatomical results can often be obtained by removal of this additional blood. Two procedures have been used successfully and are described.

MATERIALS AND METHODS

Through 1982, the full time faculty of the Bascom Palmer Eye Institute performed 66 vitreous cavity washout procedures for vitreous cavity hemorrhage with attached retinas confirmed by echography which developed following diabetic vitrectomy. Six month follow-up information was available on 62 (94%) cases with 1 patient having died, 1 eye having been enucleated for neovascular glaucoma, and the remaining 2 cases having been lost to follow-up.

In 1983 and 1984, 27 additional eyes with postvitrectomy hemorrhage and attached retinas were managed with an outpatient air fluid vitreous cavity exchange. Six month follow-up information was available on 19 of these cases as the remaining 8 were performed within the last 6 months.

Information regarding the patients' general characteristics, past ophthalmic and medical histories, best corrected visual functions, and ophthalmic findings with slit lamp microscopy, gonioscopy, funds contact lenses, and indirect ophthalmoscopy were recorded at the preoperative and 6 month follow-up examination. Data regarding the operative procedures, complications, and findings were also recorded. All of the findings were computerized.

VITREOUS CAVITY LAVAGE TECHNIQUE

The postvitrectomy lavage of the vitreous cavity was performed as described by Machemer (1). The procedure was performed in the operating room with retrobulbar anesthesia. Small conjunctival and Tenon's incisions were made over the 10 and 2 o'clock pars planas, and the globe was entered through these sites with a myringotomy blade. Two 20 gauge hypodermic needles were then inserted with each connected to a short segment of infusion tubing with one being connected to an infusion line and elevated bottle of infusion fluid. The infusion fluid entered the vitreous cavity through one hypodermic needle allowing vitreous cavity fluid and blood to egress through the other. Once the egressing vitreous cavity fluid was clear, the infusion line was switched to the egressing needle and tubing permitting subsequent vitreous cavity fluid to egress from the original infusing needle allowing better washing of the opposite wall of the vitreous cavity. Once the egressing vitreous cavity fluid was clear, the fundus was examined with a fundus contact lens and a 20 gauge fiberoptic light source which replaced the egressing 20 gauge needle.

Transvitreal diathermy and/or photocoagulation can be used to treat any apparent source of hemorrhage. Once hemostasis has been obtained, the instruments are removed and the sclerotomy sites closed with interrupted absorbable suture. Conjunctiva and Tenon's are closed, a sterile dressing is applied, and the patient is instructed to keep his head elevated in hope of preventing further bleeding.

POSTVITRECTOMY VITREOUS CAVITY HEMORRHAGE AIR/FLUID EXCHANGE

In the outpatient clinic under topical or retrobulbar anesthesia, a lid speculum is inserted and the patient is placed on their side with the temporal pars plana being most dependent. A 10cc syringe with a 23 gauge 5/8 inch needle is partially filled with 5cc of filtered air. The surgeon is comfortably positioned beneath the patient's head, and the globe is entered by inserting the 23 gauge needle through conjunctiva-sclera-pars plana 3mm peripheral to the limbus in a direction towards the optic disc.

One-half cc of air is injected into the vitreous cavity, and 1/2cc of bloody vitreous fluid is aspirated into the syringe accumulating in the more dependent portion of the syringe with the air rising superiorly. The exchange proceeds with alternating injections of 1/2cc of air and aspiration of 1/2cc of bloody fluid with the needle slowly being withdrawn from the dependent temporal pars plana until a complete exchange has been accomplished. A sterile dressing is applied, and the patient returns home with instructions to keep the head elevated. A follow-up examination the next day reveals a large single vitreous cavity air bubble (usually about 75% of the vitreous cavity) through which panretinal laser photocoagulation with a Rodenstock panscopic fundus contact lens can be accomplished.

VITREOUS HEMORRHAGE - LAVAGE RESULTS

The best corrected visual acuity before and 6 months after vitreous cavity lavage are shown in Table 1 with good ambulating acuity being obtained in the majority of cases, and 40% having 6/60 or better acuity.

Unfortunately, 16% of the eyes became blind from further problems such as neovascular glaucoma and presumed retinal detachments.

The anatomical results of the anterior segments are compared in Table 2 and of the posterior segments in Table 3. Extensive peripheral iris neovascularization was present in 32% of the cases with 18% having neovascular glaucoma before the procedure, and was a common finding 6 months following the lavage procedure. Non-clearing

Table 1. *Diabetic vitreous hemorrhage - Lavage visual acuities (62 cases)*

	Preop	6m postop
6/6 - 6/12		8%
6/15 - 6/60		32%
6/90 - 1/60	5%	15%
H.M. - L.P.	95%	29%
N.L.P.		16%

Table 2. *Diabetic vitreous hemorrhage - Lavage anterior segment (62 cases)*

	Preop	6m postop
Iris neovascularization		
None	58%	39%
Pupil	10%	11%
Peripheral	32%	50%
Neovascular glaucoma	18%	21%
Lens		
Clear	43%	16%
Minor cataract	21%	10%
Opaque	13%	6%
Aphakic	23%	68%

Table 3. *Diabetic vitreous hemorrhage - Lavage posterior segment (62 cases)*

	Preop	6m postop
Obscured		24%
Vitreous		
Clear		64%
Opaque	100%	12%
Retina		
Attached	100%	55%
Paramac detach		7%
Total detached		2%

vitreous cavity blood is much more common in the phakic eye than in the aphakic eye as indicated in Table 2, and 45% of the eyes had lens removal through the pars plana in conjunction with the lavage procedure to try and improve the spontaneous clearing rate of any additional vitreous cavity hemorrhage. Unfortunately, many of the eyes had corneal and anterior segment opacification during the 6 month postoperative follow-up period which prevented visualization of the vitreous cavity and retina (Table 3). However, most of the vitreous cavities were clear, and the retinas attached at the 6 month examination.

VITREOUS HEMORRHAGE - AIR EXCHANGE RESULTS

Occasionally, the air/fluid exchange procedure was repeated on several occasions before the vitreous cavity remained clear. Only one air/fluid exchange was required for 12 of the 19 cases with 4 having two exchanges, 2 having three exchanges, and 1 requiring four exchanges.

The best corrected pre-exchange and 6 months post-exchange visual acuities are shown in Table 4 with the procedure only being performed when there was marked loss of vision, and good visual results being obtained in the majority of cases.

Table 4. *Diabetic vitreous hemorrhage - Air exchange visual acuities (19 cases)*

	Pre exch.	6m post exch.
6/6 - 6/12		5
6/15 - 6/60		7
6/90 - 1/60	5	3
H.M. - L.P.	14	2
N.L.P.		2

Pre-exchange peripheral iris neovascularization was present in 5 of the eyes (2 phakic and 3 aphakic), and in 7 of the eyes 6 months following the exchange. Neovascular glaucoma had occurred in 4 of the 7 eyes during the 6 months following exchange.

Of the 19 cases, 3 were aphakic, and the remaining 16 had relatively clear lenses. Six months following the exchange, 10 of the 16 lenses remained clear, 3 had developed moderate opacities, and the remaining 3 could not be visualized because of corneal and anterior segment opacities.

Before the exchange all of the vitreous cavities were opaque preventing fundus examinations by indirect ophthalmoscopy, but 6 months following the exchange 14 of the vitreous cavities were clear, 2 remained opaque with vitreous hemorrhage, and anterior segment opacities obscured the vitreous cavity in the remaining 3 cases. Prior to the exchange, all of the retinas had been confirmed to be attached by echography. Six months following the exchange 14 of the retinas were completely attached with the remaining 5 being obscured by vitreous cavity and anterior segment opacities and presumed posterior retinal detachments.

DISCUSSION

The vitreous cavity lavage and vitreous blood/air exchange procedures can only be performed following pars plana vitrectomy. The presence of significant formed vitreous makes it impossible to evacuate the vitreous cavity blood, and could result in extensive retinal tears and detachments from traction by incarcerating the formed vitreous into the egressing needles. Both of the procedures result in significant clearing of the vitreous cavities, but the irrigating effect of the infusion fluid during the lavage procedure tends to wash out more of the blood layered against the inner retinal surface and around the residual vitreous cavity skirt. The air/fluid exchange does not have this irrigation effect and thus may need to be repeated on several occasions to obtain a clear vitreous cavity, but extensive panretinal photocoagulation can be performed with a Rodenstock panscopic fundus contact lens through the large air bubble the day after the exchange in both the phakic and aphakic eyes.

The iris neovascularization was directly related to aphakia (2, 3) and retinal detachments (4) which occurred following both the lavage and exchange procedures. Panretinal laser photocoagulation following the procedures probably prevented a much larger number of eyes from developing iris neovascularization and associated neovascular glaucoma.

The retinal detachments which followed both the lavage and exchange procedures could have been caused by several factors such as the entry sites being located posterior to the ora serratas, or more likely incarceration of the adjacent formed vitreous in the entry sites at the end of the procedure with subsequent contraction of the formed vitreous producing adjacent retinal tears as described by Michels (4).

An obvious source for the hemorrhage which occurred following vitrectomy was not apparent in any of the cases although it was presumed to be from the preoperative iris neovascularization in some cases, and probably from the original vitrectomy sclerotomy sites, or neovascularization on the posterior iris surface and adjacent ciliary body in the remaining cases.

REFERENCES

1. Machemer R, Aaberg TM (1979): Vitrectomy: A Pars Plana Approach, ed. 2. New York, Grune and Stratton, p. 82.
2. Blankenship GW (1980): The lens influence on diabetic vitrectomy results: report of a prospective randomized study. Arch Ophthalmol, 98:2196-2198.
3. Rice TA, Michels RG, Maquire MG, Rice EF (1983): The effect of lensectomy on the incidence of iris neovascularization and neovascular glaucoma after vitrectomy for diabetic retinopathy. Am J Ophthalmol, 95:-11.
4. Michels RG (1976): Vitreoretinal and anterior segment surgery through the pars plana. Part I. Ann Ophthalmol, 8:1353-1381.

Basic and advanced vitreous surgery
G.W. Blankenship, M. Stirpe, M. Gonvers, S. Binder (eds.)
Fidia Research Series, vol. II,
Liviana Press, Padova © 1986

RETROLENTAL FIBROPLASIA:
PATHOGENESIS OF LATE STAGES

Robert Machemer

Duke University, Dept of Ophthalmology, Durham. North Carolina
(Reported by Severino Fruscella)

The late stages in retrolental fibroplasia have been described by several authors from the clinical point of view. They have been classified as:

Grade IV - Entailing vessel tortuosity in the posterior pole, equatorial retinal folds and partial detachment of the retina.

Grade V - Total and organized retinal detachment with fibrovascular proliferation

Since there is not a great deal to be found on the description of the pathogenic mechanism in the late stages of the disease, the different forms of retinopathy are to be classified according to their location and proliferative degree. The premature newborn eye shows mesenchymal tissue which develops in the shunt area posterior to the ora serrata. The tissue proliferates and gradually contracts, producing traction on the adjacent retina. The proliferation area can be differently located pre-equatorially, equatorially and post-equatorially, probably depending upon the time of oxygen exposure. The more premature the newborn, the more posteriorly is the shunt area located.

The premature retina can be subdivided into an anterior non-vascularized and a posterior vascular part. The two retinal segments respond differently to traction. The vascular retina stretches and grows gradually thinner without detachment, while the vascular retina submitted to traction usually detaches as the vascular tree offers resistance to stretching. Consequently, the clinical pictures will be quite different according to the location and the degree of stretching upon the retina. When the proliferative tissue is limited to only one quadrant, generally located on the temporal side, stretching will be exerted on the nasal avascular retina. Retinal detachment will not occur, but the temporal retina will show all the non stretchable vessels. If the mesenchymal tissue effects the whole circumference, traction will affect the whole posterior vascular retina, which cannot stretch, so that a detachment will occur (Figure 1). The avascular periphery, however, can stretch toward the centre, up to the extreme situation shown in Figure 1.

Another very important pathogenic factor is the intravitreal proliferation of mesen-

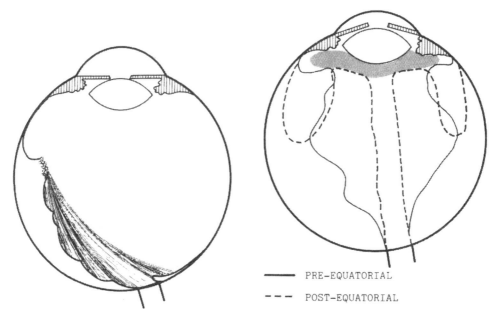

PRE—EQUATORIAL

POST—EQUATORIAL

Figure 1. If the mesenchymal tissue exerts traction on the posterior vascular retina, a detachment will occur.

Figure 2. Various stages of seriousness according to different sites of the proliferations.

chymal tissue which acts as any other connective tissue. After the usual cell-proliferating and contraction stages, it begins to deposit collagen which will give the tissue a dense white aspect. The latter is the scar stage of retrolental fibroplasia. It should be noted that for some unknown reasons, proliferation occurs towards the anterior part of the vitreous cavity, while a progressively lower density of the tissue is found toward the posterior pole. The factors affecting the development of the disease as well as the different clinical pictures are closely related to the location and the amount of proliferation of the mesenchymal tissue originating in the shunt area. Whenever the proliferation occurs in the anterior vitreous cavity, it will also affect the anterior segment because the contraction of the tissue produces a forward push of the lens and iris with subsequent shallowing of the anterior chamber, causing closed-angle glaucoma. If, on the contrary, the proliferation is located posteriorly, only a posterior retinal detachment will occur.

Basic and advanced vitreous surgery
G.W. Blankenship, M. Stirpe, M. Gonvers, S. Binder (eds.)
Fidia Research Series, vol. II,
Liviana Press, Padova © 1986

RETROLENTAL FIBROPLASIA: SURGICAL THERAPY

Robert Machemer

Duke University, Dept. of Ophthalmology, Durham, North Carolina
(Reported by Severino Fruscella)

A group of children between 5 months and 2 years of age with retrolental fibroplasia underwent closed eye vitrectomy. They had a very advanced stage of retrolental fibroplasia with severe peripheral retinal detachment and retrolental membranous formation together with fibrovascular tissue proliferation into the vitreous. When the reddish fundus reflex is detectable on ophthalmoscopic examination, a shallow posterior detachment of the retina is generally present. The retina maintains its concave structure and therefore the red reflex of the fundus is still visible to ophthalmoscopic examination.

The surgical technique entails a peritomy at the limbus and two sclerotomies; one is performed 1 mm behind the limbus on the nasal side in order to allow the insertion of two instruments. The fiberoptic infusion needle is placed on one side and the vitreous cutter on the other. The lens aspiration is then carried out prior to the superior sector iridectomy which enables better visibility of the posterior structures.

The proliferative retrolental tissue is quite hard and under tension so that a pointed knife is usually more suitable for the first cut. The opening is later enlarged with the vitreous cutter. Vitreous scissors are used for radial cuts of the fibrovascular membrane. Neovascularization must undergo bipolar diathermy coagulation in order to minimize risks of haemorrhage during the operation. The deeper the instruments go, the clearer is the vitreous, so that vitrectomy and the removal of possible remnants of the hyaloid artery are made easier.

After the surgical procedure is completed there is a replacement of infusion liquid by air or by a mixture of sulfur hexafluoride (SF_6) and air. Cryotherapy is rarely applied to the peripheral retina and must take place close to the equator in order to avoid possible cyclocryotherapy even if rare. A 2 mm silicone band is tightly pulled around the eye so as to allow better retinal reattachment. Drainage of subretinal fluid is usually not implemented.

We know that spontaneous regression can occur in the early stages of retrolental fibroplasia. The problem arises regarding the exact moment when surgery should be undertaken. When only a localized retinal detachment is present, surgery is not the chosen treatment, provided that a careful surveillance of the cases is made with biweekly control examinations. There are authors who believe that it is better to place a buckle even if the retinal reattachment is likely to occur spontaneously. Whenever the peripheral retinal detachment is found circumferentially and there is membrane formation, surgery should be performed.

In order to avoid damage to the peripheral retina, the sclerotomy has to be performed close to the limbus and practically anterior to the ciliary body. Since this procedure entails the passage of the instruments through the lens, the lens must be removed even though it is transparent. Lens removal is almost always unavoidable because proliferative tissue is in immediate contact with the lens capsule.

Since the vitreous body in the newborn has a tight retinal adhesion, the vitrectomy is more difficult to perform and calls for higher precision than in adult patients in whom a posterior vitreous detachment often occurs and the vitreous is separated from the retinal plane. In the newborn eyes the remnants of the hyaloid artery are often present and are to be removed along with the surrounding vitreous.

Subretinal fluid drainage is usually useless since the retina, following the releasing of traction, reveals a natural propensity to reattach. As long as retinal holes are not present, the fluid is spontaneously reabsorbed.

The value of cryotherapy is doubtful and consequently it is not always carried out but when performed one should consider the size and anatomy of the newborn eyes in order not to affect the ciliary body.

The value of intraocular gas tamponade is also questionable, since the retina, when vitreous tractions are released and retinal holes are not present, usually reattaches spontaneously.

Fifteen eyes were operated upon with the above technique: seven had retinal reattachment with 3 to 34 months follow-up. The cases listed above had definite improvement of vision, though a precise assesment of visual acuity was impossible because of the young age of the patients, but it is likely to be low. No complications occurred in the successfully operated cases and no eye has ever shown phthisis even after unsuccessful interventions.

Basic and advanced vitreous surgery
G.W. Blankenship, M. Stirpe, M. Gonvers, S. Binder (eds.)
Fidia Research Series, vol. II,
Liviana Press, Padova © 1986

INDICATIONS AND TIMING OF VITRECTOMY IN TRAUMA

Klaus Heimann

Department for Vitreo Retinal Surgery,
University Eye Clinic, Cologne, FRG

An exact statistical evaluation and comparative investigations are exceedingly difficult in posterior segment trauma due to the large number of diverse parameters which vary from case to case. Examples of these are the extent and localization of the injury, the quality of the first repair, the distance in time between the accident event and adequate treatment of sequelae in the posterior segment, increasing negative selection of the patients, etc. The diversity of the clinical pictures resulting from this is confusing. Clinical observations in vitrectomy as well as on different injury models in animal experiments have been of decisive assistance in understanding the principles of normal and disturbed wound healing and its clinical correlates. They have enabled inferences to be made from these principles for an appropriate specific therapy.

What happens when the posterior segment suffers a penetrating injury? Animal experiments carried out mainly in Miami (Abrams, Topping and Machemer, 1979) and Los Angeles (Cleary and Ryan, 1981) give information on this. For a better overall appraisal, I should like to give a simplified description of the results of these animal experiments.

Immediately after perforation of the region of the pars plana or the retina, there is an inflammatory reaction in the vicinity of the wound. This disappears and passes into a relatively quiet phase of proliferation in which cells grow in the vicinity of the wounds and along the injury canal in the vitreous. These cells may derive from the choroid, pigment epithelium of the retina, and may form strands and membranes. These can then in turn contract by a "cell-mediated process" and lead to the feared picture of traumatic PVR retinal detachment, in which above all the proliferative alterations in the region of the base of the vitreous play a role. They lead to an annular and anterior-posterior contraction with a corresponding funnel shaped form of the retinal detachment. This feared proliferative process is stimulated above all by vitreous hemorrhages.

In animal experiments, this process can be successfully interrupted when vitrectomy is carried out in time and the scaffold for the proliferations along vitreous structures is eliminated.

We know from further animal experiments of Paulmann and Behrendt (1979) that massive vitreoretinal proliferations with corresponding deleterious consequences can also be elicited by intravitreous copper implantations.

The prognostically unfavorable traction detachment in the clinical picture of proliferative vitreoretinopathy is a threat in the clinical course of every posterior segment injury, stimulated by intraocular hemorrhages, incarcerations of the vitreous, toxic action of metal ions, chronic and acute infections, tissue contusions and inadequate wound care.

GOALS OF PARS PLANA VITRECTOMY
IN TERMS OF SURGICAL TECHNIQUE

Depending on the nature and extent of the injury, as well as the time between vitrectomy and the accident, the following objectives of the surgical technique are:

1. Removal of coaxial opacities, i.e. of traumatic cataracts or vitreous hemorrhages, in order on the one hand to improve the visual acuity and on the other hand to obtain an exact appraisal of the retinal situation with regard to retinal injuries or remaining intraocular foreign bodies. If precise measures are to be performed in these cases for prophylaxis or reattachment of a retinal detachment or removal of the foreign body under optical control, vitrectomy must be carried out beforehand. In addition, vitreous hemorrhages are to be removed in massive hemophthalmus with hemolytic glaucoma or threat of hemosiderosis (ERG control).

2. Removal of vitreoretinal proliferations, the development of which can be prevented in some cases in the vitreal space when the vitrectomy is carried out in time, so that the scaffold for the fibrous proliferations to be expected, e.g. along the trajectory canal of a foreign body, is eliminated.

3. Treatment of traumatic PVR detachment in combination with "membrane peeling", gas and possibly silicone oil injection. This is also not rare in the sense of a revitrectomy.

4. Reconstructive measures in the region of the anterior segment, removal of a traumatic cataract, prolapsed vitreous can be carried out in an elegant and safe way by means of the pars plana technique.

TIMING OF THE PARS PLANA VITRECTOMY

Clinical experience and animal experiments clearly show how decisive the choice of the correct timing of vitrectomy is for the final result. The most favorable time is generally between the first and second week after the accident. Then, a posterior vitreous detachment has mostly developed, and the vitreous itself displays a better cuttability. Moreover, the risk of an uncontrolled intraoperative hemorrhage is much less at this time than in the first week. In terms of the surgical technique, pars plana vitrectomy is hence easier to perform technically and has less risk than in the first days after the injury (Heimann et al., 1983).

However, if there is danger of bacterial contamination, e.g. after wooden foreign bodies, agricultural accidents or an acute chalcosis, vitrectomy must be carried out without delay. Postponement of the vitrectomy past the second week after the accident entails the risk of PVR detachment; when this has occurred, there is still a very unfavorable prognosis despite pars plana vitrectomy. In eye injuries which are accompanied by severe contusion damage to the intraocular tissue (ruptures, gunshot injuries), an appreciable risk of uncontrollable intraoperative hemorrhages is to be found even after two weeks, so that sometimes we exceed the two-week limit in such cases. Spontaneous resorption of a post-traumatic, noncompact vitreous hemorrhage can be waited for when the retina is attached echographically, the peripheral retina can be seen by indirect ophthalmoscopy and ERG controls exclude the danger of hemosiderosis. If the hemorrhage is still present after four months, vitrectomy must be carried out. Recently, we have gone over to performing a pars plana vitrectomy simultaneous with silicone oil filling in primary treatment in the most severe injuries (multiple gunshot injuries, air rifle bullets, ruptures with extensive scleral wounds) with practically hopeless prognosis. This is in order to stop hemorrhages and to avoid an early detachment. Experience so far reveals exceedingly positive courses in situations which were previously regarded as hopeless.

REFERENCES

1. Abrams GW, Topping TM, Machemer R (1979): Vitrectomy for injury: the effect on intraocular proliferation following perforation of the posterior segment of the rabbit eye. Arch Ophthalmol 97:743-748.
2. Cleary PE, Ryan SI (1981): Vitrectomy in penetrating eye injury. Arch Ophthalmol 99:287-292.
3. Heimann K, Paulmann H, Tavakolian U (1983): The intraocular foreign body. Principles and problems in the management of complicated cases by pars plana vitrectomy. Int Ophthalmol 6:235-242.
4. Paulmann H, Behrendt K (1979): Glaskörper und Netzhautverhalten bei experimenteller Chalcosis. Sitzungsber Rhein-Westf Augenärzte 136:43-49.

Basic and advanced vitreous surgery
G.W. Blankenship, M. Stirpe, M. Gonvers, S. Binder (eds.)
Fidia Research Series, vol. II,
Liviana Press, Padova © 1986

PENETRATING INJURIES

Ronald G. Michels, M. D.

The Vitreoretinal Service, Wilmer Ophthalmological Institute,
Johns Hopkins University School of Medicine, Baltimore, Maryland.

Principles of surgical management of posterior segment penetrating injuries are based on an understanding of the pathophysiology of secondary intraocular complications. Penetrating injuries cause varying amounts of initial mechanical damage, and this damage may be so severe that the eye cannot be salvaged. In other cases loss of vision is due mainly to secondary pathologic processes.

Secondary pathologic processes include infective endophthalmitis that can occur after any penetrating injury, including about 10% of those associated with magnetic intraocular foreign bodies. Faulty wound healing may be associated with secondary complications due to improper apposition of the wound edges or incarceration of intraocular tissue in the wound or both. The major source of severe secondary complications, however, is intraocular fibrocellular proliferation and contracture which can result in cyclitic membrane formation and/or retinal detachment.

Clinical studies have shown that penetrating injuries involving the posterior segment and combined with vitreous hemorrhage have the worst prognosis and are most likely to be followed by intraocular fibrocellular proliferation and contracture (1). Experimental animal models have also shown that penetrating injuries involving the vitreous and dense vitreous hemorrhage are the important factors followed by fibrocellular ingrowth and secondary structural complications (2-3). The main area of fibrocellular proliferation and secondary structural damage is in the region of the ciliary body and peripheral retina (Fig. 1). Efforts are made to minimize complications in this area using vitreous surgery and scleral buckling, as discussed later.

PRIMARY REPAIR OF PENETRATING INJURIES

The objectives of primary management of penetrating wounds are to: 1) provide optimum anatomic reapposition of the wound margins, 2) prevent intraocular infec-

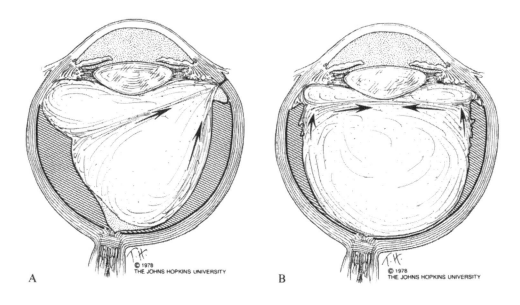

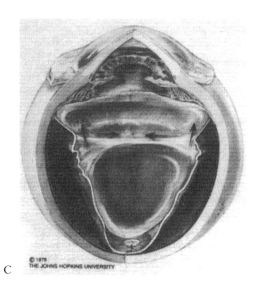

Figure 1. Pathogenetic mechanism causing total traction retinal detachment after posterior segment penetrating injury in Rhesus monkey eyes as demonstrated by Cleary and Ryan (2, 3). *A* and *B*, Condensed vitreous membrane extends to pars plana wound, and anterior portion of retina becomes detached by circumferential and posteroanterior traction from adjacent cortical vitreous and epiretinal proliferative membrane. *C*, This process may result in total funnel shaped traction retinal detachment, shown here in an aphakic eye.

tion, 3) obtain a clear pupillary space and maintain proper depth of the anterior chamber, 4) remove any reactive intraocular foreign body material and 5) minimize secondary structural complications due to fibrocellular ingrowth. Cultures are done of the conjunctiva, excised tissue, and any intraocular foreign body removed. Broad spectrum systemic antibiotics are given to reduce the risk of infection.

Thorough exploration of the globe is done at the time of initial wound repair. The conjunctiva is reflected surrounding any scleral laceration to expose the full length of the wound. The wound margins are repaired in an anteroposterior direction with 6-0 or 7-0 polyglycolic acid sutures. Sometimes larger diameter sutures are needed at selected points along the wound length to assist in reapproximating the edges if there is prominent gapping of the margins. If the wound extends to a rectus muscle insertion, careful exploration beneath and posterior to the muscle is necessary to identify and repair the full extent of the laceration.

Exogenous pressure on the globe is avoided to prevent further prolapse of intraocular tissue. It is rarely necessary to excise ciliary body or choroidal tissue which is reposited as the scleral wound is repaired. Prolapsed vitreous gel is excised, and the specimen is sent for pathologic study to determine whether retinal tissue is present.

In eyes with corneoscleral lacerations and disruption of the lens, the lens material may be removed using a vitrectomy probe through a limbal or pars plana approach after watertight closure of the laceration. However, intraocular surgery to deal with vitreous complications in either the anterior or the posterior segment is usually delayed for five to ten days after the injury. Iris tissue, vitreous gel and lens materal incarcerated in an anterior segment wound are reposited or excised by conventional methods or by using a small diameter vitrectomy instrument introduced through a limbal incision. Removal of all extraneous tissue from the posterior surface of a cornal wound is an important objective and may constitute an indication for a separate operation if this is not achieved at the time of initial repair. Air is injected into the anterior chamber at the end of the operation to minimize the possibility of recurrent adhesions to the cornea because of wound leakage during the first 24 hours.

MAGNETIC INTRAOCULAR FOREIGN BODIES

Reactive intraocular foreign bodies are usually removed at the time of initial repair of the wound. Foreign bodies located in the anterior chamber are removed through the original entry site before repair of the laceration or through a separate limbal incision. Foreign bodies within the lens and associated with significant opacities are removed by intracapsular or extracapsular cataract extraction.

Magnetic foreign bodies of small size are usually removed with a magnet. Foreign bodies of small size located in the posterior segment are removed through the adjacent sclera if the foreign body is imbedded in the retina and choroid in an accessible location further than 30 degrees from the disc or macula. Other foreign bodies are removed with a magnet through the pars plana on the opposite side of the eye to avoid possible laceration of the retina if the foreign body is extracted through the pars plana in the same meridian.

Reactive nonmagnetic intraocular foreign bodies, foreign bodies encased in a fibrous capsule, and certain other foreign bodies of unusual size, shape, composition or location may be removed with intraocular forceps, as discussed later. Alternatively, foreign bodies located in or near the eyewall anterior to the equator can be removed through the adjacent sclera using a direct grasping technique or expression by counter pressure after exact localization and creation of a proper scleral flap and incision of the uveal tissue.

VITRECTOMY

When a posterior vitrectomy is needed, a pars plana approach is used and the lens is removed if necessary. Because the lens is often soft, lens removal is usually performed without difficulty using a vitrectomy probe. Ultrasonic emulsification is used to assist in lens removal if firm material is encountered. When the anterior chamber is clear, the lens is removed only if it is cataractous or dislocated or if removal is required to permit excision of damaged anterior vitreous gel. Hyphema is usually permitted to clear spontaneously before vitrectomy to avoid sacrificing a clear lens.

The primary objectives of vitrectomy for damaged hemorrhagic vitreous gel are to clear all vitreous opacities and to remove all cortical vitreous posterior to the equator. If the posterior vitreous surface has spontaneously separated from the retina, this makes the operation easier. However, the cortical vitreous may remain adherent to the retina. In these cases a hooked needle or vitreoretinal pick is used to separate the vitreous from the retina. This may be difficult if the underlying retina is detached, and these efforts are abandoned if excessive traction seems likely to cause retinal damage. When a posterior perforation site is present, the incarcerated vitreous is cut and the surrounding cortical vitreous is removed to divide any connections between the perforation site and the retina or vitreous base elsewhere.

Intraoperative bleeding sometimes occurs in these cases, especially if vitreous surgery is perfomed during the first several days following the original injury. Active bleeding may be managed by temporarily increasing the intraocular pressure and later washing out the blood with the vitrectomy instrument. However, when possible, bleeding sites are immediately treated by intraocular diathermy. If bleeding occurs from a site that cannot be identified, it often can be stopped by performing simultaneous fluid-gas exchange to fill the vitreous cavity with a bubble and thereby tamponade the bleeding site. Later the air can be removed and replaced by irrigating solution, and the operation can proceed.

REMAINING INTRAOCULAR FOREIGN BODIES

When the mechanical objectives of vitrectomy have been achieved, any remaining intraocular foreign bodies are removed. Foreign bodies are first mobilized by removing the surrounding vitreous and lysing adhesions to the retina. If an inflammatory capsule is present, this is incised with a vitreoretinal needle or knife. If the foreign body is small and magnetic, it can be removed with a magnet through the pars plana. However, this is dangerous because the foreign body is likely to lacerate the retina if it is dropped after the vitreous is removed.

Most remaining foreign bodies, including large magnetic and reactive nonmagnetic foreign bodies, are removed with intraocular forceps (Fig. 2). After grasping the foreign body, any remaining adhesions to the retina and vitreous are cut with the vitrectomy instrument. The pars plana incision may have to be enlarged somewhat to permit withdrawal of the forceps (4). Alternatively, medium sized foreign bodies in aphakic eyes can be removed through the limbus (5). The foreign body is held in the anterior chamber and grasped with forceps introduced through a 90° limbal incision or simply passed out through the limbal wound.

RETINAL BREAKS AND DETACHMENT

Retinal breaks are treated after the vitreous gel and any intraocular foreign bodies have been removed. Retinal breaks near the macula or optic nervehead can be treated by transvitreal cryotherapy or photocoagulation or treated postoperatively by laser photocoagulation. Other retinal breaks are usually treated by transscleral cryotherapy. We prefer transvitreal drainage of subretinal fluid to flatten the retina when detachment is associated with posterior retinal breaks. Transvitreal drainage of subretinal fluid is combined with simultaneous fluid-gas exchange in aphakic eyes to fill the vitreous

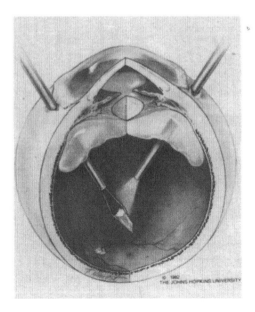

Figure 2. Removal of foreign body from posterior segment using Machemer foreign body forceps. Vitrectomy instrument is used to first remove opacities and mobilize foreign body.

cavity completely with gas in order to provide internal tamponade. In phakic eyes a smaller bubble is used because of reduced visualization during fluid-gas exchange and to avoid postoperative damage to the lens.

A scleral buckle is placed under all retinal breaks located anterior to the equator and under posterior retinal breaks associated with persistent vitreous traction or incomplete removal of the surrounding cortical vitreous. Posterior retinal breaks without persistent traction are treated with cryotherapy or photocoagulation and temporary intraocular gas tamponade.

An encircling scleral buckle is used in most cases with severe penetrating injuries involving the posterior segment. This is done to reduce the possibility of later traction or rhegmatogenous retinal detachment because of retinal breaks or fibrocellular proliferation and contraction in the area of the vitreous base (Fig. 3). A broad scleral buckle is used to support the retina between the equator and the ora serrata. This minimizes the likelihood of posterior retinal detachment due to structural complications in the anterior part of the posterior segment.

CASE SELECTION FOR VITRECTOMY

Vitreous surgery is reserved for eyes with injuries that have a poor prognosis when managed by conventional methods (6). These cases include eyes with: 1) vitreous gel, iris tissue and/or lens material incarcerated in a corneal wound, 2) a disrupted lens and mixed lens material and vitreous gel, 3) reactive, nonmagnetic foreign bodies or cer-

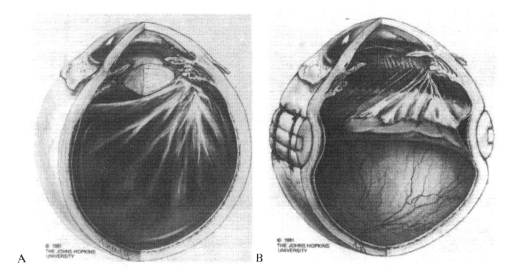

A   B

Figure 3. Combination of lensectomy, vitrectomy and peripheral scleral buckle to treat severe penetrating injury of posterior segment with dense vitreous hemorrhage, *A. B,* Broad scleral buckle supporting retina between equator and ora serrata minimizes likelihood of posterior retinal detachment due to traction from remaining anteroperipheral vitreous and secondary fibrous proliferation.

tain magnetic foreign bodies that cannot be safely removed with a magnet, 4) penetrating injuries of the posterior segment with vitreous prolapse and dense intravitreal hemorrhage, and 5) traction and/or rhegmatogenous retinal detachment with vitreous hemorrhage or severe vitreous traction. The timing of vitreous surgery is also important (7, 8). Since the objective is to minimize secondary complications, surgery should be done before these complications cause permanent structural damage. Immediate vitrectomy, performed at the time of repair of the penetrating wound, is performed when vitreous surgery methods are needed to remove reactive intraocular foreign bodies, when infective endophthalmitis is present, and when it is necessary to excise vitreous gel and extracapsular lens material from the anterior segment and pupillary space after repair of the corneal laceration.

In other cases, vitreous surgery is performed as a secondary procedure five to seven days after the injury if vitreous gel remains incarcerated in a central corneal wound or if lens material and vitreous gel in the pupillary space are likely to cause a secondary membrane. Posterior vitrectomy is performed five to 10 days after the injury in eyes with severe penetrating injuries of the vitreous and vitreous hemorrhage, double perforating injuries with severe vitreous hemorrhage, and cases with dense vitreous opacities and retinal detachment.

Delaying vitreous surgery for five to 10 days, rather than performing the operation at the time of initial repair of the penetrating wound, permits further diagnostic evaluation and allows the operation to be performed under optimum conditions. Also during this interval spontaneous separation of the posterior cortical vitreous from the retina may occur because of vitreous hemorrhage and inflammation. This permits excision of the cortical vitreous posterior to the equator with minimal risk. The likelihood of active intraoperative bleeding may also be reduced by delaying posterior vitrectomy several days.

REFERENCES

1. Eagling EM (1976): Perforating injuries of the eye. Br J Ophthalmol 60:732.
2. Cleary PE and Ryan SJ (1979): Method of production and natural history of experimental posterior penetrating eye injury in the rhesus monkey. Am J Ophthalmol 88:212.
3. Cleary PE and Ryan SJ (1979): Histology of wound, vitreous, and retina in experimental posterior penetrating eye injury in the rhesus monkey. Am J Ophthalmol 88:221.
4. Michels RG (1975): Surgical management of nomagnetic intraocular foreign bodies. Am J Ophthalmol 93:1003.
5. Hanscom TA and Landers MB (1979): Limbal extraction of posterior segment foreign bodies. Am J Ophthalmol 88:777.
6. Conway BP and Michels RG (1978): Vitrectomy techniques in the management of selected penetrating ocular injuries. Ophthalmology 85:560.
7. Coleman DJ (1982): Early vitrectomy in the management of the severely traumatized eye. Am J Ophthalmol 93:543.
8. Brinton GS, Aaberg TM, Reeser FH, et al (1982): Surgical results in ocular trauma involving the posterior segment. Am J Ophthalmol 93:271.

Basic and advanced vitreous surgery
G.W. Blankenship, M. Stirpe, M. Gonvers, S. Binder (eds.)
Fidia Research Series, vol. II,
Liviana Press, Padova © 1986

TREATMENT OF DOUBLE PERFORATING INJURIES

Klaus Heimann

Department for Vitreo Retinal Surgery,
University Eye Clinic, Cologne, FRG

Double perforating injuries involve a classical trauma situation which has also been repeatedly imitated in animal experiments. They are mainly caused by foreign bodies which penetrate the eye at high velocity.

As we know, there is danger of proliferation from the wound surfaces. This can grow along the missile channel as well as on the adjacent retinal surface. Circumscribed or total retinal detachments are the results. The degree of fibrotic reaction depends on the known factors. It can only be prevented or limited when a pars plana vitrectomy is carried out in good time in appropriately predisposed cases. It is self-evident that precisely in these cases preoperative diagnosis is of crucial importance: it should give us information on the situation of the retina, the question of vitreous incarceration and the position of the foreign body. For the further surgical procedure, it is of course decisive whether the foreign body is located intrabulbarly or extrabulbarly.

Basically, we can distinguish three situations in double perforation due to passage of a foreign body through the eye. These can be treated surgically according to the following principles:

Situation I: Foreign body exit in the region of the anterior or equatorial sclera, vitreous hemorrhage (Fig. 1).

Surgical procedure: Exposure of the exit site, possibly removal of the foreign body, wound closure under microsurgical conditions, cryopexy and buckling of the sclera, possibly associated with an encircling procedure. In dense vitreous hemorrhages, vitrectomy is carried out subsequently in the same or in a second sessions.

Situation II (Fig. 2): Foreign body exit at the posterior pole, vitreous hemorrhage. Here, it is to be recommended that the vitrectomy be carried out first of all in order to expose the exit site and to sever any vitreous incarcerations present. If the splitter is unequivocally extrabulbar, then wound treatment and removal of the foreign body

318

from the outside is not necessary. An endocoagulation and gas filling for prophylaxis of detachment may possibly be carried out.

Situation III (Fig. 3): Passage of a very large foreign body with exit at the posterior pole. Here, the wound treatment of the sclera must first of all be performed externally, since infusion fluid drains away in the subsequent vitrectomy required and extensive wound surfaces are an enormous stimulus for invasion of connective tissue into the vitreous. If the foreign body is apposed to the wall of the globe, it can be removed. However, further inspection of the orbit for localization of the foreign body is usually not necessary. Pars plana vitrectomy is carried out according to conventional principles.

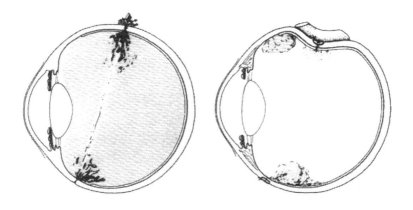

Double perforating injury (I)

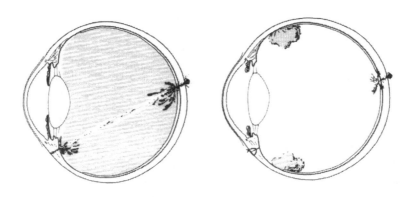

Double perforating injury (II)

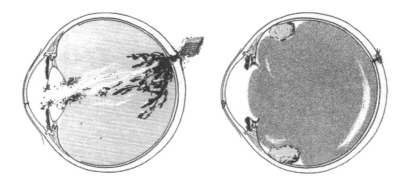

Double perforating injury (III)

Figures 1, 2, and 3. Different situations in double-perforating injuries by penetrating foreign bodies. For explanation see text.

We have reviewed 42 cases (Tab. 1).

In accordance with the very unfavorable prognostic composition of the patients, in whom gunshot injuries by shot, air rifle bullets and brass parts of cartridge cases were involved in practically half of the cases, blinding could not be avoided in 19 patients, i.e. 45% of the cases (Tab. 2). Nevertheless, the visual acuity was at least 20/20 in 11 cases. In the remaining 12 eyes, an orientative visual capacity could be preserved; the cause was mostly a destruction of the central retina by the foreign body. Compared with other injury categories, e.g. intraocular foreign-body perforations of the posterior segment, a deviant positive or negative behavior of double perforations could not be discerned.

Table 1. *Kinds of foreign bodies causing double-perforating injuries*

Double perforating injuries (n. = 42 eyes)	
buck-shot	9
BB	2
brass FB's	10
ferromagnetic FB's	16
others	5

Table 2. *Pre-operative and post-operative visual acuity in vitrectomy after double-perforating injuries.*

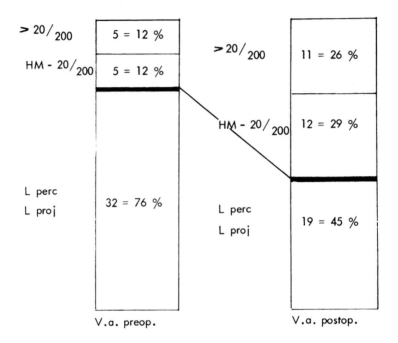

Basic and advanced vitreous surgery
G.W. Blankenship, M. Stirpe, M. Gonvers, S. Binder (eds.)
Fidia Research Series, vol. II,
Liviana Press, Padova © 1986

PROGRESS IN FOREIGN BODY EXTRACTORS

Jean-Marie Parel, Ing.ETS-G

The Bascom Palmer Eye Institute,
Department of Ophthalmology, University of Miami
School of Medicine, Miami, Florida, USA

It has been reported that over 80% of the trauma cases involving penetrating injuries are caused by magnetic foreign bodies (1). Surprisingly for the past 10 years, the surgical removal of intraocular foreign bodies has been mostly performed with specialized forceps rather than electromagnets. Before presenting a new modality, I believe it is important to analyse the recent advances made with the others.

FORCEPS

The Neubauer foreign body forceps is the world standard ophthalmic surgical instrument for trauma cases. Many variations of this instrument have been fashioned. In time and with the acceptance of the pars plana approach to vitreous surgery, the size of the foreign body forceps was reduced to 20 gauge as described by Zivojnovic and various jaw designs were introduced. In order to remove smooth glass-like foreign bodies, Hutton added a silicone rubber coating to Neubauer's invention. This softer surface would more easily take the shape of the foreign body and improved the gripping action (2). Wilson further reduced the overall size of the forceps and introduced a fully retractable, three hooked-shaped jaws designed for better gripping of irregularly shaped foreign bodies (3). Using modern technology as developed by the space research program, fine diamond crystals were later impregnated into the surface of the jaws of the foreign body forceps (4).

Diamond crystals are the hardest material known to man. This quality, in addition to their pyramidal shape and ability to penetrate all other materials, provided the perfect grip for all types of foreign bodies, thus offering the best gripping action for foreign body forceps. To ease the surgeon's manipulative, three dimentional motions during foreign body extraction, Hickingbotham also introduced the spring loaded self-closing mechanism concept to maintain a constant, uniform gripping force on foreign bodies, regardless of their composition.

ELECTROMAGNETS

The use of the electromagnetic principle for the removal of ferrous foreign bodies was introduced in 1879 (5). Larger electromagnets were later produced to increase the magnetic pull-force, thus improving the foreign body extraction success ratio. By the late 1940's, some of the electromagnets designed for and used by ophthalmologists weighed a few tons. These devices were ceiling suspended, mounted on tracks, and needed powerful electrical motors for adequate positioning over the patient's head. Others were operated by gimballed cranes which were mounted on rails and were usually manually positioned over the patient's head with the help of geared cranking mechanisms. These large devices were commonly known as Giant Magnets. During extraction, continuous electrical power was applied to these electromagnets by a foot-switch operated by the surgeon.

The limitation of these electromagnets were many, and besides their bulk, they tended to heat rapidly thereby loosing their magnetic efficiency. The surgeon then had to wait for the electromagnet metallic body to cool before re-energizing it. In some instances, this process had to be repeated many times prior to successful removal of the foreign body. These large electro/magnets were powered by a high intensity, continuous direct current wave (6).

In the late 1960's, modern technology allowed for a rapidly pulsed direct current wave to be incorporated into the electromagnet power console. This technological advance permitted the generation of higher instantaneous magnetic forces and allowed a reduction in heat dissipation. The pulsatil electromagnet body was thus reduced in size and hand-held probes were made. These devices weighed over 2 kg and had a magnetic efficiency comparable to that of the older one ton Giant Magnets (7).

In surgery, the pulsatil electromagnets are positioned externally at a very close distance to the eye. In most instances, the magnetic axis is oriented along the direction of the track made by the penetrating intraocular foreign body. Upon energizing, the foreign body is pulled backwards and follows its entrance path. For those foreign bodies located at the posterior segment of the eye, in some instances the external wound is closed and a pars plana sclerotomy is performed. In either case, the externally located magnetic pole piece is directed towards the new opening made in the eye. The pulsatil electromagnetic devices were more successful at removing foreign bodies than were the Giant Magnets. For the most part, this is due to the ease with which the hand-held devices could be oriented. Until the advent of pars plana vitreous surgery, the hand-held pulsated electromagnet was the instrument of choice for the removal of all ferrous intraocular foreign bodies. With either of the above electromagnetic instruments, the magnetic pole is external to the eye (the magnetic pole is the source of the mechanical pull-force acting on the foreign body). Once the foreign body is dislodged, it will travel with increasing speed toward the magnetic pole. Thus, a secondary incarceration will occur if the

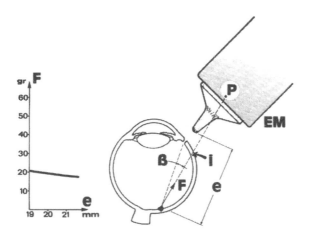

Figure 1. Diagrammatic representation of forces involved using the standard electromagnet. When the magnetic pole (P) and the foreign body are not aligned with the wound, the line of force is angled (B) and a secondary incarceration of the foreign body is possible at (i). The force field graph F = f (e) demonstrates the near constancy of the pull-power of the electromagnet (EM) equipped with a short extraocular tip. The flatness of the slope mathematically explains the "jumping" effect observed with all electromagnets.

magnetic axis is not exactly aligned with the eye wound (Figure 1). Secondary incarcerations are sometimes difficult to manage, especially if the ciliary body is involved.

In an effort to ease the capture of ferrous intraocular foreign bodies and to prevent secondary incarceration, we modified our hand-held Bronson electromagnet. A 32 mm long cylindrically shaped needle made of magnetic steel was machined and press-fitted into a hole made in the center of the existing pole piece. The blunt needle had a tip diameter of 1.65 mm (16 gauge). A maximum pull-force of 35 g was measured with the tip in contact with a steel ball. In July 1981, Dr. Mark Blumenkranz of the Bascom Palmer Eye Institute used this modified electromagnet to successfully remove a small foreign body incarcerated in the posterior retina. It was later found that secondary incarceration of a foreign body was still possible with this modified instrument. If the electrical power is applied to the magnet before physical contact with the foreign body and if the magnetic axis is slightly misaligned, the foreign body will travel directly toward the externally located magnetic pole (Figure 2).

The teachings of Dr. Robert Machemer to remove all intraocularly located foreign bodies with forceps relegated the above electromagnetic instruments to our museum shelves. Although modern foreign body forceps are light-weight and inexpensive compared to hand-held electromagnets, they still have a disadvantage: their moving jaws are not well suited for the removal of foreign bodies laying on or incarcerated in the retina. In some instances, the moving jaws will catch and pull delicate tissue and cause iatrogenic tears and holes in the retina.

The anterior segment of the eye has a relatively small volume compared to the posterior segment. Instruments designed for the removal of foreign bodies located in the vitreous cavity do not easily lend themselves to use in the anterior segment. There too, moving forcep jaws might catch iris or damage the corneal endothelium.

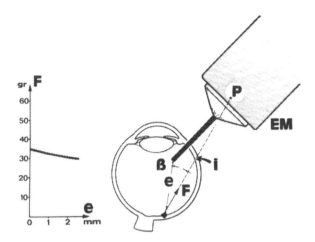

Figure 2. Diagrammatic representation of forces involved with the modified electromagnet. The addition of a thin extension to the pole piece does not prevent a secondary incarceration at (i) if power is applied to the electromagnet (EM) before contact is made with the foreign body. Note the slight increase in the slope and intensity of force-field obtained with the new intraocular tip. The added extension does not eliminate the "jumping" effect.

LODESTONES

In ancient times, lodestones were used for the removal of iron foreign bodies. It has been reported that over two thousand years ago, these natural permanent magnets were used to remove foreign bodies by Indian surgeons (6). The higher magnetic forces generated by the electromagnets invented in the early 1800's, have relegated the use of permanent magnetism in foreign body removal to oblivion.

THE RARE-EARTH IOM

The magnetic field generated by permanent magnets are inferior to those obtained with modern electromagnets. It had always been assumed that permanent magnets could not be used for the successful removal of intraocular foreign bodies. As reported by Duke-Elder, a good magnet has to comply with Lancaster's rules: "... Unless a giant magnet can pull a steel ball 1 mm in diameter with a force of over 50 times its weight at a distance of 20 mm, and unless a hand magnet will pull such a ball in contact with its tip with a force over 5000 times its weight, they are not ophthalmologically effective" (6). The above dicta ignores the properties of the foreign body. In the opinon of many vitreo-retinal surgeons, electromagnetic instruments cause foreign body secondary incarceration and associated complications, and are thus inferior to the forceps. As demonstrated in both Figures 1 and 2, secondary incarceration is due to the misalignment of the magnetic pole, the wound and the foreign body. The major complication associated with secondary incarceration is actually a by-product of the electromagnet's power: the higher the electromagnetic force field, the higher the acceleration force, thus the greater the damage made by the impacting foreign body.

If the magnetic pole is introduced *within* the eye, the above mentioned disadvantages would vanish. Furthermore, if the magnetic pole is in direct contact with the foreign body, Lancaster's dicta no longer holds, as to lift and *pull* a 1 mm steel ball *through* the vitrous requires less than 5 g of force.

Using this knowledge, I designed a unique instrument based on the theory of permanent magnetism. A highly polished, cobalt alloyed magnetic bar 75 mm in length and 1.60 mm in diameter was encased in an anodized aluminum handle. The mounted magnetic bar was then subjected to an intensely polarized 1 Mega Gauss magnetic field for 10 seconds, permanently magnetizing this new surgical instrument. The Intraocular Magnet (IOM) weighs only 10 g and is small when compared to the hand-held electromagnet it replaces (Figure 3). The first clinical prototype IOM was fabricated by David Denham in the BPEI Ophthalmic Biophysics Laboratory and was able to lift a 10 mm diameter steel ball.

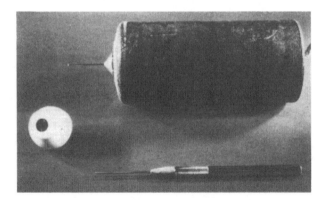

Figure 3. Comparative photograph of the electromagnet and the rare-earth intraocular magnet. The Bronson-Storz electromagnet handpiece shown here has a modified intraocular tip attached to its pole piece and weighs 2.5 kg. Although the pencil shaped prototypal Rare-Earth IOM weighs only 10 g, it delivers an equal pull-force when in contact with a ferrous foreign body.

In December 1981, Dr. Guy O'Grady, Chief Ophthalmologist at the VA Hospital in Miami, was first to use the IOM in a 10 day old trauma case involving penetrating injuries. After repairing the corneal wound and performing a total vitrectomy with the VISC-X, Dr. O'Grady successfully removed a 6.5 mm long steel splinter incarcerated in the posterior fundus. Our IOM first prototype had a pull-force of only 18 g, yet it had no difficulty in pulling this large foreign body which had fully penetrated both the retina and the choroid and was partially imbedded in the sclera.

We immediately began to further improve our first prototype and were quickly able to produce devices capable of generating a 40 g pull-force. A product of the tremendous technological advances made in the last decade are the rare-earth permanent magnets (8). With these new materials, the Rare-Earth IOM pull-force was further increased to 90 g. The permanent magnetic energy imparted to the rare-earth IOM is long lasting. We have found experimentally that the instrument loses about 15% of its energy per year. It can easily be recharged by speciality laboratories such as ours. The Rare-Earth IOM is sterilizable by flash autoclaving or by ETO gas. The use of high temperature heat sterilization is not advised. Rare-earth materials should never be subjected to flames.

It is sometimes convenient for the surgeon to release a foreign body caught by the Rare-Earth IOM tip. Such situations arises most frequently when elongated foreign bodies present themselves sideways to an insufficiently enlarged sclerotomy site. As the X-rays and ultrasound tests detect this type of foreign body prior to surgery, this situation can be avoided. Using a disposable, thin-walled catheter of appropriate size, the surgeon can fashion a simple coaxial cannula fitting the IOM tip. This cannula permits easy and safe unimanual intraocular manipulation of the foreign body. If the smallest dimension of the foreign body is such that it fits into the cannula, it can then be trapped by merely sliding the cannula over the IOM tip, then extracted through a thigh wound. This method was devised by Billy Lee at the Bascom Palmer Eye Institute. The 16 gauge Rare-Earth IOM was designed to fit into the VISC-X's coaxial fiber optic light pipe. The latter can serve as the protecting cannula described above.

Although toxicology tests conducted in live rabbits proved the selected materials safe to use in the eye, all of our prototype Rare-Earth IOMs were heavily gold plated for added patient safety: pure gold is the only material proven non-toxic as a long term implant (9).

When electromagnets placed in front of the wound are energized, it is sometime possible to observe the foreign body "jumping" towards the magnet tip. In opposition to early beliefs, with the Rare-Earth IOM, no foreign body "jumping" effect is observed as the instrument is introduced into the vitreous cavity. As the graph of Figure 4 demonstrates, the pull-force becomes significant only at a distance of 1 mm or less. The greatest pull-force is obtained only when a direct contact with the foreign body is achieved (10).

Other Rare-Earth IOM tip sizes were fabricated. A 14 gauge instrument was found useful for the removal of foreign bodies imbedded in the cornea. This larger 3 mm diameter Rare-Earth IOM can easily lift a 30 mm diameter steel ball. To accommodate surgeons using the 3-port vitrectomy technique, a 19 gauge model was made. The pull-force of this smaller model is 15 g. As the average foreign body dimension is larger than 1 mm, the sclerotomy site often has to be enlarged prior to extraction. This 19 gauge device was also found useful for the removal of foreign bodies present in the anterior segment of the eye.

Thirteen prototypes were fabricated in our laboratories and, early in 1982, were sent to different medical centers around the world for clinical testing (11). Only when the Rare-Earth magnet was improperly utilized (e.g., attempts at direct removal of long standing encapsulated ferrous foreign bodies in non-vitrectomized eyes or the use of the magnet on non-magnetic foreign bodies) were failures reported. When using the

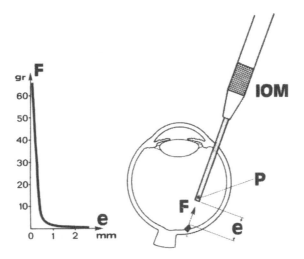

Figure 4. Diagrammatic representation of forces involved with the rare-earth IOM. The magnetic pole (P) of the rare-earth IOM is located at the tip of the instrument and is always closest to the foreign body. Secondary incarceration is thus impossible. The force-field diagram is strongly sloped. Very large pull-forces exist only at close proximity to the foreign body, making the IOM free of the "jumping" effect characterizing electromagnets.

Rare-Earth IOM, as with forceps or electromagnets, the foreign body should always be freed of encapsulating tissues. This is perhaps most important with intraretinal foreign bodies. To prevent intraoperative intraocular bleeding, we further suggest the prior cauterization of surrounding tissues before the extraction of encapsulated foreign bodies.

CONCLUSION

The Rare-Earth Intraocular magnet is a simple but powerful instrument that replaces the older and bulkier electromagnets commonly used for the removal of intraocular ferrous foreign bodies. This instrument does not work at large distances from the eye and therefore *cannot* be used externally.

ACKNOWLEDGMENTS

I would like to thank Professor Pierre Kock, Ph.D. for his teachings in magnetic sciences. David Denham, M.S., William Lee and Willi Aumayr provided many of the technical refinements and fabricated the many rare-earth intraocular magnet prototypes. Barbara French, B.A., prepared the illustrations and Marilyn Maxwell, M.B.A., wrote this paper in English. I am especially indebted to Professor Gerard Crock, M.D., who supplied the clinical film which I presented. I am grateful to Professor E.W.D. Nor-

328

ton, M.D. for his continued support and to the following physicians: Geroge Blankenship, Harry Flynn, Guy O'Grady, Donald May, Joseph Young, Scott Jaben, Michel Gonvers, Robert Machemer, Mark Blumenkranz, Professor Chang Shiao-Fang, Frits Treffers, Julian Heintz, Philippe Sourdille, Professor Akia Yamanaka and all of the other surgeons who have used the Rare-Earth IOM and shared their surgical experiences with me.

REFERENCES

1. François P, Asseman R and Constantinides G (1966): Les Corps Etrangers Intraoculaires Non-Magnetiques. Bulletins et Memoires de la Societé Française. 79:307-318.
2. Hutton WL (1977): Vitreous Foreign Body Forceps. Am J Ophthalmol 83:430-431.
3. Wilson DL (1975): A New Intraocular Foreign Body Retriever. Opthalmic Surg 6:64.
4. Hickingbotham D, Parel J-M and Machemer R. (1981): Diamond-Coated All-Purpose Foreign Body Forceps. Am J Ophthalmol 91(2): 267-268.
5. Hirschberg J: (1879): Die Electromagnet in die Augenheilkunde. Berlin Klin Wschr 16:681.
6. Duke-Elder (1972): System of Ophthalmology. Vol XIV, part 1, pp. 617-647. CV Mosby Co.
7. Bronson NR (1968): Practical Characteristics of Ophthalmic Magnets. Arch Ophthalmol. 79:22-27.
8. Robinson AL (1984): Powerful New Magnet Material Found. Science. 223:920-922.
9. Sen SC and Ghosh A (1983): Gold As an Intraocular Foreign Body. Brit J Ophthalmol 67:398-399.
10. Parel J-M, Blumenkranz M, O'Grady G, Blankenship G, Nose I, Denham D and Norton EWD (1982): Advances in Vitreoretinal Microsurgical Instrumentation. Ophthalmology, 89 (9s): 186.
11. Crock GW and Janakiraman P (1985): The Intra Ocular Magnet of Parel. Aust Med J (in press).

Basic and advanced vitreous surgery
G.W. Blankenship, M. Stirpe, M. Gonvers, S. Binder (eds.)
Fidia Research Series, vol. II,
Liviana Press, Padova © 1986

REMOVAL OF INTRAOCULAR FOREIGN BODIES

G. Santarelli *, P. Ducoli and S. Fruscella

Fondazione Oftalmologica 'G.B. Bietti', Piazza Sassari, 5, Roma
* Divisione Oculistica, C.T.O., Via Nemesio, Roma

The surgeon, when having to deal with an intraocular foreign body (F.B.), will be facing the problems related to the pathology and the surgery of perforating lesions as well as the extraction of the foreign body (2). Naturally, the problems will be different every time, and will mainly depend on the kind of perforating lesion, on its location and extent, on the position of the F.B. and on its nature, shape and dimensions. Both the pre-operative period and when to proceed with surgery must be determined with extreme accuracy. During the pre-operative period, after having performed the necessary examinations, the surgeon must decide what procedure is to be followed and when to perform surgery. Even though an early operation may partly prevent inflammatory reactions, vitreo-retinal proliferations, and prolonged hypotonicity, it may on the other hand cause hemorrhages and choroidal detachments.

PRE-OPERATIVE EVALUATION

During the pre-operative period, an accurate anamnesis is gathered in order to determine the nature of the F.B. Ophthalmoscopic examination is performed, but in case the transparency of the media does not allow it, echography and an X-Ray of the orbit must be carried out in order to determine the exact location, shape, dimensions, point of entry, and trajectory of the F.B. inside the bulb. Computerized axial tomography may be useful only if the F.B. is in contact with the scleral wall (2).

TIMING OF SURGERY

The appropriate moment for the removal of a F.B. is determined by two factors: (a) Complications caused by the trauma, (b) Nature of the foreign body.

Surgery must be performed immediately if dealing with a non-magnetizable F.B. that can provoke serious inflammatory reactions (bakelite, casein plastics) or if the F.B. is believed to be made of iron or copper. Immediate surgery should also be performed when faced with endophthalmitis, a reactive inflammatory condition, or retinal detachment, particularly if it is followed by hemorrhage into the vitreous chamber (Table 1).

Table 1. *Reaction to the various kinds of intraocular foreign bodies*

Non-magnetizable F.B.	+ + +
Fe	+ +
Cu	+ + +
F.B. of large dimensions	+ +
F.B. with endophthalmitis	+ + +
F.B. with retinal detachment	+ +
F.B. with hemorrhage	+ + +
Pb	+
Glass	+
Plastic: Polyethylene, Polymethylmethacrylat	
Bakelite, Casein plastics	+ + +

Lead, aluminium, steel and glass are much less toxic and for this reason the eye may tolerate them for a longer period of time. Sometimes, iron and copper foreign bodies may be incapsulated with substances deriving from fiber proliferation. In this case, surgery can be postponed, provided there are no symtoms of evident toxicity caused by the foreign bodies. Choroidal congestion contraindicates immediate surgery. The possibility of vitreo-retinal proliferation must also be considered. Frequently, this type of complication becomes evident 15-30 days after the trauma. Vitrectomy should be performed in order to isolate the proliferation at the initial stage, that is, before it can further damage the internal ocular structures.

SURGICAL TECHNIQUE

The most appropriate surgical technique is determined according to the localization, nature, dimensions and shape of the F.B. Those located in the anterior chamber can be extracted through the breach of entry if it has been observed a short time after the trauma, that is, before the natural process of scarring has begun or after suture. However, it is better to perform the extraction through a limbal aperture if the initial lesion is at the point of scarring and involves the central cornea.

Located in the lens, the F.B. may be extracted by performing an extracapsular lens extraction if the posterior capsule has not been damaged. In the case of a transparent lens with a small F.B., the lens is to be left "in situ". The F.B. located in the vitreous chamber can be extracted only through an intraocular surgical procedure. As much vitreous as is necessary to allow visualization of the F.B. should first be removed. The F.B. will then be freed from the vitreous or from any other membrane-like structure that hampers its mobilization. If the F.B. is encapsulated by reactive tissue, it is necessary to open the capsule by means of an appropriate instrument (2) (Fig. 1).

This surgical manoeuvre is very dangerous because frequently the capsule, caused by inflammatory proliferation, is firmly attached to the retina; during this surgical step hemorrhages and retinal lacerations can occur.

The sclerotomy at the pars-plana is to be widened in order to allow the forceps and the F.B. to pass. A T-shaped scleral incision may facilitate the extraction (3). Otherwise, when the F.B. and the forceps pass through the sclerotomy, there is the risk of the latter losing its grip and of the F.B. dropping onto the underlying retina. If the F.B. is of large dimensions, a limbal aperture must be made and after having extracted the lens "in toto", the surgeon must grasp the F.B., move it through the pupillar foramen to the anterior chamber, and extract it through the limbal aperture (1) (Fig. 2).

Magnetizable F.Bs situated near the ocular wall on the pre-equatorial side may be extracted through an aperture of the scleral wall utilizing a magnet. The extraction must be preceded by accurate scleral localization of the F.B. and followed by cryo treatment at the sclerotomy in order to assure adequate adhesion (3). This method should be avoided when dealing with a F.B. situated near the posterior wall of the bulb unless it is of small dimensions, in inframural localization or is anyhow situated on the extramacular side. In any case, one should know exactly when to use a magnet, because this technique is difficult to control and may further damage the internal ocular structures.

The extraction of pellets poses another particular problem. A pellet may be made of

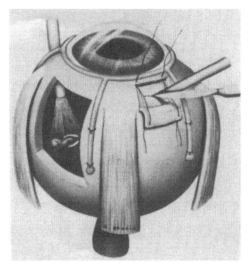

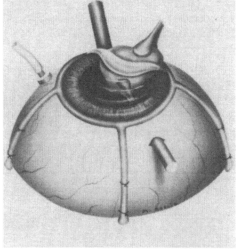

Figure 1. Removal of foreign bodies located posteriorly.

Figure 2. Removal of foreign bodies of large dimension through the anterior chamber.

332

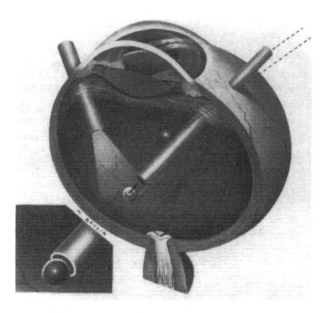

Figure 3. Removal of pellet with a cannula.

lead or of steel: in the first case, it should be extracted by means of a 3-tip forceps, in the second case, a magnet should be used (Fig. 3).

In order to facilitate removal and make it less traumatic, we have also used a third technique: the use of a series of cannulas of different diameters. The cannula which has a diameter slightly smaller than the diameter of the pellet's equator is chosen for the extraction. After having removed the vitreous, the cannula is inserted into the pars-plana and the pellet is aspirated through its opening. The depression inside the cannula will block the pellet in order to make the extraction possible.

CONCLUSION

The surgical technique to be performed depends on the location, composition, dimensions, and shape of trhe F.B.

Most F.B. are extracted by an intraocular surgical procedure: this procedure is not used for F.B. of small dimensione located near the scleral wall or a F.B. situated on the pre-equatorial side.

It is particularly important to determine the most appropriate moment for the surgical procedure; this depends also on the nature of the F.B. and on the complications that follows the trauma.

REFERENCES

1. Charles S (1981) In: Vitreous Microsurgery, Williams and Wilkinson, Baltimore, pp. 143-154
2. Michels RG (1981) In: Vitreous Surgery, C V Mosby Company, St. Louis, pp. 257-284
3. Machemer R (1978): Vitrectomy, 2nd ed, Grune and Stratton New York, pp. 102-108

Basic and advanced vitreous surgery
G.W. Blankenship, M. Stirpe, M. Gonvers, S. Binder (eds.)
Fidia Research Series, vol. II,
Liviana Press, Padova © 1986

VITRECTOMY IN THE MANAGEMENT
OF INFECTIOUS ENDOPHTHALMITIS

Harry W. Flynn, Jr., M.D.

The Bascom Palmer Eye Institute, Department of Ophthalmology,
University of Miami School of Medicine, Miami, Florida.

Infectious endophthalmitis remains a devastating ocular complication, often resulting in complete loss of vision. The use of topical, periocular, and systemic antibiotics is well established in the treatment of endophthalmitis (1-3) and intraocular antibiotics have also been commonly used in recent years (4-6). Vitrectomy has been employed in selected cases, both to obtain a vitreous specimen and to remove infectious material from the vitreous cavity (7-12). The use of vitrectomy instruments in this disease has remained controversial and is not indicated in all cases. This review will summarize the clinical features of endophthalmitis, the decision making process regarding treatment approaches, preparation for and technique of vitreous surgery, culture techniques, recommended antibiotics, and overall visual results in endophthalmitis.

CLINICAL FEATURES OF ENDOPHTHALMITIS

Endophthalmitis must be considered when the intraocular and periocular inflammatory response of an eye is greater than the usual clinical course. Suspicious signs and symptoms for bacterial endophthalmitis include excessive pain, edema involving the conjunctiva and lids, corneal clouding, and a marked intraocular inflammatory reaction with vitritis and often with a hypopyon (7). There may be a marked decrease in vision, seemingly out of proportion to the inflammatory reaction, often declining to the light perception level. Retinal periphlebitis has been described as an early sign of bacterial endophthalmitis (13). Fungal endophthalmitis, on the other hand, may cause only minimal visual impairment after a prolonged course of progressive intraocular inflammation.

Endophthalmitis occurs in four major clinical categories (7). The most common type of endophthalmitis occurs during the recent postoperative period following cataract or other anterior segment surgery. Gram positive organisms are most often involved in this recent postoperative type of endophthalmitis. Post-traumatic endophthalmitis may occur following a penetrating ocular injury. Almost any organism gaining access to the eye in sufficient quantity during such an injury seems capable of causing endophthalmitis. Endogenous endophthalmitis occurs in intravenous drug abusers, debilitated patients, and patients with immune deficiency diseases. These cases may be bilateral or unilateral, and often are caused by fungal organisms. Finally, spontaneous endophthalmitis may occur in eyes with filtering blebs resulting from previous glaucoma or cataract surgery. These spontaneous cases are often caused by Gram positive organisms, especially the Streptococcus species.

TREATMENT APPROACHES

The clinical examination at the time of presentation may be used to dictate the treatment approach. Vitrectomy instrumentation is not required in all cases, especially those with a relatively mild clinical presentation (defined as hand motion or better visual acuity with the ability to view fundus details or obtain symmetric red reflex). In this mild setting, the initial approach includes aspiration of aqueous and anterior vitreous for culture, injection of antibiotics directly into the vitreous cavity, and use of topical, periocular, and systemic antibiotics. When there is a low index of suspicion for fungi, periocular steroids may be administered during the initial treatment.

The results of initial cultures and the follow-up clinical course determine the subsequent approach. If the culture results indicate a relatively benign organism (e.g. Staphylococcus epidermidis) and if the clinical course is one of gradual improvement, appropriate antibiotic therapy is continued without further intraocular intervention. If a virulent organism is isolated (e.g. Gram negative) or if the eye is developing progressive inflammation despite initial antibiotic therapy, vitrectomy should be considered.

In eyes presenting initially with more severe inflammation (defined as less than hand motion vision, with an inability to view fundus details or absence of a red reflex), initial vitrectomy is usually recommended. Although the prognosis for useful vision in these eyes is generally poor, vitreous surgery offers the theoretical advantage of draining the vitreous abscess, thus removing active infectious organisms as well as bacterial toxins and proteolytic enzymes. Further treatment in these eyes is also dictated by the clinical course and by the organism cultured from the vitreous specimen. If the organism isolated is relatively benign and the inflammation is gradually subsiding, a full course of antibiotics is given. In eyes clinically deteriorating, consideration can be given to repeat vitreous tap and reinjection of antibiotics.

Injection of intravitreal antifungal agents combined with systemic therapy may not be effective in eradicating fungal proliferation. In cases of probable fungal endophthalmitis from endogenous or exogenous sources, vitrectomy is advised initially (14-15). Vitreous surgery will yield the best specimen for positive culture results and appropriate antifungal medications can be injected after the vitrectomy into the mid-vitreous cavity. Removal of the majority of formed vitreous will allow better distribution of the antifungal medication throughout the eye.

PREPARATION FOR VITRECTOMY IN ENDOPHTHALMITIS

The operating room is alerted that an endophthalmitis case is being scheduled in order that appropriate precautions are taken. These precautions include isolation of the patient with endophthalmitis from other surgical patients and meticulous postsurgical clean-up of instruments used during the vitrectomy.

Except in the presence of wound dehiscence from previous surgery, local with sedation anesthesia is used more commonly than general anesthesia. A routine intravenous line is established during local with sedation anesthesia, but intravenous antibiotics should be started only after the vitreous specimen has been obtained for culture and sensitivity.

The rationale (7) for using vitrectomy in endophthalmitis is the following:
1. To obtain an adequate specimen for culture, sensitivity, and special stains.
2. To remove infectious material (drain abscess).
3. To allow better distribution of intraocular antibiotics.
4. To clear opaque debris from the visual axis.

The theoretical advantages of vitrectomy must be balanced against potential complications caused by vitreous surgery. In advanced endophthalmitis cases, retinal necrosis may occur. Aggressive vitrectomy with irrigation in areas of necrotic retina may create retinal breaks and irreparable retinal detachment results. The visual prognosis is very poor when retinal detachment occurs during the management of eyes with endophthalmitis (9-16). Other potential complications of vitrectomy are retinal dialyses, intraocular hemorrhage from sclerotomy sites, and delayed postoperative cystoid macular edema. In spite of these possible complications, vitrectomy has become a frequently used diagnostic and therapeutic modality in endophthalmitis.

VITRECTOMY TECHNIQUES IN ENDOPHTHALMITIS

Vitrectomy instruments can be used by way of a limbal or pars plana route in eyes with endophthalmitis. The technique selected depends on the degree of corneal clouding, the extent of purulent intraocular material, and the overall experience of the individual surgeon. In some cases, corneal edema and infiltrate may limit the view necessary to perform a pars plana vitrectomy. Dense purulent material may fill the anterior chamber and mid-pupillary space, necessitating an initial limbal approach before a pars plana approach can be undertaken. The anterior segment surgeon may feel uncomfortable with pars plana vitrectomy and perform a limited anterior vitrectomy. No controlled studies are available to compare the efficacy of a limited anterior vitrectomy versus a more complete pars plana vitrectomy in endophthalmitis.

The pars plana approach is often preferable because a greater portion of the vitreous abscess can be drained and traumatic irrigation of the compromised corneal endothelium can be avoided. Using this approach, excision of the anterior vitreous gel, combined with removal of a major portion of the central core of vitreous, can be performed in most aphakic eyes. If vitrectomy is to be performed in phakic patients with endophthalmitis, the pars plana route is mandatory and a clear lens can be preserved (17).

The presence of an intraocular lens may limit visibility, and therefore limit the ability to perform a posterior vitrectomy. When the patient is placed in the supine position, the hypopyon may spread out to form a thin opaque film on the anterior surface of the implant. Irrigation of the anterior chamber may be necessary to remove this film on the intraocular lens prior to attempting pars plana vitrectomy. In cases of severe intraocular inflammation, a limited posterior vitrectomy through the peripheral iridectomy can be considered. No attempt is made to perform a complete vitrectomy in the presence of an intraocular lens because of the limitations of visibility. Since a posterior chamber intraocular lens usually remains positioned in the ciliary sulcus or in the capsular bag during a pars plana vitrectomy, there is no need for implant removal in spite of opening the posterior capsule during the vitrectomy.

Controversy exists as to whether the intraocular lens should be removed in pseudophakic eyes with endophthalmitis. At the Bascom Palmer Eye Institute, the intraocular lens is not usually removed unless there is threatened extrusion of the implant through a wound dehiscence or spontaneous dislocation of the implant during vitrectomy. Most infected eyes can be sterilized even though the IOL is not removed. In the rare case which can not be sterilized, as documented by persistent positive intraocular cultures, the implant should probably be removed.

ANTIBIOTIC TREATMENT IN ENDOPHTHALMITIS

After removal of the vitreous specimen using vitrectomy instrumentation, Gram and Giemsa stains can be immediately performed by the Microbiology Department. The results can be forwarded to the operating room and the surgeon can select appropriate antibiotics. The entire vitreous specimen can be passed through a membrane filter in order to concentrate the infectious material, which may increase chance for positive culture results (7). Pieces of the membrane filter with concentrated specimen are placed on individual culture plates. Organisms are often identified within 24 hours, and adjustment of antibiotics can be made if necessary.

The following antibiotic regimen is currently used at the Bascom Palmer Eye Institute in the management of suspected bacterial endophthalmitis:

A. Intraocular
   1. Gentamicin 0.1 mg in 0.1 cc solution
   2. Cefazolin 2.25 mg in 0.1 cc solution

B. Periocular (subconjunctival)
   1. Gentamicin 40 mg
   2. Cefazolin 100 mg

C. Topical
   1. Gentamicin 9.0 mg/ml q1h
   2. Cefazolin 50 mg/ml q1h, or Bacitracin 5000 units/ml q1h, or Carbenicillin 4.4 mg/ml q1h

D. Systemic
   1. Cefazolin 1 gram IV STAT, then 1 gram q6h

2. Gentamicin 1 mg/kg/IM (or IV) q8h. (Caution - Nephrotoxicity)

Using a tuberculin syringe, intraocular antibiotics can be injected into the mid-vitreous space after vitreous surgery has been completed. The bolus of concentrated antibiotic solution insures that the desired dosage will be administered to the eye. The pharmacist may assist in preparation of intraocular antibiotics in order to arrive at the correct concentration of medications (18-19). The following technique is used to arrive at the correct dosage of intraocular antibiotics:

A. Gentamicin 0.1 mg/0.1 ml
   1. Withdraw 0.1 ml (4 mg) from a fresh vial of gentamicin sulfate for injection (40 mg/ml).
   2. Add to this 3.9 ml sterile (not bacteriostatic) saline.
   3. 4 ml of this solution contains 4 mg gentamicin sulfate; thus, 1 ml contains 1 mg and 0.1 ml contains 0.1 mg.
   4. Slowly inject 0.1 ml of this solution into the vitreous cavity.

B. Cefazolin 2.25 mg in 0.1 ml
   1. Reconstitute the powder in a 500 mg vial using 2 ml sterile (not bacteriostatic) saline. This will result in a concentration of 500 mg/2.2 ml or 225 mg/ml.
   2. Withdraw 1 ml of this solution and dilute with 9 ml of sterile saline. Since 10 ml of this solution contains 225 mg, 1 ml contains 22.5 mg, and 0.1 ml contains 2.25 mg.
   3. Slowly inject 0.1 ml of this solution into the vitreous cavity.

C. Amphotericin-B 0.005 ml
   1. A 50 mg vial with 10 cc sterile (non-bacteriostatic) water equals 50 mg in 10 cc (.5 mg in 0.1 cc).
   2. Take 0.1 cc of solution and add 9.9 cc of water, giving 10 cc with .5 mg (0.1 cc = .005 mg).
   3. Slowly inject 0.1 ml (.005 mg) of Amphotericin-B into the vitreous cavity.

In suspected fungal endophthalmitis, intraocular injection of Amphotericin 0.005 mg is given initially. Systemic Amphotericin, 5-Flurocytocine, or Ketaconazole may also be used in fungal endophthalmitis. Topical and periocular antifungal agents are ineffective due to poor intraocular penetration.

CULTURE MEDIA FOR ENDOPHTHALMITIS CASES

Although a variety of culture media are available, the standard blood agar plates at room and body temperature are the most useful. The following culture media are most commonly employed at the Bascom Palmer Eye Institute:

1. *Blood agar* - at 25 and 37° (both bacterial and fungal infections).

2. *Chocolate agar* - (Hemophilus and Neisseria).

3. *Thioglycolate media* - (anaerobic bacteria).

4. *Sabouraud's media* - (fungi and yeast).

POST-VITRECTOMY MEDICATIONS

Concentrated topical antibiotics, using hourly administration, are started on the morning after initial treatment. Selection of individual topical antibiotics is based on the results of the Gram and Giemsa stains and positive culture results. These concentrated antibiotic solutions are prepared in the following manner:

1. *Gentamicin 9 mg/ml (Garamycin)*
   Withdraw 1 cc of a gentamicin injectable vial (80 mg/ 2 cc).
   Add the 1 cc to a gentamicin ophthalmic solution vial (5 ml) to give a 9 mg/cc solution.

2. *Cefazolin Solution 54 mg/ml (Ancef)*
   Add 9.2 cc of Tears Naturale to a vial of Cefazolin 1 mg (powder for injection). Dissolve. Take 5 cc of this solution and add it to 5 cc of Tears Naturale.

3. *Bacitracin Solution 5,000 units/ml*
   Add 9 cc of Tears Naturale to a vial of Bacitracin 50,000 units (powder for injection). Dissolve. Empty the remainder of the solution in the Tears Naturale bottle. Once the Bacitracin powder is dissolved in the vial, withdraw the resulting solution and inject it into the empty Tears Naturale container to give 5,000 units/ml solution.

4. *Carbenicillin Solution 4.4 mg/ml*
   Add 3.6 cc of Tears Naturale to a 1 gram vial of Carbenicillin. Let it dissolve. Add 0.2 cc of the resulting solution to 11 cc of Tears Naturale Solution to give 4.4 mg/ml solution.

Subconjunctival antibiotics are usually given daily for three days to supplement the concentrated topical antibiotics. Other topical medications include cycloplegics and steroids. Cycloplegics are started on a twice daily schedule. Topical steroids are used hourly except in the presence of known fungal endophthalmitis or organisms resistant to currently used antibiotics.

Systemic steroids are often utilized to decrease intraocular inflammation. They may be started either at the time of initial treatment or after the initial culture results have been obtained (7, 19). Depending on the patient's general systemic status, Prednisone 60 mg daily by mouth is a frequently used dosage. The systemic steroids are tapered after a one week course of treatment.

RESULTS OF ENDOPHTHALMITIS TREATMENT

The final visual result is dependent on a number of factors, including the virulence of the infecting organism, the promptness of therapy, and any secondary complications during or after treatment. Staphylococcus epidermidis is the most frequent organism causing postoperative endophthalmitis and usually has a better visual prognosis than other organisms (7, 9). O'Day et al reported successful management of 18 postsurgical cases caused by this organism without intravitreal antibiotics or vitrectomy (21). The clinician, however, is unable to distinguish endophthalmitis caused by this organism, from more visually devastating types of infection caused by more virulent organisms. Endophthalmitis caused by Staphylococcus aureus and Gram-negative organisms has a poor visual prognosis, and the use of intraocular antibiotics combined with vitrectomy may improve this prognosis.

A delay in diagnosis and initiation of therapy may be an adverse factor in the final visual result of endophthalmitis treatment. Although there are no randomized prospective studies to confirm this clinical impression, it is essential that the clinician consider the possibility of infectious endophthalmitis in order to initiate early treatment or prompt referral. In general, the individual virulence of the infecting organism may determine the rate of onset of visual symptoms. The more virulent organisms usually have an acute course with a poor prognosis, as opposed to the more benign organisms, like Staphylococcus epidermidis, which has a more protracted course with a better visual prognosis.

Secondary complications may occur during or after treatment. The most significant complications involve the posterior segment. In a recent review of 40 cases of postoperative endophthalmitis at the Bascom Palmer Eye Institute, four cases of retinal detachment occurred during the follow-up course (9). Two of these cases were reattached by scleral buckling techniques and two could not be reattached. Also, four patients without retinal detachment and with clear media have reduced visual acuity attributed to widespread retinal atrophic changes and pigment clumping at the level of the retinal pigment epithelium. Although these retinal changes could have been caused by the intraocular infection itself, intraocular antibiotic toxicity may cause similar changes (22).

These three factors (specific infecting organism, promptness of therapy, and secondary complications) play an important role in the final visual results for each of the major categories of endophthalmitis. Recent postoperative endophthalmitis is the most commonly observed type seen in clinical practice. A retrospective review of culture-proven postoperative endophthalmitis cases at the Bascom Palmer Eye Institute indicated that 52% of eyes (31 of 65) achieved a final visual acuity of 20/400 or better (9). In this series, the treatment approach was generally guided by the initial clinical presentation and by the individual physician preference for treatment. Milder cases with better visual acuity were usually treated with intraocular and conventional antibiotics alone, reserving vitrectomy for the more severe cases. In these milder cases not requiring vitrectomy, 67% (16 of 24 eyes) achieved 20/400 or better. In the more advanced endophthalmitis cases, with hand motion to light perception vision and no view of fundus details because of purulent material in the pupillary axis, vitrectomy combined with intraocular and conventional antibiotics was the most common treatment. Forty-one percent (15 of 36 eyes) in this group achieved 20/400 or better. Because the vitrectomy group of endophthalmitis eyes generally had a more advanced clinical presentation, poorer presenting visual acuity, and usually more virulent organisms, the poor visual results in the vitrectomy group could be expected. Since cases were not randomly assigned to a treatment approach, this retrospective series of cases does not help to settle the controversial role of vitrectomy in the management of postoperative endophthalmitis.

Post-traumatic endophthalmitis has a poorer visual prognosis than recent postoperative endophthalmitis because of multiple secondary complications induced by trauma and by the introduction of variable quantities of virulent organisms into the eye from penetrating injuries. A recent retrospective review by Affeldt et al (23) of post-traumatic endophthalmitis cases seen by referral at the Bascom Palmer Eye Institute found that 15% (43 of 279 eyes) were of traumatic origin. Using follow-up data on

34 of these cases, a final visual acuity of 20/400 or better was achieved in only 24% (8 of 34 eyes) and 35% (12 of 34 eyes) were no light perception. Brinton et al (24) reported 19 culture-proven post-traumatic endophthalmitis cases, in which a final visual acuity of 20/200 or better was achieved in 42% (8 of 19 eyes). In eyes involved in an intraocular foreign body injury, endophthalmitis occurred in 10.7% (11 of 103) of cases reviewed by Brinton. Virulent organisms, retinal breaks, or retinal detachment seen at the time of primary trauma repair indicated a poor visual prognosis in these series.

The endogenous or metastatic category of endophthalmitis is relatively less frequent than recent postoperative and post-traumatic cases. Depending upon the virulence of the infecting organism, retinal involvement, and host resistance, treatment by vitrectomy and intravitreal injection of appropriate medication may salvage useful vision in many cases.

In late onset endophthalmitis associated with filtering blebs, the visual prognosis is generally poor. Streptococcus species are most frequently involved. Hemophilus influenzae are the second most frequent gram negative organisms isolated in these patients. Both streptococcal and Hemophilus endophthalmitis in eyes with filtering blebs have a rapid course of progressive inflammation and vitrectomy should be considered in the initial management of these cases because of this poor prognosis.

Bacterial endophthalmitis after vitreous surgery is very rare and the visual prognosis is poor in reported cases (25-26) In spite of intensive antibiotic therapy, most eyes lose all vision in this setting. The usual post-vitrectomy inflammatory reaction may mask important clinical indicators of endophthalmitis and a delay in the initiation of therapy may result.

CONCLUSION

This review has summarized the current approaches in the management of infectious endophthalmitis, with special emphasis on the role of vitrectomy. Although vitrectomy is not recommended in all cases, its use may be helpful in selected cases.

REFERENCES

1. Allen HF, Mangiaracine AB (1964): Bacterial endophthalmitis after cataract extraction: A study of 22 infections in 20,000 operations. Arch Ophthalmol. 72:454-462.
2. Allen HF, Mangiaracine AB (1973): Bacterial endophthalmitis after cataract extraction: II. Incidence in 36,000 consecutive operations with special reference to preoperative topical antibiotics. Trans Am Acad Ophthalmol Otolaryngol. 77:581-588.
3. Theodore FH (1965): Bacterial endophthalmitis after cataract surgery. Int Ophthalmol Clin. 5:59.
4. Forster RK (1974): Endophthalmitis: Diagnostic cultures and visual results. Arch Ophthalmol. 92:387-392.
5. Peyman GA, Vastive DW, Crouch ER, Herbst RW (1974): Clinical use of intravitreal antibiotics to treat bacterial endophthalmitis. Trans Am Acad Ophthalmol Otolaryngol. 78:862-875.

6. Peyman GA: Antibiotic administration in the treatment of bacterial endophthalmitis (1977): II. Intravitreal injections. Surv Ophthalmol. 21:332-346.

7. Forster RK (1978): Endophthalmitis. IN: Duane TD (ed) Clinical Ophthalmology. Hagerstown, MD, Harper and Row, Vol. 4. Ch. 24: 1-20.

8. Cottingham AJ, Forster RK (1976): Vitrectomy in endophthalmitis: Results of study using vitrectomy, intraocular antibiotics, or a combination of both. Arch ophthalmol 94:2078-2082..

9. Olson JC, Flynn HW, Forster RK, Culbertson WW (1983): Results in the treatment of postoperative endophthalmitis. Ophthalmology 90:692-699.

10. Diamond JG (1981): Intraocular management of endophthalmitis: A systematic approach. Arch Ophthalmol. 99:96-99.

11. Puliafito CA, Baker AS, Haaf J, Foster CS (1982): Infectious endophthalmitis: Review of 36 cases. Ophthalmology, 89:921-928.

12. Rowsey JJ, Newson DL, Sexton DJ, Harms WK (1982): Endophthalmitis: Current approaches. Ophthalmology 82:1055-1065.

13. Packer AJ, Weingeist TA, Abrams GW (1983): Retinal periphlebitis as an early sign of bacterial endophthalmitis. Am J Ophthalmol. 96:66-71.

14. Doft BH, Clarkson JG, Rebell G, Forster RK (1982): Endogenous Aspergillus endophthalmitis in drug abusers. Arch Ophthalmol. 98:859-862.

15. Snip RC, Michels RG (1976): Pars plana vitrectomy in the management of endogenous Candida endophthalmitis. Am J Ophthalmol. 82:699-704.

16. Charles S (1981): Vitreous Microsurgery. Baltimore, MD, Williams and Wilkins, pp. 155-158, 1981.

17. Gelender H, Flynn HW, Mandelbaum SH (1982): Bacterial endophthalmitis resulting from radial keratotomy. Am J Ophthalmol. 93:323-326.

18. Smith RE, Nozika RA (1983): Uveitis: A Clinical Approach to Diagnosis and Management. Baltimore, MD. Williams and Wilkins, Chapter 209, pp. 94-98.

19. Mandelbaum SM, Forster RK (1983): Infectious endophthalmitis. Clinical modules for ophthalmologists. The American Academy of Ophthalmology, Module 9.

20. Jeglum EL, Rosenberg SB, Benson WE (1981): Preparation of intravitreal drug doses. Ophthalm Surg. 12:355-359.

21. O'Day DM, Jones DB, Patrinely F, Elliott JH (1982): Staphylococcus epidermidis endophthalmitis. Ophthalmology. 89:354-360.

22. D'Amico DJ, Libert J, Kenyon KP, Hanninen LA, Caspers-Velu L (1984): Retinal toxicity of intravitreal gentamicin. Invest Ophthalmol Vis Sci. 25:564-572.

23. Affeldt JC, Forster RK, Mandelbaum SM: Traumatic endophthalmits (in preparation).

24. Brinton GX, Topping TM, Hyndiuk RA, Aaberg TM, Resser FH, Abrams GW (1984): Post-traumatic endophthalmitis. Arch Ophthalmol. 102:547-550.

25. Blankenship GW (1977): Endophthalmitis after pars plana vitrectomy. Am J Ophthalmol. 84:815-817.

26. Ho PC, Tolentino FI (1984): Bacterial endophthalmitis after closed vitrectomy. Arch Ophthalmol. 102:207-210.

Basic and advanced vitreous surgery
G.W. Blankenship, M. Stirpe, M. Gonvers, S. Binder (eds.)
Fidia Research Series, vol. II,
Liviana Press, Padova © 1986

COMPLICATIONS OF VITREOUS SURGERY

Ronald G. Michels, M. D.

The Vitreoretinal Service, Wilmer Ophthalmological Institute,
Johns Hopkins University School of Medicine,
Baltimore, Maryland

Various complications are associated with vitreous surgery, ranging from mild non-progressive abnormalities that do not affect the vision to severe complications resulting in blindness, discomfort and/or a cosmetically unacceptable appearance. Intraoperative complications are usually caused by mechanical or toxic damage to intraocular tissues. Postopertive complications result from: 1) late effects from intraoperative damage, 2) progressive changes due to structural alterations caused by the operation, and 3) changes in the balance of biologically active substances that, in turn, cause abnormalities such as iris neovascularization. Any ocular tissue can be involved by these complications, either separately or in combination with others. The type, incidence and severity of complications depend on several factors, including: 1) the clinical condition for which the operation was performed, 2) whether or not the objectives of the operation were achieved, and 3) whether iatrogenic damage occurred. The overall incidence and severity of complications have been reduced by improved instrumentation and surgical techniques and by better understanding of the factors causing complications.

CORNEAL COMPLICATIONS

Corneal complications usually occur postoperatively, although they are caused by intraoperative mechanical and/or toxic damage. Intraoperative corneal edema only rarely causes enough opacification to interfere with visualization. However, posterior stromal folds occur if the epithelium is removed, and this may be a problem during fluid-gas exchange in aphakic eyes because the combination of posterior corneal folds and air in the anterior chamber markedly reduces visualization.

Postoperative corneal complications are mainly limited to persistent or recurrent epithelial defects and/or stromal and epithelial edema. Troublesome epithelial defects occur almost exclusively in diabetic patients when some of the epithelium was removed intraoperatively. Therefore, removal of the epithelium is avoided whenever possible.

Both the occurrence of inadvertent epithelial defects and aspects of delayed postoperative healing can be caused by the abnormal physiologic and ultrastructural features of the diabetic cornea. In these eyes there is a loose adhesion between the basal epithelial layer and Bowman's membrane, due to marked thickening of the interposed basement membrane material which is characterized by multiple laminations and contains aberrant anchoring fibrils (1). Therefore, relatively minor trauma with the operating corneal contract-lens can cause an epithelial defect.

An epithelial defect is first covered by reparative sliding of adjacent epithelial cells, and this has been shown to be normal even though the neurotropic influences of the diabetic cornea are not normal (2,3). However, a more important feature is the additional time required to form a new basement membrane layer and to develop anchoring fibrils attached to the superficial stroma. During this time, recurrent epithelial defects can occur. Semi-pressure bandaging is used postoperatively to encourage healing of an epithelial defect, and this can usually be achieved within three days. Topical medications are not used until the epithelial layer is intact.

Corneal edema persisting after the epithelial layer is intact is due to endothelial damage. This may be caused by a combination of factors, including: 1) the composition, volume, and turbulence of flow of the intraocular irrigating solution, 2) mechanical damage to the endothelium by ultrasonic energy, lens fragments, or surgical instruments during the operation, 3) toxic damage from topically-applied phenylephrine used while an epithelial defect is present (4) or from use of intracameral epinephrine in a high concentration (5, 6), and perhaps 4) mechanical damage from an intraocular bubble. Severe endothelial damage is rare. This occurs most commonly in eyes with preexisting corneal damage or eyes in which combined pars-plana lens removal and vitrectomy is complicated by flattening of the anterior chamber and/or anterior displacement of lens fragments.

Improved irrigating solutions with additional constituents such as glucose for cell metabolism, calcium and glutathione for cell-membrane stability, and a physiologic buffer system have reduced the amount of endothelial damage (7-9). Also, the volume of irrigating solution used has been reduced by the use of automated devices to produce the suction force. Special techniques such as segmentation of stiff pupillary membranes with scissiors, and ultrasonic emulsification of firm lens material, reduce the need for strong suction force which is associated with high volume flow.

Corneal endothelial damage may also occur from toxic effects of other pharmacologic agents. Phenylephrine seriously damages the endothelium if applied topically while an epithelial defect is present (4). Therefore, this drug is not used intraoperatively or postoperatively when a portion of the epithelium has been removed. Epinephrine can also have a damaging effect on the endothelium when used in the anterior chamber to redilate the pupil. This depends on the concentration of the drug, and therefore only a dilute solution of 1:10,000 or higher is used in the anterior chamber (5). Even then caution is required to be certain that the ph and osmolarity are in a physiologic range and that no toxic preservatives are present (6).

The rate of important postoperative corneal complications was high during the early days of vitreous surgery, and it ranged from 50% in diabetic eyes to nearly 75% if lens removal was combined with vitrectomy (10, 11). The current incidence of these complications is not known, although permanent corneal opacification is rare. This improved situation is the result of efforts to: 1) avoid epithelial defects during the operation, 2) encourage rapid postoperative healing of inadvertent epithelial defects, 3) avoid direct mechanical damage to the endothelium, 4) use only physiologic irrigating solutions, and 5) prevent toxic effects from topical phenylephrine and intracameral epinephrine in certain circumstances and concentrations.

LENS COMPLICATIONS

Lens complications include cataract formation and also intraocular inflammation or mechanical damage to other tissues from lens remnants. Cataract formation may occur because of direct mechanical damage by the vitrectomy instruments, toxic effects from the irrigating solution, and/or prolonged postoperative contact with an intravitreal bubble. Direct contact between the surgical instruments and the lens is rare, and this is most likely to occur while excising portions of the retrolenticular and/or anteroperipheral vitreous gel. This contact is avoided by using caution when working near the lens and by use of retroillumination while excising anteroperipheral vitreous gel using a two-instrument method (Fig. 1).

The composition of the irrigating solution seems to be an important factor in maintaining lens clarity, especially if the operation is prolonged. Fern-like posterior subcapsular opacities occur intraoperatively in some diabetic eyes when a balanced salt solu-

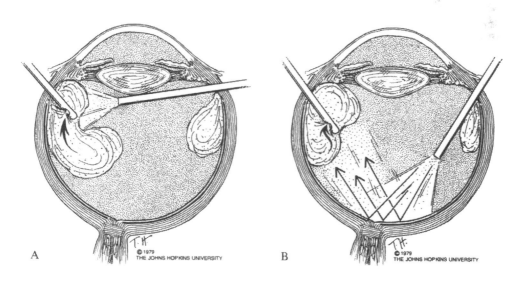

Figure 1. *A*, Damage to posterior lens capsule by illuminating probe while cutting anteroperipheral vitreous on opposite of eye using divided-system instrumentation. *B*, Lens damage avoided with light reflected off posterior retinal surface to illuminate area of vitrectomy probe tip and anteroperipheral vitreous.

tion is used for irrigation (12), whereas this does not occur if a suitably enriched solution is used containing added constituents, as mentioned before. A similar effect was demonstrated when the lens from rhesus monkey eyes was incubated in various irrigating solutions (13).

When an inert intravitreal gas bubble is used, special postoperative posturing is required to avoid prolonged contact between the bubble and the posterior lens capsule (Fig. 2). Fern-like opacities and vacuoles in the posterior lens cortex occur after about 24 hours of contract between the lens and an intravitreal bubble (14). These changes become irreversible soon thereafter.

Visually significant lens opacities now occur postoperatively in about 20% of eyes undergoing vitrectomy for posterior segment indications when the lens is not removed. The exact incidence of this complication, and the cause-and-effect relation in each case, are difficult to analyze because several factors are involved, including: 1) the patient's age and health, 2) the length of the operation and the type and volume of irrigating solution used, 3) the presence of preexisting lens opacities, 4) use of an intravitreal bubble and/or other accessory techniques such as retinal cryotherapy, and 5) the occurrence of other complications such as glaucoma, hemorrhage, or retinal detachment.

Lens material remaining after incomplete pars-plana lens removal can cause serious postoperative complications depending on the amount, location, and type of residual material. Cortical material remaining behind the iris becomes quite swollen and opaque, and it may temporarily obstruct the pupil. However, swollen cortical material usually absorbs spontaneously, and the eye is treated with steroids by topical application or subconjunctival depot injection. Retained nuclear material may cause prolonged inflammation and/or secondary mechanical damage to the retina or the cornea if the fragment(s) are freely mobile. Therefore, every effort is made to remove these fragments

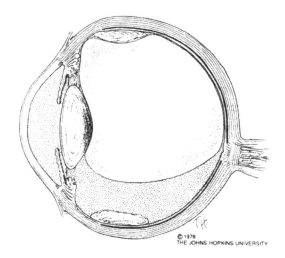

© 1978
THE JOHNS HOPKINS UNIVERSITY

Figure 2. Posterior subcapsular lens opacities from prolonged contact between intravitreal gas bubble and posterior lens surface. Face-down posture is chosen to prevent prolonged contact between gas bubble and posterior lens capsule.

during the initial operation, using intravitreal ultrasonic emulsification after excising portions of the vitreous gel and retrieving the fragments. The same methods can be used during a second operation when necessary.

Premature rupture of the posterior lens capsule and displacement of some lens material into the vitreous cavity occur in about 25% of eyes undergoing combined pars-plana lens removal and vitrectomy. However, most often this is cortical material, and rupture of the posterior capsule occurs when the peripheral cortical material is being separated from the equatorial capsule after the lens nucleus has been removed. The soft cortical material is readily removed with the vitrectomy probe or with the ultrasonic needle before the lens material falls further posteriorly. This reduces the risk of retinal damage associated with retrieval of lens fragments from the posterior part of the vitreous cavity.

SCLEROTOMY COMPLICATIONS

Complications related only to the pars plana incisions are infrequent. Damage to the adjacent retina can occur if the incision is located too far posterior, if there is excessive traction on the adjacent vitreous base, or if retinal detachment is present and the peripheral retina becomes incarcerated in the wound when the surgical instruments are withdrawn. Fibrovascular ingrowth from the incision occurs postoperatively in some eyes, and this can cause traction on the adjacent peripheral retina and perhaps cause recurrent vitreous hemorrhage (Fig. 3) (15-18).

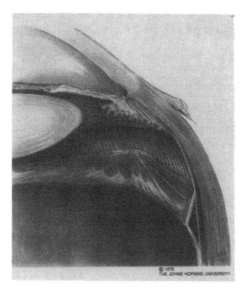

Figure 3. Vitreoretinal traction causing retinal detachment along posterior vitreous base because of postoperative contraction of anteroperipheral vitreous incarcerated in pars plana sclerotomy.

Direct retinal damage from preparing the incisions or introducing instruments is rare because the incisions are made 3.0 to 4.0 mm posterior to the limbus, which means they are near the pars plana ciliaris and safely anterior to the ora serrata and the anterior part of the vitreous base. Bleeding from the pars plana uveal tissue is rare when the incisions are made, although limbal-parallel incisions transect the radially-oriented vessels in the pars plana zone.

Incarceration of detached peripheral retina in the pars plana incision can usually be avoided by lowering the intraocular pressure before withdrawing the surgical instruments. However, if this complication occurs, or if vitreous gel is incarcerated in the sclerotomy and causes marked traction on the adjacent retina, simultaneous fluid-gas exchange is used to free the tissues. The incarcerated retina and/or vitreous gel is first disengaged from the wound with the vitrectomy probe or a bunt needle. Then a bubble is injected, and the expanding bubble flattens the peripheral vitreous gel and retina against the eyewall while displacing subretinal fluid posteriorly. This prevents further prolapse of tissue into the incisions when the instruments are again withdrawn (Fig. 4).

Some fibrous proliferation occurs within every pars plana incision as part of the normal wound-healing process, and this tissue may grow into the scaffold of adjacent vitreous fibers incarcerated in the incision. However, clinically significant fibrovascular ingrowth is infrequent, in the absence of other complications such as generalized intraocular neovascular proliferation as seen in some diabetic patients with postoperative rubeosis iridis (19). Still, neovascular tissue is visible in some eyes extending from the pars plana incision, and this may cause recurrent vitreous hemorrhage. In such cases, the neovascular tissue extending from the internal aspect of the sclerotomy can be treated with transvitreal bipolar diathermy in suitable aphakic eyes. Fibrovascular tissue growth can also cause peripheral retinal detachment that may require a scleral buckling operation if traction detachement is progressive or if a rhegmatogenous component occurs.

VITREOUS HEMORRHAGE

Intraoperative bleeding can be a serious complication during vitreous surgery, and recurrent hemorrhages can also occur postoperatively. Intraoperative bleeding is the only major complication that has become more frequent despite improvements in vitreous surgery instrumentation and technique. The increased occurrence of bleeding is probably due to changes in case selection and operative technique. Surgery is now performed in some eyes with severe intraocular neovascularization, and more extensive dissection of this tissue is performed than in the past. Intraoperative bleeding occurs most frequently from the retina and/or from neovascular tissue in the posterior segment. This may occur when vascularized tissue is cut with the vitrectomy instrument or intraocular scissors, or it may be due to traction on vitreoretinal attachments when vitreous sheets and/or proliferative tissue are manipulated.

The possibility of bleeding is reduced by use of scissors to minimize traction on vitreoretinal attachments when adjacent tissue is cut, and by use of diathermy to coagulate abnormal vessels before or immediately after vascularized tissue is cut (Fig. 5). Despite these efforts, some bleeding occurs frequently, and clotted blood often remains on the retina at the end of the operation. Residual blood becomes dispersed throughout the vitreous cavity postoperatively, and it may take a prolonged time to clear in phakic eyes.

Some fresh blood remaining in the vitreous cavity is present postoperatively in about 75% of eyes with proliferative diabetic retinopathy, whereas this complication is rare

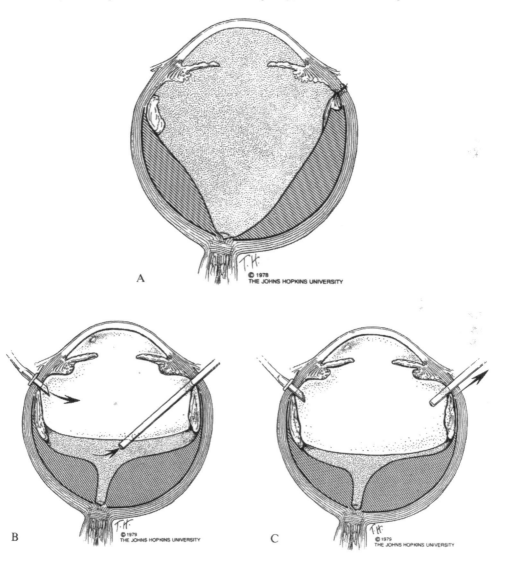

Figure 4. A, Treatment of peripheral retinal distortion due to incarceration of vitreous in pars plana sclerotomy at end of vitrectomy procedure. *B* and *C*, After disengaging vitreous from incision with blunt needle tip, fluid-gas exchange is performed to flatten peripheral retina against pigment epithelium. This displaces subretinal fluid posteriorly and an intraocular bubble prevents recurrence of retinal or peripheral vitreous prolapse into sclerotomy site as instruments are withdrawn.

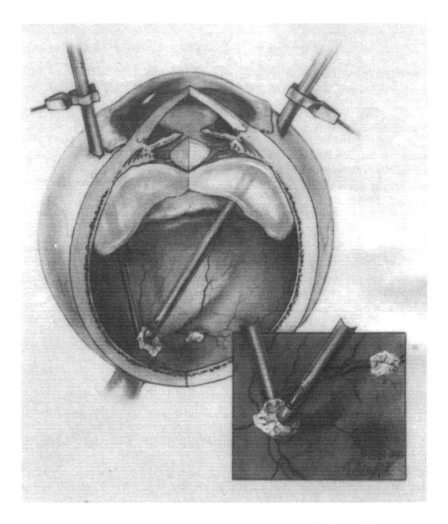

Figure 5. Bimanual bipolar diathermy used to treat the cut edges of epiretinal fibrovascular membrane. Fiberoptic probe and vitrectomy instrument serve as electrodes to apply diathermy after cutting the tissue.

in other conditions when fibrovascular tissue is not cut or manipulated. Postoperative hemorrhage is also common in eyes with proliferative diabetic retinopathy, and some bleeding occurs in up to 50% of cases. However, this is most common during the initial postoperative period. Early postoperative hemorrhages tend to be small in amount, and the blood usually clears spontaneously in 4 to 12 weeks depending on whether the eye is aphakic or phakic.

Later bleeding occurs in about 20% of diabetic patients, and this is rare in other conditions. The exact origin of late postoperative hemorrhage usually cannot be determined, and possibilities include: 1) residual neovascular tissue in the posterior segment,

2) fragile retinal or ciliary-body blood vessels damaged by the underlying disease, 3) fibrovascular ingrowth from the sclerotomy site(s), and 4) abnormal blood vessels on the iris. The latter is probably not a common cause of recurrent bleeding, because this complication seems to occur with equal frequency in phakic and aphakic eyes, and hyphema is rarely present in the involved phakic eyes. Still, eyes with abnormal iris vessels seem to have a higher incidence of later vitreous hemorrhage, although the iris changes may only be evidence of more widespread vascular abnormalities.

Photocoagulation is used to treat areas of residual retinal neovascularization in eyes with recurrent vitreous hemorrhage. Nonclotted blood can be removed by later lavage in the phakic eyes if spontaneous clearing does not occur. The timing of further surgery depends on several factors, including: 1) the status of the fellow eye, 2) the visual potential in the eye with recurrent hemorrhage, 3) the amount of vitreous blood as judged by clinical and ultrasonic examination, and 4) the presence of other complications such as retinal detachment or rubeosis iridis. Lavage of vitreous blood, and retinal reattachment surgery, are done immediately if progressive detachment is demonstrated by ultrasonography. Also, eyes with progressive postoperative rubeosis iridis may be treated by lavage of nonclotted blood and intraoperative scatter retinal photocoagulation to treat the anterior segment neovascularization. In other eyes, secondary lavage is performed only if spontaneous clearing does not occur after 3 to 6 months. If repeated episodes of bleeding occur, lens removal through the pars plana may be performed at the time of vitreous lavage to permit more rapid clearing of any further hemorrhages.

RETINAL DAMAGE

Retinal tears and detachment are serious and relatively frequent complications of vitreous surgery. Retinal tears can occur from direct damage by the surgical instruments or from traction on areas of vitreoretinal attachment. These tears occur mainly along the posterior margin of the vitreous base or adjacent to areas of posterior vitreoretinal attachment.

Retinal tears from traction along the posterior vitreous base are infrequent when small amounts of suction force are used, and this complication now occurs in only 1 to 2% of cases (12). Posterior retinal tears rarely occur from direct damage by the vitrectomy probe or vitreoretinal scissors, although this is more likely when cutting opaque tissue near an area of retinal detachment. Posterior retinal breaks occur most commonly from traction on areas of vitreoretinal attachment when preretinal membranes are cut or epiretinal tissue and/or cortical vitreous is dissected from the retina (Fig. 6). This complication now occurs in about 20% of diabetic eyes with complicated vitreoretinal anatomy. Posterior retinal tears are treated with cryotherapy or photocoagulation, combined with an intraocular bubble if all traction on the area has been relieved. A localized scleral buckle supporting the break is added if anteroposterior or tangential traction persists.

Postoperative retinal detachment can occur from iatrogenic retinal breaks, or new breaks occurring postoperatively, or just from traction by residual vitreous gel and/or epiretinal membranes. New retinal breaks can occur from persistent traction by remaining

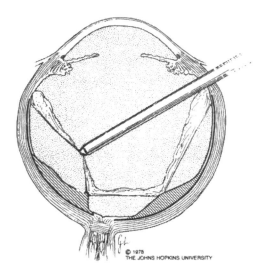

Figure 6. Posterior retinal break caused by traction on area of vitreoretinal attachment while resecting adjacent posterior vitreous surface. Retinal breaks are especially likely to occur in areas of previous traction detachment where retina is thin and atrophic.

vitreous gel or fibrovascular tissue, or the breaks can occur in other, less involved areas. In the latter case the pathogenesis of the break is unknown. Scleral buckling, together with intraocular gas injection, is used to treat postoperative rhegmatogenous detachments. Often the retinal break is quite small, and careful preoperative evaluation with a contact lens is needed to identify the defect. Further vitreous surgery can also be used to treat persistent traction detachment if a cleavage plane is visible between the contracted membranes and the inner retinal surface.

Rhegmatogenous detachment occurs postoperatively in 5 to 10% of eyes with diabetic retinopathy, and about one-half of these cases can be successfully treated by further surgery (20-23). Also, small areas of postoperative traction detachment are common in these eyes because of tangential traction from remaining epiretinal tissues. However, residual traction detachment is rarely of clinical significance if the original objectives of the operation were achieved. Postoperative retinal detachment is rare in other conditions, except in eyes with previous detachment complicated by proliferative vitreoretinopathy (PVR). In these cases, recurrent detachment occurs in about 50% of eyes because of further epiretinal membrane growth (24).

RUBEOSIS IRIDIS

Growth of neovascular tissue on the iris (rubeosis iridis) and in the anterior-chamber angle is the most frequent postoperative complication causing failure of an otherwise successful vitrectomy procedure. This complication is limited almost entirely to eyes with preexisting retinal vascular disorders characterized by extensive areas of capillary nonperfusion. Also, the incidence of rubeosis iridis is considerably higher in aphakic than in phakic eyes (25-27). The mechanism causing this complication is unproven, but it is presumed to be caused by an angiogenic substance elaborated by ischemic retinal tissue and capable of producing a neovascular response in adjacent and remote ocular locations.

Rubeosis iridis results in glaucoma due to obstruction of the anterior-chamber angle by neovascular tissue in some eyes (neovascular glaucoma). This usually occurs 2 to 12 weeks after the vitrectomy operation. This type of angle-closure glaucoma is especially difficult to treat after extensive obstruction of the anterior-chamber angle occurs. Therefore, frequent postoperative observation is necessary to detect early changes, because prompt treatment with scatter retinal photocoagulation causes regression of the anterior segment neovascularization in some eyes (20, 28). However, the natural history of iris neovascularization is variable, and not all untreated eyes progress to neovascular glaucoma (26). Therefore, the effect of treatment with scatter retinal photocoagulation is difficult to evaluate. Still, treatment is recommended in suitable cases when neovascular tissue is visible in the anterior-chamber angle and before extensive peripheral anterior synechiae develop.

Abnormal iris vessels have been observed in up to 44% of eyes after vitrectomy for complications of proliferative diabetic retinopathy (20, 25, 27). However, this high incidence of vascular abnormalities includes both cases of benign dilation of normal iris vessels (iris hyperemia) and also aphakic eyes with total retinal detachment and neovascularization. Diabetic eyes with retinal detachment after vitrectomy are consistently complicated further by rubeosis iridis and neovascular glaucoma or phthisis bulbi (20). Therefore, in some of these eyes the abnormal iris vessels are benign, whereas in others it is a predictable secondary complication superimposed on another blinding condition. Visual loss caused only by rubeosis iridis now occurs in less than 10% of all cases (21-23).

The incidence of rubeosis iridis is also strongly influenced by whether or not the crystalline lens is present, and rubeosis occurs at least twice as often in aphakic eyes as in phakic eyes (25, 27, 29). Therefore, a clear crystalline lens is preserved whenever possible in eyes with proliferative retinopathies. This is done to preserve a more physiologic optical system and to reduce the risk of postoperative anterior-segment neovascularization.

PHTHISIS BULBI

Phthisis bulbi characterized by hypotony, intraocular scarring, and disorganization and shrinkage of the globe is the final complication in some eyes after vitreous surgery. This occurs most commonly in diabetic patients with retinal detachment and rubeosis iridis, or after severe penetrating injuries, or after surgery for retinal detachment complicated by proliferative vitreoretinopathy. When the vitreous surgery operation is initially successful, phthisis bulbi rarely occurs. However, phthisis happens sometimes after seemingly successful vitrectomy for infective endophthalmitis with severe enzymatic retinal and uveal damage and in eyes with chronic intraocular hemorrhage and hemosiderosis. Therefore, phthisis bulbi is usually a secondary complication. The incidence of phthisis bulbi is probably 15 to 20% of all vitreous surgery procedures, but much of this high rate is due to the fact that many of these eyes are high-risk cases with a poor prognosis.

REFERENCES

1. Kenyon KR (1979): Recurrent corneal erosion: Pathogenesis and therapy. Int Ophthalmol Clin 19 (19): 169.
2. Snip RC, Thoft RA, Tolentino FI (1980): Similar epithelial healing rates in the corneas of diabetic and nondiabetic patients. Am J Ophthalmol 90:463.
3. Hyndiuk RA, Kazarian EL, Schultz RO et al (1977): Neurotrophic corneal ulcers in diabetes mellitus. Arch Ophthalmol 97:937.
4. Edelhauser HP, Hine JE, Pederson H et al (1979): The effect of phenylphrine on the cornea. Arch Ophthalmol 97:937.
5. Hull DS, Chemotti TM, Edelhauser HF et al (1975): Effect of epinephrine on the corneal endothelium. Am J Ophthalmol 79:245.
6. Edelhauser HF, Hyndiuk RA, Zeeb A et al (1982): corneal edema and the intraocular use of epinephrine. Am J Ophthalmol 93:327.
7. Edelhauser HF, van Horn DL, Hyndiuk RA et al (1975): Intraocular irrigating solutions: Their effect on the corneal endothelium. Arch Ophthalmol 93:648.
8. Edelhauser HF, van Horn DL, Schultz RO et al: Comparative toxicity of intraocular irrigating solutions on the corneal endothelium. Am J Ophthalmol 81:473.
9. Edelhauser HF, Gonnering R, van Horn DL (1978): Intraocular irrigating solutions: A comparative study of BSS-Plus and lactated Ringer's solution. Arch Ophthalmol 95:516.
10. Perry HD, Foulks GN, Thoft RA et al (1978): Corneal complications after closed vitrectomy through the pars plana. Arch Ophthalmol 96:1401.
11. Brightbill FS, Myers FL, Bresnick GH (1978): Postvitrectomy keratopathy. Am J Ophthalmol 85: 651.
12. Faulborn J, Conway BP, Machemer R (1978): Surgical complications of pars plana vitreous surgery. Ophthalmology: 85: 116.
13. Christiansen JM, Kollarits CR, Fukui H et al (1976): Intraocular irrigating solutions and lens clarity. Am J Ophthalmol 82:594.
14. Fineberg E, Machemer R, Sullivan P et al (1975): Sulfur hexafloride in owl monkey vitreous cavity. Am J Ophthalmol 79:67.
15. Tardif YM, Schepens CL, Tolentino FI (1977): Vitreous surgery. XIV. Complications from sclerotomy in 89 consecutive cases. Arch Ophthalmol 95:229.
16. Tardif YM, Schepens CL (1977): Closed vitreous surgery. XV. Fibrovascular ingrowth from the pars plana sclerotomy. Arch Ophthalmol 95:235.
17. Pulhorn G, Teichmann KD, Teichmann I (1977): Intraocular fibrous proliferation as an incisional complication in pars plana vitrectomy. Am J Ophthalmol 83:810.
18. Buettner H, Machemer R (1977): Histopathologic findings in human eyes after pars plana vitrectomy and lensectomy. Arch Ophthalmol 95:2029.
19. Rice TA, Michels RG (1980): Long-term anatomic and functional results for diabetic retinopathy. Am J Ophthalmol 90:297.
20. Michels RG (1978): Vitrectomy for complications of diabetic retinopathy. Arch Ophthalmol 96:237.
21. Michels RG, Rice TA, Rice EF (1983): Vitrectomy for diabetic vitreous hemorrhage. Am J Ophthalmol 95:12.
22. Rice TA, Michels RG, Rice EF (1983): Vitrectomy for diabetic traction retinal detachment involving the macula. Am J Ophthalmol 95:22.
23. Rice TA, Michels RG, Rice EF (1983): Vitrectomy for diabetic rhegmatogenous retinal detachment. Am J Ophthalmol 95:34.
24. Machemer R, Laqua H (1978): A logical approach to the treatment of massive periretinal proliferation. Ophthalmology 85:584.

25. Blankenship G, Cortez R, Machemer R (1979): The lens and pars plana vitrectomy for diabetic retinopathy complications. Arch Ophthalmol 97:1263.
26. Madsen PH (1971): Rubeosis of the iris and haemorrhagic glaucoma in patients with proliferative diabetic retinopathy. Br J Ophthalmol 55:368.
27. Rice TA, Michels RG, Maguire MG et al (1983): The effect of lensectomy on the incidence of iris neovascularization and neovascular glaucoma after vitrectomy for diabetic retinopathy. Am J Ophthalmol 95:1.
28. Little HR, Rosenthal AR, Dellaporta A et al (1976): The effect of panretinal photocoagulation on rubeosis iridis. Am J Ophthalmol 81:804.
29. Blankenship GW (1980): The lens influence on diabetic vitrectomy results. Report of a prospective randomized study. Arch Ophthalmol 98:2196.

Basic and advanced vitreous surgery
G.W. Blankenship, M. Stirpe, M. Gonvers, S. Binder (eds.)
Fidia Research Series, vol. II,
Liviana Press, Padova © 1986

FLUID/GAS EXCHANGE IN VITREOUS SURGERY

Maurice B. Landers III, David Robinson, Karl R. Olsen and Jeff Rinkoff

Department of Ophthalmology, Duke University Medical Center,
Durham, North Carolina 27710

In the past decade there have been many innovations and improvements in the field of vitreo-retinal surgery. New vitrectomy instruments, along with the intraocular SF_6 and C_3F_8 gas and silicone oil, have permitted surgical correction of vitreo-retinal diseases previously felt untreatable. However, as a result we are now faced with increasingly complicated operations, with more complicated postoperative courses.

Because of the complexity of these surgical problems, a patient's eye will often have to be reoperated upon multiple times to obtain the best possible visual result. Nevertheless, the need to avoid excessive re-operation is also present, as they are expensive, involve prolonged hospitalization, and may present additional hazards to the patient's health.

We are now using several techniques of fluid/gas exchange in an examining room setting outside of the operating room in an attempt to deliver optimum postoperative care and to treat several postoperative complications. Following are detailed descriptions of fluid/gas exchange techniques and some other procedures we have found to be effective, both in successfully treating postoperative complications and in avoiding re-operations. If done cautiously and carefully, these procedures also appear to have a very low incidence of complication.

FLUID/GAS EXCHANGE OUTSIDE THE OPERATING ROOM

In the postoperative period following vitrectomy, fluid/gas exchange is often helpful in the management of vitreous cavity hemorrhage. While postoperative hemorrhage is common and despite the fact that most blood will clear spontaneously over several weeks to months, a clear view of the fundus may be necessary for correct diagnosis and management of potential complications. Not only will the fluid/gas exchange provide a clear view of the fundus, it may also have a secondary effect of causing cessation of bleeding. In cases of postoperative pressure elevation where red blood cells are obstructing aqueous outflow, fluid/gas exchange may be useful in decreasing the red blood cell concentration in aqueous and thereby increasing aqueous outflow and lowering the intraocular pressure. In persistent or recurrent postoperative retinal detachments, an intraocular gas bubble may be augmented, thereby providing a buoyant force to re-attach the retina. If necessary, cryo or laser therapy can then be used to treat the appropriate retinal pathology. Fluid/gas exchange can be carried out safely outside the operating room if a few precautions are taken. Below is an outline of an approach to the procedure.

Anesthesia

Safe intraocular injection of gas outside the operating room may require retrobulbar anesthesia. However it is not always necessary, particularly when injecting gas into the eye is through the limbus. In cooperative patients topical anesthesia with 0.5% pro-paracaine HC1 often provides adequate anesthesia. Topical anesthesia can also be supplemented with application of a cotton pledget soaked with 4% Xylocaine to the area where the needle is to be injected, but this is rarely necessary. Should retrobulbar anesthesia be required, we generally use 2% xylocaines along with hyaluronidase.

Antibiotics

It is our practice to apply a topical antibiotic such as gentamycin eye drops to the cornea and conjunctiva prior to and immediately following intraocular gas injection, and one drop of 5% povidone-iodine solution.

Exposure

In order to eliminate the need for manual lid retraction, and to maximize the view of the entry site, the anterior segment, the vitreous cavity and fundus, a lid speculum is routinely used, and the patient's pupil is widely dilated prior to starting the procedure.

Entry site

In aphakic eyes following vitrectomy, a spontaneoulsy sealing shelved entrance through the 9 o'clock limbus in the right eye and the 3 o'clock limbus in the left eye is the safest and easiest approach. However, when the eye is phakic, the injection of gas into the vitreous cavity must be carried out through the pars plana. In this case the needle is placed through the conjunctiva, sclera and pars plana at a point 3.5 mm posterior to the limbus with a single, controlled stab incision into the central vitreous cavity.

Needle size

A disposable 30 gauge needle can be easily placed through the pars plana or corneal limbus, but may not be large enough to remove blood from the eye, particularly if any of the blood is clotted. A 25 gauge needle is sufficiently large to remove most blood-stained fluid, but may leave a small hole, especially at the limbus, through which some of the gas can escape. We have found a 5/8 inch long 27 gauge needle to be satisfactory in most cases. Generally a 5 or 10 cc syringe is used containing the gas, usually sterile air, to be injected into the eye. It is helpful to fill the syringe only 80% with gas, allowing for movement of the syringe plunger outward to extract fluid from the eye prior to injecting gas into the eye.

Position of patient

It is possible to carry out fluid/gas exchange with the patient in many different positions. It can be done with the patient lying in the prone position on an examining table or with the patient kneeling in the face-down position on an examining chair. We have found it practical to carry out fluid/gas exchange procedures in the postoperative period at the slit lamp in essentially all of our aphakic patients, and many of our phakic patients as well.

Slit lamp technique

In this technique, the patient is seated at the slit lamp and the fluid/gas exchange carried out under slit lamp visualization. Either topical or retrobulbar anesthesia may be used, and a lid speculum is put in place. It is extremely helpful to have an assistant available to support the patient's head position and to aid in the manipulation of the syringe plunger.

A 5 cc syringe is desirable for use at the slit lamp. A much larger syringe is difficult to manipulate safely. A much smaller syringe will usually have a narrower internal lumen, and subsequently will not allow the aspirated fluid to run down the barrel of the syringe and away from the needle. A 22 micron millipore filter is placed on the 5 cc syringe, and then the syringe is partially filled with the air or air/gas mixture to be used. The filter is removed and replaced with a 27 gauge needle. Under direct visualization, the primary surgeon places the needle through the temporal limbus into the anterior chamber of the aphakic eye (Fig. 1A), or through the conjunctiva, sclera, and pars plana into the vitreous cavity behind the lens of the phakic eye. The assistant slowly retracts the plunger, withdrawing a small amount of fluid (Fig. 1B). The primary surgeon then manipulates the barrel of the syringe downward so that this fluid will run away from the needle into the proximal syringe leaving the distal syringe filled with the air/gas mixture. At this point, close attention must be paid to the position of the tip of the needle within the eye.

After maneuvering the needle to fill the distal syringe with air, the assistant injects a small amount of gas into the eye (Fig. 1C). The primary surgeon then manipulates the needle tip back into the intraocular fluid and the cycle is repeated as necessary, with additional gas injected into the eye with each cycle (Figs. 1D and 1E). Ultimately, it is possible to inject a large volume of gas into the eye.

In most cases it is possible to completely fill the vitreous cavity with air or gas using this technique. When the patient has had only topical anesthesia, it is often helpful to have the patient slowly and carefully look down so the residual intraocular fluid will flow from the inferior aspect of the vitreous cavity over the iris and into the anterior chamber where it can be easily removed by the needle in the anterior chamber. To aspirate the last small amount of liquid from the eye, the iris sphincter can be depressed at the six o'clock position (Fig. 1F), allowing fluid to flow from the posterior chamber into the anterior chamber, from which it can be aspirated (Fig. 1G). However, this may be slightly painful to the patient unless retrobulbar anesthesia has been used.

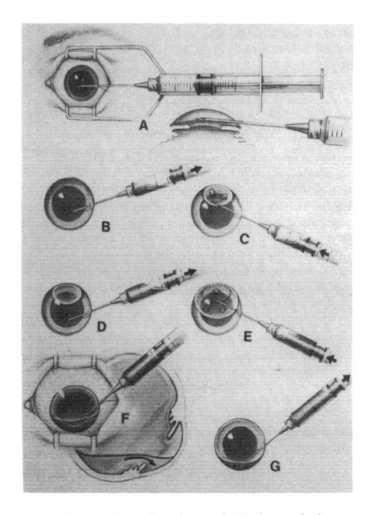

Figure 1. Fluid/gas exchange at the slit-lamp in an aphakic vitrectomized eye.
A. Pupil is widely dilated, lid speculum placed, and needle placed through the limbus. Note syringe is not completely full of air/gas mixture.
B. Fluid withdrawn from anterior chamber.
C. Syringe lowered to allow fluid to run away from needle leaving the distal syringe with air. A small amount of air is then injected into the anterior chamber.
D. The needle tip is then lowered back into the fluid layer and more fluid removed.
E. The needle tip is then placed within the existing bubble and more air injected. This method will avoid "fish-eggs" in the anterior chamber.
F. The patient looks down and the iris depressed with the needle to allow the remaining vitreous cavity fluid to draw anteriorly.
G. This remaining fluid is then drawn from the inferior anterior chamber.

Using this slit lamp technique, it is possible in the vast majority of cases to remove essentially all of the liquid or blood-stained fluid from the aphakic eye and replace it with a large air bubble. In some cases it may be difficult to safely carry out a complete fluid/gas exchange in the phakic eye using the slit lamp technique, and for that reason we occasionally use a face down technique or a horizontal technique (Blankenship, 1984 - personal communication) when attemping *complete* fluid/gas exchange in the phakic eye.

Face down technique

In this technique the patient is placed in the kneeling position on the examining chair facing backwards with his head resting on the headrest of the examining chair. The examining chair is elevated to the highest position and the surgeon sits on a stool in the lowest position. The surgeon positions himself in such a way as to be looking up into the patient's eye. This technique is aided by the surgeon wearing an indirect ophthalmoscope to illuminate the patient's eye. After administering retrobulbar anesthesia as described above it is possible to place a sharp needle through either the corneal limbus in aphakic eyes or through the pars plana in phakic eyes. Fluid/gas exchange is then carried out in a similar fashion as described above, often with the aid of an assistant manipulating the syringe plunger. The face down method has the advantage of being a desirable technique when total fluid/gas exchange is needed in the phakic eye, since it is relatively easy using this technique to remove all or nearly all of the intraocular fluid from the eye and replace it with gas. Minimal manipulation of the needle is required within the eye. However, the disadvantage of this technique is that the visualization is only fair compared with the slit lamp technique, and many small gas bubbles ("fish-eggs") are often produced, making visualization of the fundus difficult for as long as 24 to 36 hours.

Horizontal position

In this technique the patient is positioned in such a way that the temporal pars plana is in the dependent position. With the syringe partially filled as described above with sterile gas, the needle is pushed through the conjunctiva and sclera approximately 3.5 mm posterior to the limbus in the most temporal position (Fig. 2A). The surgeon again uses an indirect ophthalmoscope to illuminate the patient's eye. Approximately 1/2 cc of fluid stained with blood is removed. The blood-stained fluid is allowed to run down the barrel of the syringe and away from the needle. Following this, a small amount of gas, approximately 1/2 cc, is injected into the eye. This is repeated several times until the eye is moderately firm and essentially completely filled with gas. To remove as much blood-stained liquid from the eye as possible, it is helpful to exert gentle traction on the plunger of the syringe as the needle is slowly withdrawn from the eye (Fig. 2D). Thus, it is possible to get almost the last drop of blood-stained liquid out of the eye.

In most cases, using any of the above three techniques, the 27 gauge needle can simply be withdrawn from the eye and the tract will be self-sealing. The limbal entrance will seal spontaneoulsy in most cases because of the valve effect of a shelved puncture. In some cases, it can be helpful to hold a Q-tip sponge against this tract momentarily to ensure that it remains closed. Rarely iris tissue will become incarcerated in the inner

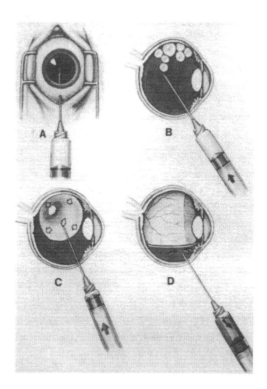

Figure 2. Horizontal position fluid/gas exchange in a phakic vitretomized eye.
A. Pars plana approach in a widely dilated, well exposed eye.
B. Slow injection of gas will cause multiple small bubbles, "fish-eggs", to occur.
C. Rapid injection of approximately 1 1/2 cc of gas will avoid "fish-eggs", with the resulting gas bubble being under pressure.
D. As fluid is withdrawn from the eye this bubble will expand to fill the vitreous cavity.

opening in the cornea. This can usually be released by a simple message of the cornea with a blunt instrument externally over this area of iris incarceration. Also, it is possibile that the needle may be pulled out of the eye prematurely. If this is done and if the corneal tract has sealed itself, it is usually desireable to use a new needle which is sharp and sterile and place it back into the anterior chamber through the limbus at a new place in the cornea. Placing it through the previously used corneal opening will often stretch this opening so that it subsequently leaks.

Complications

"Fish-egg" gas bubbles

One problem encountered during any of the above three maneuvers is that as gas is injected into the eye the gas tends to move upward and away from the tip of the needle. This produces multiple small bubbles of gas within the eye ("fish-eggs") (Fig. 2B). These can make the visualization of the fundus and laser treatment of the retina extremely difficult immediately following the fluid/gas exchange, particularly when the lens is in place. One way to minimize the development of these "fish-eggs" is to use a technique in which air is injected into the eye under pressure. This can only be done safely and comfortably when retrobulbar anesthesia has been used. In this situation gas is first injected into the eye in an amount of approximately 1 1/2 cc. This immediately raises the pressure in the eye and compresses the gas bubble within the eye (Fig. 2C). At this point, fluid can now be removed fairly quickly from the vitreous cavity with the syringe, allowing the gas bubble to expand within the eye, filling the eye completely with the bubble (see Fig. 2D). If the globe feels firm in response to delicate manipulations of the needle where it passes through the sclera, some gas can be removed from the eye through this same needle at this time.

Another method of avoiding "fish-eggs" is to position the needle tip such that it is initially within any small bubble already within the eye (see Figure 1E). Then, as the gas is injected, the pre-existing bubble will simply enlarge rather than having multiple small bubbles forming at the tip of the needle. This technique is especially applicable in the slit lamp technique described above. However, it is somewhat dangerous and should generally be avoided in phakic patients using the face down or horizontal position. If necessary, it is possible to cause these "fish-eggs" to coalesce rapidly into a large bubble by using a laser focused into the eye onto the interfaces of these bubbles (de Juan E., 1984, personal communication). However, this does pose certain hazards to the retina. Occasionally, gentle tapping on the cornea of the anesthetized eye will cause multiple small gas bubbles to coalesce into one large bubble (Rodiquez A., 1984, personal communication).

Other complications

More serious complications are possible, as with any time the eye is entered. The phakic eye can develop a cataract if the lens capsule is touched by the needle. Other complications include wound leak, iris incarceration in the corneal wound, elevated intraocular pressure, corneal endothelial injury, and possible endophthalmitis. Endophthalmitis following a fluid/gas exchange procedure outside of the operating room has been seen in the Duke Eye Center one in approximately 1,000 such procedures. Fortunately, this was recognized early and treated with complete recovery.

NEEDLE ASPIRATION FOR POSTOPERATIVE ELEVATION OF INTRAOCULAR PRESSURE

Although it is often necessary to augment a gas bubble in postoperative vitreoretinal surgery, another frequent problem in these cases is a postoperative elevation of intraocular pressure. Maximal medical therapy is initiated when necessary. However, the intraocular pressure often cannot be adequately controlled secondary to the nature of expanding gases now being used in surgery. In such cases it may be necessary to place a needle into the eye to withdraw some of this gas.

It is important to recognize the different values obtained when comparing Shiotz to applanation tonometry in eyes filled with a gas bubble. Shiotz tonometry will tend to under-estimate the actual pressure in these eyes (1), and therefore applanation tonometry should be used to obtain the most accurate value. We generally attempt to reduce intraocular pressure by needle aspiration of gas or fluid when it is persistently above 40 mm Hg despite medical therapy, measured by applanation tonometry. Variations of the techniques described above are used for this procedure.

In the vitrectomized, aphakic eye, the limbal approach is used. Often, the anterior chamber is shallow or flat, and special care must be used to avoid damaging the iris. In the phakic eye a pars plana approach is used. Anesthesia, antibiotics, and exposure are similar to those mentioned above. A 30 gauge needle is generally used, since often no fluid needs to be drawn out, and a smaller needle is less likely to create a wound which will leak.

With the patient sitting at the slit lamp, the 30 guage needle on a 1 cc TB syringe is placed into the eye under biomicroscopic view. Although this can be done alone, an assistant is often helpful to work the syringe plunger while the tip of the needle is kept in view through the slit lamp. The small syringe allows for better control of the amount of gas removed. Generally, removal of .2 to .3 cc of gas will sufficiently lower the intraocular pressure to an acceptable level. With the aid of an assistant it is possible to measure the pressure by applanation tonometry with the needle inside the eye, but this is not routinely done.

By gentle manipulation of the needle at the point where it enters the eye, it is often possible to judge whether the intraocular pressure is markedly elevated, close to the normal range, or very soft. This procedure can be repeated as necessary to reduce pressure, but we have found a single aspiration is usually sufficient. In some cases in which the intraocular pressure is elevated and the eye is partially filled with a gas bubble and partially with fluid, it may be desirable to aspirate only the fluid.

Complications include those listed above for fluid/gas exchange. Additional problems include 1) wound leak, which most often can be controlled by pressure from a cotton-tipped applicator after withdrawing the needle, 2) initial removal of too much gas and subsequent re-detachment of the retina, and 3) continual wound leak over many hours or days with reduction of the gas volume in the eye and re-detachment of the retina. These complications are rare, and can usually be avoided by careful attention to proper technique.

THE USE OF SODIUM HYALURONATE FOR CORNEAL ENDOTHELIAL STRIAE

The fluid/gas procedure outlined in Part I above is extremely helpful in affording an improved view of the fundus for postoperative examinations or in those eyes requiring further laser treatment. However, in many aphakic eyes after repeated operations, or following days or weeks with a gas bubble in the eye, folds in Descemet's membrane develop. This may be from the large volume of irrigating fluid used during vitrectomy, from the effect of elevated intraocular pressure, or possibly the effect of gas on the corneal endothelial pump function. These folds in Descemet's membrane often make pan-retinal photocoagulation or even simple fundus examination difficult or impossible. This is particularly frustrating after successful fluid/gas exchange has been done but the view of the fundus is still obscured due to the optical distortion by these folds. We have used Sodium Hyaluronate (Healon[R], Pharmacie laboratories, 800 centennial Ave, Piscataway, New Jersey 08854) in the operating room to improve visualization secondary to Decemet's folds with some success (2). Recently, following fluid/gas exchange in an aphakic post-vitrectomized eye, we were able to markedly improve fundus visualization by coating the endothelial surface with sodium hyaluronate under biomicroscopic view. The following is a description of this procedure.

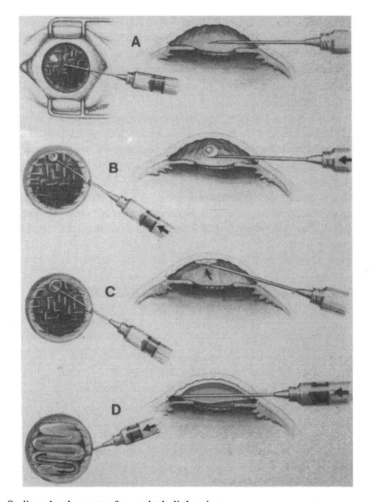

Figure 3. Sodium hyaluronate for endothelial striae.
A. Note schematic representation of Descemet's folds. The needle is placed through the limbus, bevel up, after fluid/gas exchange is completed.
B. A drop of sodium hyaluronate is expressed from the tip.
C. This drop is pressed against the endothelial surface.
D. The needle is swept back and forth, moving inferiorly with each stroke, as the sodium hyaluronate is gently expressed. Note the now smooth posterior optical surface allowing for examination of the fundus and retinal laser therapy if needed.

Anesthesia, antibiotics and exposure are the same as described previously. After complete fluid/gas exchange is performed, a separate entry wound is made at the corneal limbus, with the patient seated at the slit lamp, using a 27 gauge needle fitted on a 2 cc syringe filled with 0.4 cc of 10 mg/cc sodium hyaluronate (Fig. 3A). The tip of the needle is then directed superiorly within the anterior chamber, taking care not to allow the tip to actually invade any angle structures or touch the corneal endothelium. The plunger is pushed in slowly, either by the surgeon or an assistant, and a drop of sodium hylauronate is expressed at the tip of the needle (Fig. 3B). Starting superiorly, the surgeon then sweeps the drop of sodium hyaluronate slowly across the posterior surface of the cornea (Figure 3C), then back and forth across the endothelium with each stroke progressing inferiorly (Figure 3D). Extreme care must be taken to avoid letting the needle itself touch the corneal endothelium. Placing the bevel of the needle forward during this part of the procedure allows the Healon to contact the endothelial surface without needle contact.

Using this technique it is possible to coat the Descemet's folds and create a smooth optical surface clear enough to view the fundus, and regular enough so that laser therapy to the retina can be carried out immediately. This effect lasts for approximately one hour, followed by gradual reappearance of the folds, superiorly first, then gradually appearing inferiorly as Healon is pulled downward by gravity.

Possible complications are similar to those listed with fluid/gas exchange, along with a small risk of transient elevated intraocular pressure from Healon clogging the angel, although this was not noted in the immediate postoperative period in the case described above.

ADHERENT VITREOUS STRANDS

Vitreous incarceration in a cataract wound is a well known complication of cataract surgery, and is felt to be responsible in many cases for the development of postoperative cystoid macular edema (3-7). Recent reports have shown both anterior vitrectomy and pars plana vitrectomy to remove incarcerated vitreous are associated with significant improvement of visual acuity compared to conservative medical therapy (8-12). When there is extensive incarceration this is the procedure of choice. However, in some cases a single strand of vitreous may extend into a corneal wound (Fig. 4A). An isolated strand of vitreous up to the cornea may be the result of an accidental or even iatrogenic needle-sized perforation of the cornea. This strand may produce vitreo-retinal traction, and may even produce a retinal hole. To release such a strand, a modification of our slit lamp technique may be used as an alternative to anterior vitrectomy.

A limbal approach is used, utilizing mydriasis, topical anesthesia, and antibiotics as noted previously. In this technique, a 27 gauge needle on a 3 cc syringe containing 1/2 cc of sterile air is inserted through the temporal limbus into the anterior chamber. The bevel of the needle is brought into contact with the vitreous strand (Fig. 4B), and suction is used to draw the strand into the opening of the needle. Traction is then exerted on the vitreous strand by slightly withdrawing the needle, and the strand then pulled free from the old corneal wound. Once freed from the corneal wound, the vitreous strand still held by suction is moved back into the center of the pupil (Fig. 4C). Care must be taken not to twist vitreous around the needle at this point, resulting in increased areas of contact between the needle and vitreous. Once the strand is located in the center of the pupil, a small amount of air is refluxed through the syringe to release the vitreous strand. This usually results in a number of small bubbles forming in the anterior chamber (Fig. 4D). When the strand is released, the needle is withdrawn.

Complications arising from this procedure in addition to those listed above include failure to remove the vitreous strand and reincarceration of vitreous in the exit site. Should either of these occur, anterior vitrectomy should then be considered.

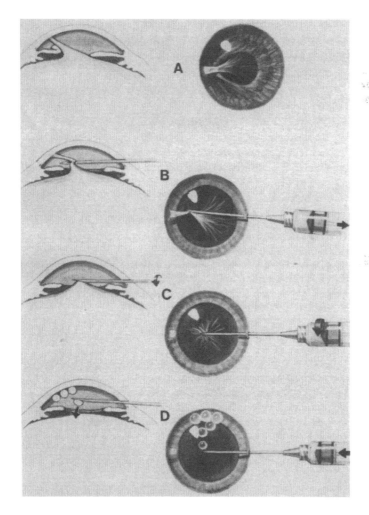

Figure 4. Slit-lamp approach to adherent vitreous strands.
A. Vitreous adherent to wound with irregular pupil.
B. A needle is placed through the limbus, and suction applied to grab the strand.
C. The needle is withdrawn slightly to center over the pupil, and rotated bevel down.
D. Air is expressed through the needle releasing the vitreous strand posteriorly.

368

CONCLUSION

Recent advances in ophthalmology now allow surgical correction of more complicated vitreo-retinal diseases, often which are commonly performed outside the operating room to effectively treat postoperative problems. Fluid/gas exchange in the postoperative vitrectomy patient done outside the operating room can be a useful aid in their management. Sodium hyaluronate can be used as an adjunct to fluid/gas exchange to improve visualization of the fundus in selected cases with Descemet's folds. Surgical removal of single strands of incarcerated vitreous can also be approached in an examining room setting in certain cases. The advantanges of not having to return the patient to the operating room have been discussed. With careful attention to detail during the procedures, along with care to insure the sterility of the instruments entering the eye, these procedures can be done safely, comfortably, and effectively with minimal risk to the patient.

REFERENCES

1. Moses RA (1966): Schiotz tonometry with an air bubble in the eye. Am J Ophthalmol 62 (2): 281-282.
2. Landers MB, III (1982): Sodium hyaluronate (Healon) as an Aide to Internal Fluid/gas exchange. Letter to the editor. Am J Ophthalmol 94 (4): 557-559.
3. Irvine SR (1953): A newly defined vitreous syndrome following cataract surgery. Interpreted according to recent concepts of the structure of the vitreous. The Seventh Francis I. Proctor Lecture. Am J Ophthalmol 36:599.
4. Gass JDM and Norton EWD (1966): Cystoid macular edema and papilledema following cataract extraction. Arch Ophthalmol 76:646.
5. Irvine AR, Bresky R, Crowder BM, Forster RK, Hunter DM and Kulvin SM (1971): Macular edema after cataract extraction. Ann Ophthalmol 3:1234.
6. Michels RG, Green WR and Maumenee AE (1971): Cystoid macular edema following cataraction (the Irvine-Gass syndrome). A case studied clinically and histopathologically. Ophthalmic Surg 2:217.
7. Norton AL, Brown WJ, Carlson M, Pilger IS and Riffenburgh RS (1975): Pathogenesis of aphakic macular edema. Am J Ophthalmol 80:96.
8. Aaberg TM (1977): Pars plana vitrectomy for persistent aphakic cystoid macular edema secondary to vitreous incarceration in the cataract wound In McPherson A (ed.): New and Controversial Aspect of Vitreo-retinal Surgery. St Louis, CV Mosby pp 230-233.
9. Taylor HR, Michels RG and Stark WJ (1979): Vitrectomy methods in anterior segment surgery. Ophthalmic Surg 10:25.
10. Federman JL, Annesdey WH, Sarin LK and Remer P (1980): Vitrectomy and cystoid macular edema. Ophthalmology 87:622.
11. Fung WE (1980): Anterior vitretomy for chronic aphakic cystoid macular edema. Ophthalmology 87:189.
12. Robinson D, Landers MB, III Hahn DK (1983): An anterior surgical approach to aphakic cystoid macular edema. Am J Ophthalmol 95 (6): 811-817.

Basic and advanced vitreous surgery
G.W. Blankenship, M. Stirpe, M. Gonvers, S. Binder (eds.)
Fidia Research Series, vol. II,
Liviana Press, Padova © 1986

SILICONE OIL: RESULTS IN 300 CASES

Klaus Heimann

Department for Vitreo Retinal Surgery,
University Eye Clinic, Cologne, FRG

Successful treatment of retinal detachment in proliferative vitreoretinopathy (PVR) by injection of silicone oil into the vitreous space to unfold and permanently reattach the detached retina was developed by P. Cibis. After Cibis's death, E. Okun and J. Scott have continued and extended this surgical technique. It has been taken up again above all in Europe (Leaver and Grey, Haut, Zivojnović) after vitrectomy in association with a temporary gas tamponade of the vitreous cavity had not provided the hoped-for positive long-term results in these unfavorable forms of retinal detachment. In the Department of Ophthalmology at the Cologne University Medical School, the silicone oil technique has been applied since 1979. Experience in operation of 300 cases will be reported below.

METHOD

In various forms of complicated retinal detachment (Table 1), silicone oil was injected into the vitreous cavity in order: 1. to unfold mobile retina, 2. to fix the retina in order to avoid or to limit recurrence of detachment and 3, to stop intraoperative and postoperative bleeding, e.g. in proliferative diabetic retinopathy. In most cases (80%), a pars plana vitrectomy was performed before injection of the oil; this permits microscopic control of the entire operation process.

The surgical procedure takes place in the following steps: first of all, a partial vitrectomy is performed to remove transvitreal strands. It is attempted to preserve the anterior vitreous in phakic eyes in order to avoid direct contact between the silicone oil and the back of the lens. If the retina is contracted together in rigid folds, it must be mobilized by means of severance and removal of epiretinal membranes, proliferatively altered and contracted vitreous base and subretinal proliferations (Fig. 1). Subretinal proliferations require circumscribed opening of the retina above them. If the retina nevertheless remains stiff and contracted, the circumscribed or extensive retinotomies are necessary

Table 1. *Indications for silicone oil injection in 300 cases of complicated retinal detachment (Oct. 1979 - April 1983)*

	n.	%
PVR detachment	143	47.7%
traumatic detachment	84	28.0%
giant tear detachment	37	12.4%
macula hole detachment	10	3.3%
prolif. diab. retinopathy	19	6.3%
phthisis	7	2.3%
	300	

in order to achieve a smooth fixation of the retina in the subsequent injection of silicone oil and to prevent retinal tears. If necessary, the ends of the retina cut free must be fixed by suture (Zivojnović) or by small plastic nails (Ando) in the sclera. Injection of silicone oil into the vitreous cavity takes place through an automatically operated silicone syringe or via the infusion tube of the vitrectomy instrument set. The intraocular fluid is drained from the preretinal space via a flute needle under microscopic control. Drainage of the subretinal space can be carried out transretinally via a hole in the retina (endodrainage) (Fig. 2) or transclerally (exodrainage). Remaining tractions on the retinal

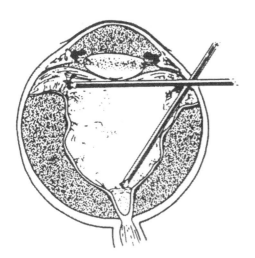

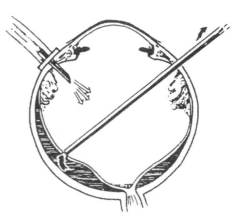

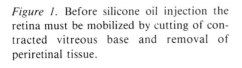

Figure 1. Before silicone oil injection the retina must be mobilized by cutting of contracted vitreous base and removal of periretinal tissue.

Figure 2. Fluid - silicone oil exchange followed by endodrainage of subretinal fluid through retinal hole.

surface or in the region of the base of the vitreous are shown up particularly clearly under the silicone oil and can be detached or severed retrospectively with appropriate instruments (vitreous scissors). These surgical measures are always associated with a slightly pre-equatorial circlage, possibly in connection with additional buckling measures in the region of peripheral tears. In centrally situated, tension-free retinal holes, it is sufficient to close the gap by endodiathermia or endocryopexy.

PATIENTS

From October 1979 to April 1983, 293 cases of complicated retinal detachments of various indications and seven eyes with prephthisis were treated by silicone oil injection, the latter at the request of the patients in order to arrest further shrinkage of the globe. With the exception of the patients with giant tears of the retina, these were in some cases eyes which had been previously operated on several times. In 54% (161/300), there was an aphakia (Tab. 1). Since the majority of the patients came from outside the region, the number of patients was reduced in the postoperative control period, so that appraisals of long-term results can only be made on the basis of ever smaller numbers of patients.

RESULTS

An anatomical reattachment of 182 patients who were checked after 12 months showed a total reattachment in 52% and a partial reattachment in 27.5%. We take partial retinal reattachment to mean a residual detachment delimited by the silicone oil bubble, mostly in the lower half of the fundus. It does not include the macular zone and does not lead to appreciable loss of function, so that re-operations do not appear to be necessary. *Functionally*, at least orientative vision (vision $\geq 1/50$) could be achieved in 54%. In contrast to the morphology, the functions deteriorate with longer postoperative control period due to the complications. For the patient, the reattainment of almost normal outer boundaries of the visual field is more important than the central visual acuity. This is above all important for patients in whom the other eye is already blind. In 75 cases, the *only eye* of the patient is involved. At a six month follow-up, a total or partial retinal reattachment could be detected in 73%, and orientative vision in 42%.

If the individual indication groups are compared, the functional results (12 months postoperatively) in the PVR detachments are better than after traumatic retinal detachments (59% as compared to 46% with at least orientative vision). In all seven phthisis cases, the silicone oil injection prevented a further painful shrinkage of the bulb under reasonably satisfactory cosmetic conditions.

REFERENCES

1. Ando F, Kondo J (1983): A plastic tack for the treatment of retinal detachment with giant tear. Am J Ophthalmol 95:260-261.

2. Cibis PA, Becker B, Okun E, Canaan S (1981): The use of liquid silicone in retinal detachment surgery. Arch Ophthalmol 68:590-592.
3. Grey RHB, Leaver PK (1979): Silicone oil in the treatment of massive preretinal retraction. I. results in 105 eyes. Br J Ophthalmol 63:355-360.
4. Haut J, Ullern M, Boulard ML, Gedah A (1978): Utilisation du silicone intra-oculaire apres Vitrektomie. Note Preliminaire. Bull Soc Ophthalmol Fr 78:361.
5. Heimann K (1980): Zur Behandlung komplizierter Riesenrisse der Netzhaut. Klin Mbl Augenheilk 176:491-492.
6. Okun E (1968): Intravitreal surgery utilizing liquid silicone. A long term follow-up. Transact Pacif Cst Otoophthalmol Soc 141.
7. Scott JD (1973): Treatment of the detached immobile retina. Transact Ophthalmol Soc UK 92:351-357.
8. Scott JD (1975): Giant tear of the retina. Transact Ophthalmol Soc UK 95:142-144.
9. Scott JD (1981): Use of liquid silicone in vitrectomised eyes. Dev Ophthlmol 2:185-190.
10. Wessing A, Lagua H, Herwig H, Meyer-Schwickerath H. (1981): Silikonölinjektion bei komplizierten Netzhautablösungen. Sitzungsber Rhein-Westf Augenärzte 140:91-94.
11. Zivojnovic R, Mertens DAE, Baarsma GS, (1980): Das flüssige Silikon in der Amotiochirurgie. I. Bericht über 90 Fälle. Klin Mbl Augenheilk 179:17-22.
12. Zivojnovic R, Mertens DAE, Peperkamp E (1982): Das flüssige Silikon in der Amotiochirurgie. II. Bericht über 200 Fälle - Klin Mbl Augenheilk 181:44-452.

Published in detail in the Klinische Monatsblätter für Augenheilkunde 185, 505, 1984.

Basic and advanced vitreous surgery
G.W. Blankenship, M. Stirpe, M. Gonvers, S. Binder (eds.)
Fidia Research Series, vol. II,
Liviana Press, Padova © 1986

LASER TREATMENT OF RETINAL DETACHMENT WITH P.V.R. AFTER VITRECTOMY IN THE PRESENCE OF SILICONE OIL

C. Villani and M. Del Duca

Divisione Oculistica C.T.O., Via Nemesio, Roma

The once skeptical attitude towards the use of silicone oil has recently given way to one of confidence, mainly due to the characteristics of this substance (transparency, stability, tamponing power unaltered in time). Its utilization, confined at first to the cases of proliferative vitreoretinopathy with possibility of relapse, has been extended to other pathologies, such as giant retinal tears, some proliferative diabetic retinopathies and perforating traumas. In all these cases, internal tamponing with silicone oil at the end of the operation, although it cannot prevent relapses, makes it possible to immobilize the membranes, to prevent the occurrence of complete detachment of the retina and to carry out an aimed removal (with silicone) of newly proliferated membranes. Intra-operative physical treatments (endocryo-cryo-transcleral, endophotocoagulation) may not be possible and must often be completed in the post-operative phase by means of the tamponing effect of silicone.

In this study we have considered treatment with Argon Laser applied to patients with a rhegmatogenous retinal detachment and proliferative vitreoretinopathy — either original or subsequent to surgery — who had been subjected to vitrectomy, encircling and internal tamponing with silicone oil (Fig. 1). Those treatments were employed to cause a steady retinal adhesion after encircling, to close holes which appeared after the first operation and block residual proliferations in view of the oil extraction operation. We carried out a circular post-equatorial treatment with an average of 4 parallel rows of 250 micron-diameter spots adjacent to one another, in addition to the treatment — varying from case to case — of holes and proliferations. 54 patients were treated over a period of 3 to 20 days after surgery. The follow-up stage is influenced by the extraction of silicone oil, which is carried out considering the state of the retina and the tolerance shown by such structures as the crystalline lens, the ciliary body and the cornea. For these reasons silicone oil may be extracted a month after the operation or may be left in the vitreous chamber for years without causing any reaction or intolerance effect. As far as the cases that we treated are concerned, we never experienced variations in the state of the retina after laser treatment in the presence of silicone oil, either immediately or some time after treatment.

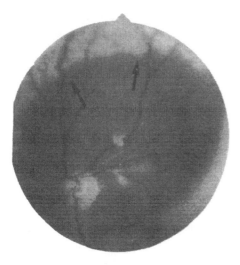

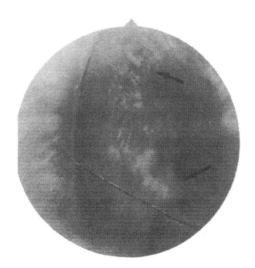

Figure 1. Picture of the ocular fundus in the presence of silicone oil with laser treatment.

Figure 2. Deviation of the laser beam due to the presence of the meniscus of the silicone oil bubble.

Thirty-two cases were subjected to the oil extraction operation. The follow-up stage lasted from 20 days to 3 years. Eight retina detachment relapses — accounting for 25% of the cases — were recorded, but this figure includes 4 cases of allergy to silicone, with extraction performed less than a month after vitrectomy, and two cases of sub-retinal proliferations, already evident during the treatment phase, with imperfect retinal adhesion.

The main problems that we faced in applying this kind of treatment were caused by the characteristics of silicone and by its V.C. structure. We constantly noticed the necessity of a 20% increase in order to obtain the impact, as compared to retinal treatments not using silicone oil. Probably, this is due partly to the partial reflection of the beam on the bubble surface and partly to defocalization phenomena occurring when crossing the bubble itself.

Furthermore, it should be noted that this power increase must be accompanied by a further one necessitated by the retinal edema subsequent to vitrectomy, and that such an increase must be as large as possible if the treatment is to be performed right after the operation. Another difficulty is caused by the structure and the size of the silicone bubble, that forms its meniscus in proximity to the encircling buckle, very often near the retinal areas to be treated. The presence of the meniscus is an obstacle to the focusing on the retina. Also, the areas adjacent to the meniscus present, as a consequence of the curvature of the bubble, a prism-like effect which deviates the beam towards the rear retinal areas.

This factor may make the treatment of adjacent retinal areas impossible, particularly in the presence of considerably marked encircling or subjected blocks. Moreover, the surgeon should be very careful in treating the area near the bubble edges in order to prevent a reflection of the laser beam and the subsequent occurrence of a second, distant impact (Figs. 2,3).

A final consideration of the characteristics of this particular treatment concerns the possible occurrence of bleeding. These bleeding phenomena are usually very limited and consist generally of small blood traces surrounding the spot (Fig. 4).

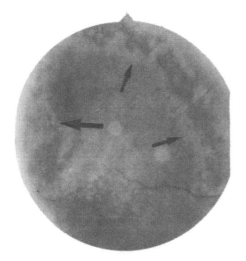 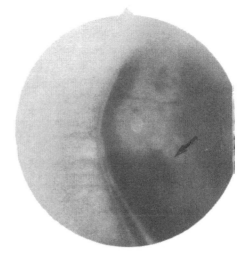

Figure 3. Duplication of the impact due to the presence of the meniscus of the silicone oil bubble

Figure 4. Bleeding subsequent to treatment

The pressure exerted by the silicone oil bubble on the underlying tissues is certainly due to a haemostatic mechanical effect, which restricts the bleeding phenomenon. In a few cases, the presence of retinal or sub-retinal proliferations made the treatment of the areas under consideration impossibile due to an imperfect retinal adhesion caused by the proliferations and to the risk of a stimulating effect of the treatment on the proliferation themselves.

Basic and advanced vitreous surgery
G.W. Blankenship, M. Stirpe, M. Gonvers, S. Binder (eds.)
Fidia Research Series, vol. II,
Liviana Press, Padova © 1986

INTERNAL TAMPONADE WITH SILICONE OIL: ECHOGRAPHIC EVALUATION

M. Del Duca

Divisione Oculistica C.T.O., Via Nemesio, Roma

Silicone oil is used as an internal tamponade after vitrectomies. We also used this method for peeling off posterior epiretinal membranes with P.R. of recent occurrence. If there is a lens or vitreous opacity after vitrectomy, echography is necessary for the postoperative controls. Blood residuals or exudates in the early post-operatory period hinder exploration, as do cataracts which form during the months after the operation. The physical properties of silicone oil make the echographic interpretation more difficult. One of the features of silicone is the reduced speed of propagation of ultrasound in this media. We know from literature that the velocity value in silicone oil is about 983 meters a second. The ratio between the velocity in silicone oil and the theoretic velocity of ultrasound through the optic axis gives a coefficient which allows us to compare the magnitudes obtained echographically with silicone with real magnitudes:

$$C = \frac{V1}{V} = \frac{983}{1550} = 0.63$$

Another feature of silicone is that of having an ultrasound absorption coefficient, linked to features such as high viscosity, which is expressed in a reduction of the echo amplitudes calculated approximately as 1 db per mm using 8 MHz probes.

Also to be borne in mind are factors such as acoustic impedence formed by the product of the velocity and density of means:

$$Z = p. \ C.$$

The considerable difference of this parameter between silicone and ocular tissues leads to a reflection coefficient R which is expressed when the ultrasounds pass from the fluid of the vitreous chamber to the silicone or vice versa:

$$R = \frac{Z2 - Z1}{Z1 + Z2} = 0.26$$

Other factors to remember are the angle of incidence or the defocalization phenomena caused by the curve of the silicone bubble. The quantitative evaluation of these factors goes beyond the possibilities of our instruments and this note is intended as an approach to a problem to be investigated more thoroughly.

In clinical practice we obtained a series of images, confirmed by surgical diagnosis, which show the possibilities, even though limited, offered by this technique. An initial feature, when there is a scleral encirclement, in eyes tamponed with silicone oil, consists of the false echographic localization of the encirclement. According to whether the silicone bubble is in front of or behind the encirclement, it appears much further back or vice versa with respect to its actual position due to the aforesaid silicone features (low ultrasound velocity) (Figs. 5, 6, 7).

The magnitude of the silicone bubble represents the most important problem in echographic diagnosis (Figs. 8, 9). If the bubble does not totally fill the vitreous chamber, the posterior echo of the bubble can be observed, as well as a space between the bubble and the rear wall. This space can either be empty or appear filled with blood or membranes or the retina itself (Figs. 10, 11, 12). It is obvious that the larger this space is, the greater the possibilities are of making a correct diagnosis. It is also possible to find blood or membranes in front of the bubble, thus confining it to the rear (Figs. 13, 14).

In some cases we succeeded in identifying the detached and contracted retina behind the bubble on the basis of the morphological features of the echographical pictures (Figs. 15, 16, 17, 18). We also obtained good pictures when there were substances behind the detached retina such as blood or silicone (Figs. 19, 20, 21, 22).

Finally there is the possibility that the silicone bubble is emulsified and that the small air bubbles inside it prevent a view of the rear structures (Fig. 23).

LITERATURE

1. Poujol J, Haut J, Fleury P (1978): Corrections à apporter dans l'examen ècographique des jeux remplis de silicone liquide. Bull Soc Opht France, 4-5, 367-369.
2. Poujol J, Massim M (1979): L'examen echographique des jeux opèrè de decollement de retinè avec injection de silicone. Diagnostica ultrasonica in ophtalmologia. SIDUO VII H. Germet, 111-115.
3. Coleman J, Lizzi F, Jack R (1977): Ultrasonography of eye and orbit. Lea and Febiger, 1977, Philadelphia.
4. Hassani SN: Real time ophthalmic ultrasonography. Springer Verlag, New York Heidelberg Berlin.

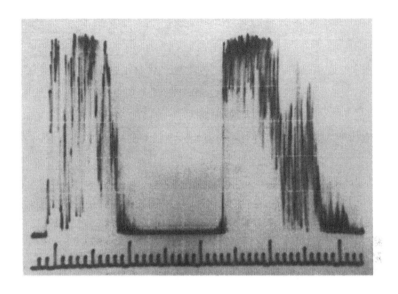

Figure 1. Scan picture of a normal eye.

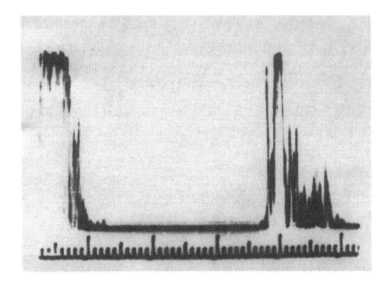

Figure 2. Scan picture of an eye with silicone oil.

380

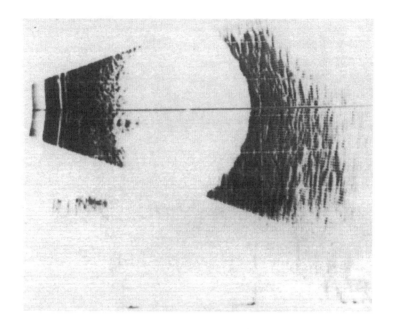

Figure 3. Scan picture of a normal eye.

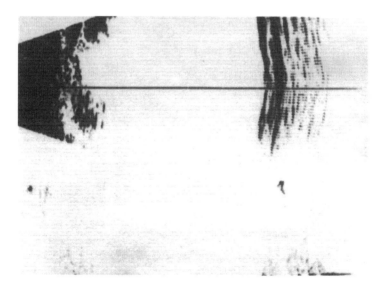

Figure 4. Scan picture of an eye with silicone oil.

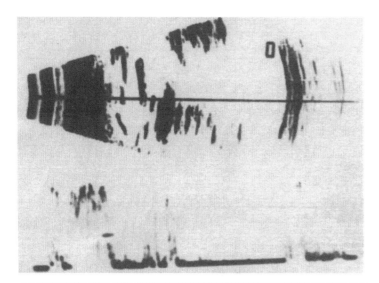

Figure 5, 6. False location of the encircling buckle because of the presence of the silicone oil bubble.

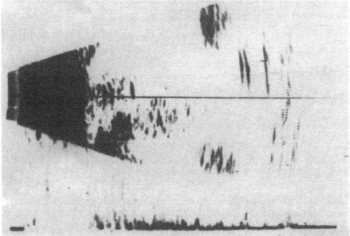

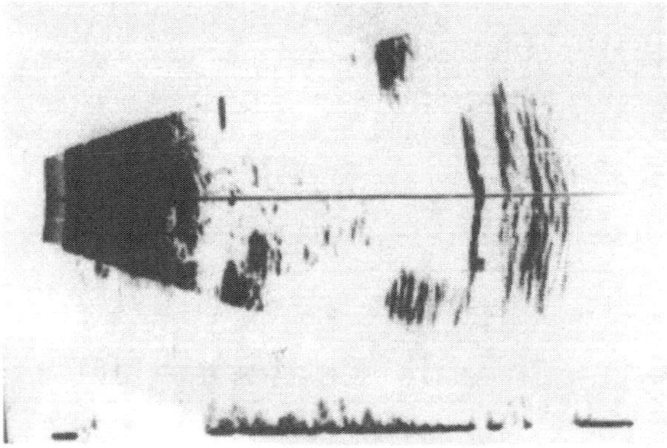

Figure 7. Echography of the ocular fundus in the presence of silicone oil.

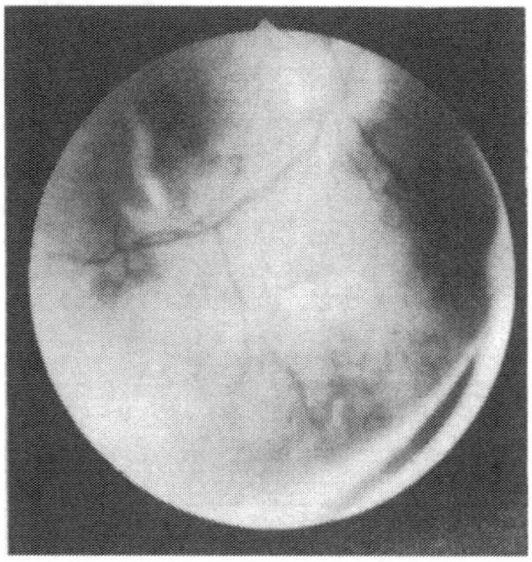

Figure 8. Picture of the ocular fundus in the presence of silicone oil.

382

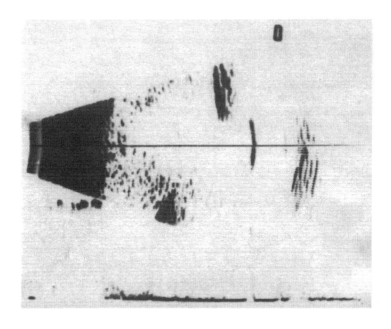

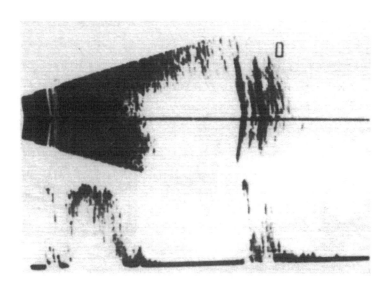

Figure 9, 10. Presence of echoes to refer to the posterior meniscus of the silicone oil bubble.

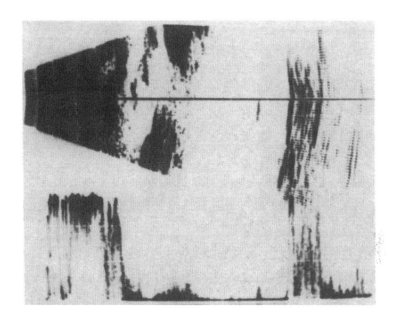

Figure 11. Presence of blood behind the silicone oil bubble.

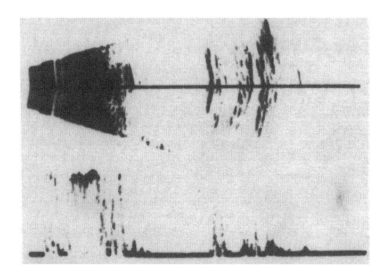

Figure 12. Presence of fibrin behind the silicone oil bubble.

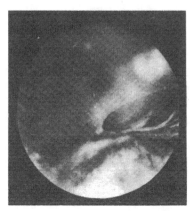

Figure 13. Picture of membranes before the silicone oil bubble.

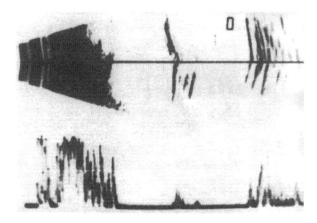

Figure 14. Echography of the same case.

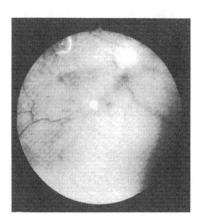

Figure 15. Picture of retinal detachment behind the silicone oil bubble.

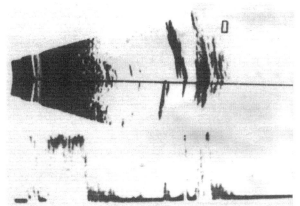

Figure 16. Echography of the same case.

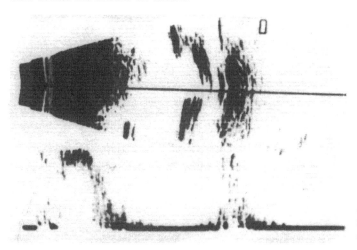

Figure 17. Retinal detachment behind the silicone oil.

385

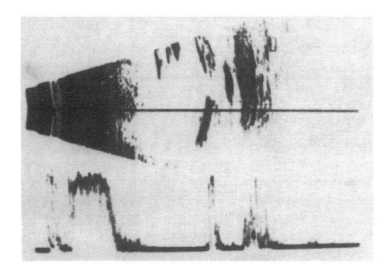

Figure 18. Retinal detachment behind the silicone oil.

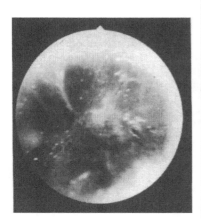

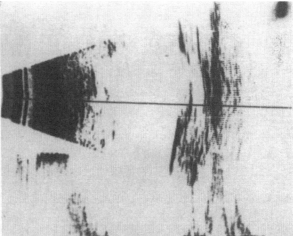

Figure 19. Presence of subretinal blood behind the silicone oil bubble.

Figure 20. Retinal detachment in the presence of silicone. Echography of the same case.

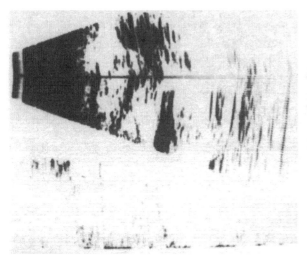

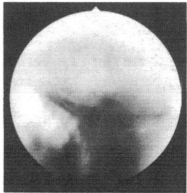

Figure 21. Retinal detachment in the presence of silicone oil behind the retina.

Figure 22. Picture of the same case.

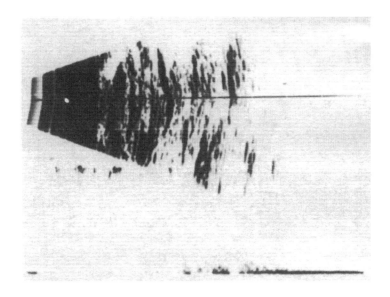

Figure 23. Emulsified silicone oil bubble.

Basic and advanced vitreous surgery
G.W. Blankenship, M. Stirpe, M. Gonvers, S. Binder (eds.)
Fidia Research Series, vol. II,
Liviana Press, Padova © 1986

Section XIV
Internal tamponade
III. Complications of silicone oil

COMPLICATIONS OF SILICONE OIL

P.K. Leaver

Moorfields Eye Hospital, City Road, London EC1V 2PD

Since the introduction by Paul Cibis of silicone-oil as an agent for intraocular tamponade in human eyes, the complications associated with its use have been widely reported.

Until recently speculation concerning retinal toxicity went largely unchallenged following the damaging reports of Schepens and his co-workers. Due largely to the work of John Scott in England silicone-oil is now widely used in several European centres for the treatment of otherwise refractory cases of complex retinal detachement.

Recent studies by workers of high integrity and scientific standing have confirmed the findings of previous authors that intraocular silicone-oil is well tolerated by the retina in primates as well as in a wide variety of mammals. There now seems little doubt that retinal toxicity is not a significant threat and that silicone-oil can be left in contact with the inner surface of the retina for long periods of time without harm.

Clinical experience suggests that while silicone oil may not be toxic to other ocular tissues its close apposition to the posterior lens capsule or corneal endothelium leads to cataract and keratopathy. Our experience at Moorfields supports this view.

Keratopathy is not a common complication of intraocular silicone-oil because it is not usual for the silicone-oil globule to be in contact with the endothelium for long periods. Such a complication arises usually in a phakic eye where silicone-oil has managed to penetrate the zonules and enter the anterior chamber as a single large globule or in an aphakic eye where the retina is not attached behind the oil globule. In a recent series of 73 eyes with giant retinal tears we found only one example of silicone keratopathy in 63 successful cases.

Okun in 1968 found nearly 60% of phakic eyes in Cibis's original series had developed cataract after 3 years or longer. Our own experience has been similar, up to 80% developing some degree of lens opacity after this period in eyes in which silicone oil was injected without undertaking vitrectomy. More recently, in reviewing the large series of eyes with giant retinal tears in which vitrectomy was always undertaken prior to silicone-oil infusion, we found that only one phakic eye retained a completely clear lens after 18 months. It is our belief that silicone-oil does cause cataract in most instances.

Raised intraocular pressure has long been associated with silicone-oil injection, often unfairly. In phakic eyes with normal anterior segments, glaucoma is very uncommon after silicone-oil injection, except where silicone-oil enters the anterior chamber in large quantities through the zonules. If no silicone-oil enters the anterior chamber or only a moderate quantity of fine emulsion is present the intraocular pressure is unaffected.

However in aphakic eyes, particularly those with previously compromised anterior segments, glaucoma is common after retinal reattachment with silicone-oil. In eyes in which the lens is removed at the time of or after silicone-oil injection, glaucoma is much less common. Nevertheless, there can be little doubt that silicone oil injection in aphakic eyes is associated with a high incidence of glaucoma.

TREATMENT

Keratopathy can be treated successfully by removal of silicone-oil and penetrating keratoplasty provided that raised intraocular pressure is not a problem.

Cataract extraction either by the intracapsular or extracapsular method or by lensectomy can be accomplished without difficulty in eyes containing silicone-oil or from which it has been removed. In most instances it is best done by the intracapsular method if silicone-oil is left in situ because silicone-oil nearly always enters the anterior chamber during the course of extracapsular extraction and when trapped in the anterior chamber will cause keratopathy and/or glaucoma. Where the silicone-oil has already been removed the lens is usually best removed by lensectomy or intracapsular extraction unless a posterior chamber intraocular lens implant is planned.

The management of silicone-oil induced glaucoma is a bigger problem. In some cases control can be achieved by medical means alone. In those eyes with completely closed angles in which maximal medical therapy fails, removal of silicone-oil and the insertion of a Molteno tube or cyclocryotherapy when the silicone-oil cannot be removed offer the best alternatives.

In our recent review of 54 successful cases with giant retinal tears treated by vitrectomy and silicone-oil injection, 16 had glaucoma after 18 months. In 8 of these eyes the intraocular pressure was controlled, 3 by medical therapy alone, 2 by trabeculectomy, 2 with a Molteno tube and 1 with a combination of medical therapy and surgical treatment. In 8 eyes the intraocular pressure was not well controlled.

In summary, the occurrence of long-term complications of intraocular silicone-oil is not disputed. Keratopathy is rarely a significant problem provided that the retina is successfully reattached while cataract though common can be treated without difficulty. We believe that intractable glaucoma in aphakic eyes represents the most serious long-term complications of intraocular silicone-oil.

Basic and advanced vitreous surgery
G.W. Blankenship, M. Stirpe, M. Gonvers, S. Binder (eds.)
Fidia Research Series, vol. II,
Liviana Press, Padova © 1986

ENDOTHELIAL CELL DENSITY IN PATIENTS WITH INTRAVITREAL SILICONE OIL INJECTION

L. Cerulli, M. Stirpe *, A. Corsi, F. Ricci

Clinica Oculistica, Università di Roma,
* Fondazione Oftalmologica 'G.B. Bietti', Piazza Sassari, 5, Roma

In 1962 Cibis introduced human eye silicone oil injection. This surgical procedure is employed in retinal detachment complicated by massive retraction, when the normal surgical techniques have failed or would presumably fail (1,2). The literature reports various complications associated with intravitreal silicone oil injection, arising either in the posterior or anterior segments, those in the anterior segment being more delayed. In particular, many authors have described corneal complications variously related to whether the silicone oil does or does not pass into the anterior chamber. This occurs more often in aphakic eyes (1,2,10). In this condition the silicone which has passed into the anterior chamber may appear either in the form of large or small bubbles (1,2,4,6,10) or as a thin emulsion (3,6). Large bubbles have been described occasionally to occur in phakic eyes too (8), even if it is more than likely that the passage of silicone through the fibers of the zonula could lead to small bubbles or vitreous silicone emulsion appearing in the anterior chamber (2).

Corneal lesions described consist of:

1) corneal opacities in the area of contact between the cornea and silicone meniscus (1);

2) band keratopathy which is associated with a discontinuity in the endothelial cell layer (3);

3) intracytoplasmic vacuoli, which probably originate from phagocytosis of the silicone (10);

4) disorganization and inhibition of the fibers at the stromal level.

In some cases, corneal lesions located in the periphery of the cornea are accompanied by the presence of a silicone oil bubble in the anterior chamber (8). However, the anterior dislocation of silicone oil doesn't always end up causing macroscopically evident complications (2,5,7). Brodrick (9) has reported a band keratopathy following silicone oil intravitreal injection in three patients all of them having corneal anaesthesia, no silicone in the anterior chamber, and calcium phosphate subepithelial deposits. Due to the numerous surgical procedures performed on the eyes, it was difficult to identify silicone oil as the only pathogenetic cause. Taking into account the above considerations, it seemed interesting to us to carry out a specular microscopy study of corneal endothelium in patients who have had silicone oil injection.

MATERIALS AND METHODS

Our study has been carried out on a sample of 23 patients (13 males and 10 females) aged between 5 and 78 years, 15 of whom phakic, 5 aphakic only in one eye, 3 in both eyes. All patients have been subjected to vitrectomy followed by silicone oil injection into one eye, from 1 to 21 months before our observation. Since these patients have been examined only after the operation, in order to record possible changes, the endothelial cell density of the operated eye was compared with that of the unoperated eye. Two cases showing silicone in the A.C. on the first observation were examined by us after 12 months (pat. n. 4) and after 12 and 24 months (pat. n. 22). All the patients were subjected to a complete ophthalmological examination; the exact localization of silicone oil was assessed and corneal endothelium in the axial part of both eyes photographed utilizing a Zeiss non contact specular microscope and Ektachrome 200 Kodak film. The evaluation of cell density was carried out with a method we have previously described (11).

RESULTS

The localization and appearance of silicone oil in the different ocular compartments was observed by means of a slit-lamp. When silicone is located in the posterior chamber only (17 patients in our sample) due to the fact that it is optically neutral, it is hardly seen by focal light observation. However, its different refractive index, compared to the vitreous and the cristalloids, allows localizing the respective interface as a very intense yellowish reflection during the specular observation, while the borders of the intravitreal bubbles are more visible by retroillumination.

In one patient silicone was present in both the posterior and anterior chambers. In two patients it was possible to locate silicone in the anterior chamber only. Two subjects who also had a complicated cataract and who did not show signs of oil in the anterior chamber, were included in a group with silicone in the posterior chamber, just like another patient who had had silicone removed before the observation. In those cases where silicone was present in the anterior chamber we examined its appearance, its mobility during ocular movements and the possibility and extent of contact with corneal endothelium.

Two other patients, one with silicone in the anterior chamber and the other in the posterior chamber were excluded from the sample owing to their unsatisfactory cooperation. Silicone in the posterior chamber looked more often like a large bubble, generally well contained in a more or less fluid vitreous.

Instead, the appearance of silicone in the anterior chamber takes on different forms: in two aphakic patients it looked like a single large bubble that occupied the upper portion of the anterior chamber (Figs. 1,2). Another phakic patient had, on the contrary,

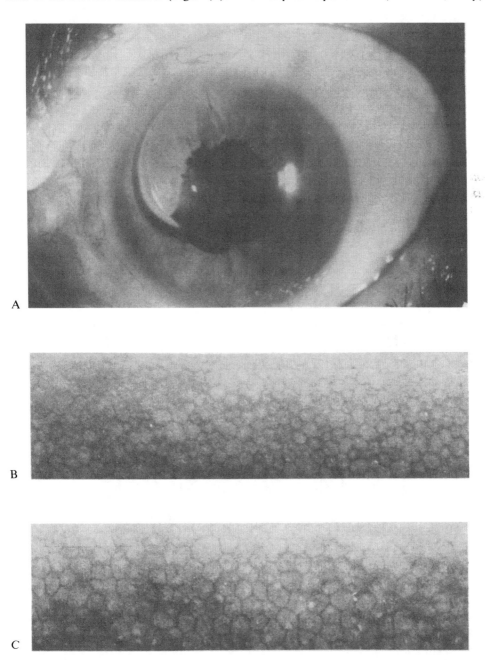

Figure 1. Patient n. 23. A) Large bubble of silicone oil in anterior chamber of aphakic patient. B) First observation: E.C.D. 2400 Cell/mq. C) Follow-up 12 months after: E.C.D. 1002 cell/mmq.

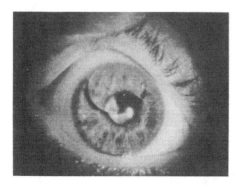

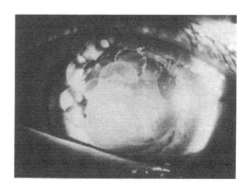

Figure 2. Patient n. 18. Large silicone bubble in anterior chamber of aphakic eye.

Figure 3. Small bubbles of silicone oil in the anterior chamber of phakic eye.

small bubbles which almost entirely occupied the anterior chamber (Fig. 3). In another patient silicone was dispersed in microspheres which, due to gravity, gathered together in the upper portion of the chamber angle and clearly separated from the aqueous humour (Fig. 4).

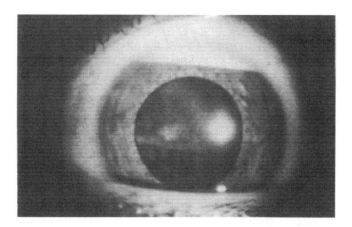

Figure 4. Patient n. 4. Presence of silicone microspheres in the upper portion of the angle.

Table 1 gives the data relative to age, the time since the operation, silicone location and the axial endothelial cell density of all patients divided into the three groups: phakic patients, one eye aphakic patients and both eyes aphakic patients. Table 2 reports the results of the Wilcoxon test on the differences in the ECD found between the operated eye and fellow healthy eye.

Table 1.

Phakic patients	Age	Follow-up (months)	Location of the Silicone	Cell Density cell/mm²	
				Normal eye	Eye with silicone
1	5	3	C.P.	3665	3653
2	8	10	C.P.	3452	3549
3	14	1	C.P.	3129	3274
4	18	3	C.A./C.P.	3132	3270
4a	19	15	C.A./C.P.	2997	2734
5	23	12	C.P.	3020	3046
6	50	10	C.P. *	2961	2613
7	52	12	C.P.	2340	2646
8	57	21	C.P.	2896	3177
9	60	3	C.P.	2871	2689
10	61	2	C.P.	2501	2621
11	64	14	C.P.	3111	2873
12	64	3	C.P.	2926	2653
13	65	6	C.P.	2663	2679
14	67	5	C.P.	3016	2813
15	68	3	C.P. *	3026	2743
One eye Aphakic					
16	6	12	C.P.	3366	3548/1918 *
17	46	12	C.P.	2893	2416
18	53	24	C.A.	2374	2952
19	74	4	C.P.	2876	2013
20	75	7	C.P.	2577	2038
Both eyes Aphakic					
21	47	12	C.P.	2093	1445
22	61	12	C.P.	2199	1349
23	77	12	C.A.	2800	2400
23a	78	24	C.A.	2919	1002
23b	79	31	C.A.	2348	1389

* Patient n. 16 perforating injury 3548 cell/mm² (peripheral area); 1918 cell/mm² (axial area).

Table 2
E.C.D. (Cell/mm²)

	Eye with injection	fellow eye
Mean	2953	2980
S.D.	351	329

Wilcoxon test
n = 15
T = 52 not significant

CONSIDERATIONS AND CONCLUSIONS

According to our data in phakic patients, it seems important to point out that the mean cell densities of the eyes with silicone, compared to that of normal healthy eyes, did not show a statistically significant difference (Tab. 2), whereas there was an important difference of this parameter in the other two groups of patients. However the decrease in the ECD found in this case might have been derived from different causes and not necessairly from the presence of silicone oil. In case n. 16 the low cell density found in the axial area (1,918 cell/mm²) compared to that of the adjacent areas (3,548 cell/mm²) is presumably due to the previous perforating corneal injury. In the remaining aphakic subjects we must consider that the cataract extraction is a notorious cause of decrease in cell density. Furthermore, these eyes with retinal detachment have undergone several operations in their clinical history (cataract extraction, lensectomy, vitrectomy). However, the 12 months follow-up from the first observation of the aphakic eye in patient n. 23 (Tab. 1, 23a) showed a decrease in cellular density of about 50% in the eye with the silicone bubble in the anterior chamber: this was certainly due to the presence of the latter (Fig. 1).

It is interesting also to note that the last control carried out 9 months after removing the silicone (Tab. 1, 23b) did not show further cell loss. On the other hand, it is impossible to state with absolute certainty that the cell density decrease being present in patient n. 18, who was aphakic too, with a silicone bubble in the anterior chamber, was exclusively due to the presence of silicone (Fig. 2). The decrease in cell density (13%) found during the follow-up of the only phakic patient (Tab. 1, 4a) who showed from the first observation the presence of silicone microspheres in the upper portion of the angle (Fig. 4), is not in our opinion so relevant as to prove, beyond any reasonable doubt, a silicone toxicity in this particular case. Finally, it seems interesting to point out that we did not find a significant difference between the mean cell density of the eyes with silicone; silicone doesn't seem to cause damage of the corneal endothelium if the normal compartimentalization of the eye chambers is preserved.

A decrease in endothelial cell density occurs if silicone oil, penetrating into the anterior chamber in the form of a large bubble, causes a continuous or intermittent mechanical trauma to the posterior corneal surface and/or a discontinuity of the endothelium-aqueous interchange. In conclusion, it seems advisable, should this event occur, to remove silicone from the anterior chamber immediately in order to avoid further damage which, in the long run, would cause corneal decompensation.

REFERENCES

1. Cibis PA, Becker B, Okun E, Canaan S (1962): The use of liquid silicone in retinal detachment. Arch Ophthal 68: 45-55.
2. Watzke RC (1967): Silicone retinopoiesis for retinal detachment. A long-term clinical evaluation. Arch Ophthal 77, 185-196.
3. Watzke RC (1967): Silicone retinopoiesis for retinal detachment. Surv Ophthal Clin Pathol Conference.
4. Cockerham W, Schepens CL, Freeman HM (1969): Silicone injection in retinal detachment. Mod Probl Ophthal 8: 525-540.
5. Rosengren B (1969): Silicone injection into the vitreous in hopeless cases of retinal detachment. Acta Ophthal 47:757-760.
6. Blodi FC (1971): Injection and impregnation of liquid silicone into ocular tissues. Am J Ophthal 71:1044-1051.
7. Kanski JJ, Daniel R (1973): Intravitreal silicone injection in retinal detachment. Brit J Ophthal 57:542-545.
8. Sugar HS, Okamura ID (1976): Ocular findings six years after intravitreal silicone injection. Arch Ophthal 94, 612-615.
9. Brodrick JD (1978): Keratophaty following retinal detachment surgery. Arch Ophthal 96: 2021-2026.
10. Leaver PK, Grey HB, Garner A (1979): Silicone oil injection in the treatment of massive preretinal retraction. II. Late complications in 93 eyes. Brit J Ophthal 63: 361-367.
11. Cerulli L, Corsi A, Cedrone C, Scuderi GL (1983): Densità cellulare dell'endotelio corneale al microscopio speculare non a contatto. Clin Oc Pat Oc 3: 187-190.

Basic and advanced vitreous surgery
G.W. Blankenship, M. Stirpe, M. Gonvers, S. Binder (eds.)
Fidia Research Series, vol. II,
Liviana Press, Padova © 1986

VITRECTOMY AND SILICONE OIL INFUSION: PATTERN OF OCULAR HYDRODYNAMICS

M.G. Bucci

Fondazione Oftalmologica 'G.B. Bietti', Piazza Sassari, 5, Roma

In many cases vitrectomy allows to resolve very severe clinical conditions with success. However in some cases vitrectomy alone is not sufficient to prevent complications or relapse.

The introduction into the vitreous chamber of some appropriate substances, as an internal tamponade, becomes advisable.

Silicone oil represents a very effective means to be used in such a procedure even if, after a variable interval of time from the infusion, it must be removed.

However, before its removal, one must be sure that any proliferative process of vitreo-retinal membranes is blocked.

Vitrectomy with the introduction of silicone oil is responsible for significant hydrodynamic changes that depend on the type of disease and may condition the postoperative evolution after silicone oil removal.

The purpose of the present study was to investigate the ocular hydrodynamic conditions of eyes operated by vitrectomy with silicone oil infusion.

METHODS

Twenty-nine patients operated by vitrectomy with silicone oil infusion by M. Stirpe were examined. The eyes were effected by:
A: Retinal detachment (R.D.) with giant breaks (4).
B: Haemovitreous with relapsing haemorrhages after vitrectomy (6).
C: Diabetic retinopathy (5).
D: R.D. with vitreo-retinal proliferations (14).

At various time intervals (1-3-6-12-24 months) the following parameters were checked:
— Ocular pressure (Goldmann aplanation tonometer) in mm Hg.

— Aqueous humour inflow (Bucci's Cup-Tonograph) expressed in mm^3/m'.
— Coefficient of aqueous outflow (Computerized Tonography) expressed in mm^3/m'/mm Hg.

Since tonography (Bucci, 1981) can investigate ocular hydrodynamics when the ocular pressure is not inferior to 12-13 mm Hg, in many cases characterized by marked hypotension, it was necessary to use cup tonography.

The technique, previously described in detail (Bucci, 1967), evaluates and graphically records the progressive increase of ocular pressure when the aqueous outflow channels (aqueous and episcleral veins) are blocked by a vacuum-cup (Fig. 1). Pressure values are transformed in the correspondent volume changes by means if the Friedenwald equation.

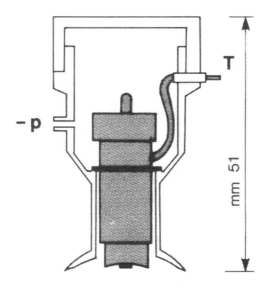

Figure 1. Schematic drawing of the Cup-Tonograph. P = Negative pressure of 50 mm Hg. T = Connection to the recorder.

RESULTS

The table reports the values of ocular pressure, coefficient of the aqueous outflow (C) and aqueous inflow (F) observed in the patients studied at the various time intervals (1-24 months).

Vitrectomy with silicone oil infusion constantly reduced the ocular pressure.

Table 1. *Group A: patients with retinal detachment, with giant breaks. Group B: Haemovitreous with relapsing haemorrhages after vitrectomy. Group C: Diabetic retinopathy. Group D: Retinal detachment with vitreo-retinal proliferation.*

	OCULAR PRESSURE (Po)						F			C		Po
Months	1	3	6	12	18	24	3	6	12	3	6	After
A	13	14	14	17	16	16	.34	.36	.68	.09	.11	12,5
Cont. eye		18					1,61			.22		
B	14,5	15	17	16	14	15	.50	.81	1,1	.11	.12	12
Cont. eye		17					1,50			.24		
C	14	14	14	13	15	15	.31	.38	.66		.10	11,5
Cont. eye		18					1,72					
D	9,6	10	11	11	13	—	.20	.13	.48			10,5
Cont. eye		16					1,83					
M	12,8	13	14	14	14,5	15	.33	.42	.73	.10	.11	11,6
Cont. eye		17					1,66			.23		

F = aqueous humour inflow; C = coefficient of outflow; Cont. eye = contralateral eye; Po = ocular pressure; after = after silicone oil removal.

The extent of this decrease depends on the kind of the ocular disease before vitrectomy. The most marked hypotension has been observed in eyes with retinal detachment and vitreo-retinal proliferations, submitted to vitrectomy with silicone oil infusion. Hypotension was evident at every check.

In general, and more evidently in the latter group of patients, ocular hypotension must be ascribed to a severe reduction of aqueous flow (mean = -80%) when compared with the contralateral normal eye. On the contrary, aqueous outflow appeared significantly decreased (-43%).

In two eyes of group D in spite of persistent marked ocular hypotension, silicone oil removal after 12 and 16 months respectively, produced an eyeball ptisis. In the remaining cases, a marked hypotension persisted after silicone oil removal.

COMMENT

Literature on the ocular hydrodynamic pattern after vitrectomy with and without silicone oil infusion, is very scanty. Only few cases of ocular hypertension have been reported as complications (Leaver et al., 1979; Haut et al., 1980; Roussat and Ruellan, 1984), even if some authors (Mukai e Schepens, 1972; Ni et al., 1983) consider glaucoma the second most common complication of silicone oil injection after cataract.

It seems to occur more frequently in aphakic eyes than in phakic ones.

The main cause of secondary glaucoma in silicone oil injected eyes was found to be infiltration of the trabecula by silicone bubbles and by silicone-laden phagocytes (Rentsch, 1981).

In selecting the patients for the present study we observed three cases of hypertension having arisen after 3-6 months from surgery. They were not considered for the present study as secondary glaucoma (lens dislocated into the anterior chamber, pupillar seclusion, sub-retinal penetration of silicone oil) and were therefore useless for our hydrodynamic investigation. In these latter cases, removal of a certain amount of silicone oil was necessary to normalize the ocular pressure.

As for the pathogenetic mechanism of ocular hypotension, two hypotheses may at present be considered:

a) Stasis of the dynamics and aqueous humour turnover with subsequent qualitative changes of the aqueous itself.

b) Membranes proliferation due to cell migration at the level of the residual peripheral vitreous, pushed by silicone oil against the ciliary epithelium so that it remains covered.

The latter hypothesis seems to be the most likely one since the most severe hypotension has been observed in eyes which, before the intervention, had shown consistent proliferative processes.

CONCLUSION

It is not surprising that silicone oil injection into the vitreous chamber both in phakic and in aphakic eyes induces significant changes of ocular hydrodynamics.

However we must distinguish two different aspects of the problem, indirectly connected with one another: The first is the possibility that long-term permanence of silicone oil in the eye might produce a secondary glaucoma; the second is the risk that after silicone oil removal, a marked ocular hypotension or ptisis might occur.

The second aspect of the problem becomes important when we consider that the incidence of secondary glaucoma increases with the duration of permanence of the oil in the eye.

Ni et al. (1983) were able to detect silicone bubbles in the trabecular meshwork of an eye in which silicone oil had been introduced twelve years previously. It therefore seems reasonable to postulate that the removal of silicone oil from the eye must take place after a not too prolonged time.

Before the removal of the oil one must be sure that any proliferative process has definitely come to an end.

According to the results of the present study it seems important to evaluate another parameter, that is ocular hydrodynamics.

In fact marked and prolonged hypotension after the removal of the oil may be responsible for many complications such as eyeball atrophy.

Before the removal of the silicone oil it is necessary that recovery of the normal ocular hydrodynamic conditions has taken place.

This can be evaluated by simply measuring ocular pressure, but much more significantly by controlling the amount of the aqueous humour inflow.

REFERENCES

1. Bucci MG (1967): Tecnica per la registrazione continua della produzione di umore acqueo. Boll Ocul 46: 359-376.
2. Bucci MG (1981): Computerized tonography: technique and first result. Glaucoma 3: 181-186.

3. Haut J, Ullern M, Chermet M, Effenterre G (1980): Complications of ocular injection of silicone combined with vitrectomy. Ophthalmologica 180: 25-35.
4. Leaver PK, Grey RHB, Garner A (1979): Silicone oil injection in the treatment of massive pre-retinal retraction: late complications in 93 eyes. Brit J Ophthal 63: 361-367.
5. Machemer R (1972): A new concept for vitreous surgery. Surgical technique and complications. Am J Ophth 74: 1022-1028.
6. Mukai N, Lee PF, Schepens CL (1972): Intravitreous injection of silicone: An experimental study: II. Histochemistry and electron microscopy. Ann Ophthalmol 4: 273-278.
7. Ni C, Wang WJ, Albert DM, Schepens CL (1983): Intravitreous silicone injection Histopathologic findings in a human eye after 12 years. Arch Ophthal 101: 1399-1401.
8. Rentsch FJ (1981): Electromicroscopical aspects of acid compartments of the ground substance and of collagen in different cases of intravitreal tissue proliferation. Dev Ophthalmol 2: 385-395.
9. Roussat B, Ruellan YM (1984): Traitement du dècollement de retine par vitrectomie et injection d'huile de silicone. JFr Ophthalmol 7: 11-18.

Basic and advanced vitreous surgery
G.W. Blankenship, M. Stirpe, M. Gonvers, S. Binder (eds.)
Fidia Research Series, vol. II,
Liviana Press, Padova © 1986

INTRAOCULAR SILICONE OIL: AN EXPERIMENTAL STUDY

M. Gonvers, M.D.

Hôpital Ophtalmologique, Lausanne

The intraocular injection of silicone oil has not only been one of the most controversial subjects in ophthalmology, but also one where passion actually won over scientific objectivity. It is striking to notice the lack of scientific rigor which characterizes publications made in the past and it seems today that polemics were a greater goal than scientific proofs. As example, in one experimental study (1) retinal toxicity to silicone oil is demonstrated as existing already a few hours after the intraocular injection. However, the described lesions look much more like traumatic lesions than retinal infiltration by silicone, and when reading carefully the experimental protocol, one realizes that vitreous was aspirated with a regular syringe. No comment has to be made on the consequences on the retina of such an aspiration. In other studies it is extrapolated from the observation of vacuoles in the retina that silicone oil had invaded the retinal layers, which was hastily considered as proof of silicone retinopathy.

Opposing these experimental studies which aimed at condemning intraocular use of silicone oil in the United States, good clinical results were described by more and more European surgeons who followed or modified Scott's technique who, himself, had adopted Cibis' idea.

It became the general feeling that new experimental works were necessary. Thus a Californian team headed by Stephen Ryan recently conducted an experimental study which seemed to demonstrate that, contrary to all other previous experiments, silicone oil had no toxic effect on the rabbit retina (2).

This conclusion seemed such an important argument in the plea for silicone oil that we decided to repeat the experimentation with minor modifications.

Our own study, however, gave us subtle conclusions or even results totally in contradiction with those of the Californian team. For this reason, we will complete the number of our cases and make a statistical analysis of the retinal lesions that could be related to silicone oil toxicity. Consequently, the results which are presented here are still incomplete and must be accepted with some prudence.

MATERIAL AND METHODS

Out of the 30 pigmented rabbits which were used, 10 went through the whole study. These 10 rabbits were vitrectomized in both eyes. One eye was kept as a control, the other one had an intraocular silicone oil injection. The lens was left in place. The vitreous cavity was filled one half to two thirds with silicone oil. The animals were killed after six weeks. This period of time was chosen on purpose, as we usually remove the silicone in our human patients one and a half month after its injection. To avoid any artifact which cannot be avoided when the rabbit retina is not immediatly fixated, the animals were perfused in vivo, glutaraldehyde being injected in the heart of the rabbit.

Electron microscopic examination of the retina of both the silicone and the control eyes was performed. Samples of superior and inferior retina were examined so that two different types of samples were obtained in the silicone group: those — the superior ones — where silicone oil was in contact with the retina, and those — the inferior ones — where the silicone bubble did not touch the retina.

RESULTS

The electronmicroscopy showed that the control retina, whatever the level the sample was taken at, was in most cases normal or presented only minor changes such as some vacuoles in the internal layer of the retina, vacuoles which are considered as artifacts by specialists of the rabbit eye. It was then observed that the inferior retinas of the eyes which were injected with silicone oil were practically as normal as the control eyes. On the other hand, in many cases, where the superior retina was in contact with the silicone, it presented some specific lesions. These were present in most of the eyes but in various degrees. The lesions were encountered essentially in the outer nuclear layer and in the outer plexiform layer. In the outer nuclear layer, an excessive number of picnotic photoreceptors were observed. The outer plexiform layer had lost most of its normal components and looked much thinner than usual.

CONCLUSIONS

Our temporary conclusion seems to be in favor of a silicone retinopathy which appears already evident after six weeks. The retinal lesions are not marked and perhaps do not show any clinical evidence. We do not know if it is a chemical toxicity or if we come up against a physical phenomenon such as a modification of metabolic changes at the surface of the retina. As yet, we do not know if this retinopathy is progressive or not, nor do we know if it is reversible when silicone is removed. We do not have a good explanation for the difference between our study and that of the Californian team. However, we think there may be a difference in the technique of the vitrectomy which could be an important factor, since a layer of vitreous left at the surface of the retina could protect the retina from silicone contact.

Another explanation could be a difference in the quality of the silicone oil, ours not being as pure. Finally, we do not know exactly where the pieces of retina which were examined by the American team were taken, did the authors examine the superior retina in contact with silicone oil, or only the mid or inferior retina which is less or not touched at all by the silicone bubble?

We have not yet proved the existence of silicone retinopathy. However, we think that a low-grade toxicity of silicone with regards to the retina exists.

REFERENCES

1. Mukai N, Lee PF, and Schepens CL (1972): Intravitreous injection of silicone: an experimental study. Ann. Ophth. 4:273-287.
2. Ober RD, Blanks JC, Ogden TE, Pickford M Minckler DS and Ryan SJ (1983): Experimental retinal tolerance to liquid silicone. Retina 3:77-85.

Basic and advanced vitreous surgery
G.W. Blankenship, M. Stirpe, M. Gonvers, S. Binder (eds.)
Fidia Research Series, vol. II,
Liviana Press, Padova © 1986

INHIBITION OF EXPERIMENTAL INTRAOCULAR PROLIFERATION AND RETINAL DETACHMENT BY VARIOUS DRUGS

Susanne Binder, Christian Skorpik, Panayote Paroussis, Rupe Menapace

First University Eye Clinic, Vienna, Austria

Animal models have been developed to study intraocular cellular proliferation and retinal detachments, and the influence of various drugs on these processes. Experimental retinal detachments in animal models have been produced with numerous agents. Retinal detachments of rabbit eyes were produced with intravitreal blood injections by Freilich (1), and with different inflammatory agents by Landholm (2). Foulds (3), and Machemer and Norton (4) produced detachments in rabbit and monkey eyes using a combination of iatrogenic retinal holes and Hyaluronidase. Kloti (5) injected plastic beads into the central retinal artery to produce detachments, and Algvere (6) combined embolization of the central retinal artery, occlusion of the vortex veins, and injection of intravitreal Hyaluronidase to produce detachments with proliferative vitreoretinopathy (PVR).

Animal models have been extensively used to investigate intraocular cellular proliferation following injection of cells into the vitreous cavity. Mueller-Jensen (7) produced intravitreal membranes similar to those of PVR following autotransplantation of pigment epithelial cells. Machemer (8) found that both retinal pigment epithelial cells and glial cells could undergo metamorphosis and produce fibroblast-like cells with extensive intraocular proliferation. Algvere and Kock (9) produced intravitreal proliferation and detachments with autologue dermal tissue and fibroblasts. Blumenkranz (10), and Fastenberg (11) used different cells to produce similar results. Sugita (12) used 250,000 autologue fibroblasts to produce a large percentage of traction detachments following intravitreal cellular proliferation without opacification of the media permitting visualization of this process. More recently, we have had similar findings of a high percentage of traction retinal detachments following intravitreal cellular proliferation of a similar number of homologue fibroblasts (13) (Figures 1, 2).

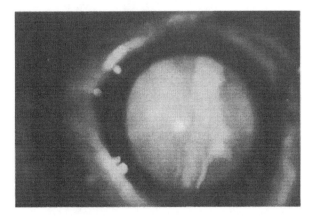

Figure 1. 48 hours after implantation of the cell suspension the fibroblasts started to form strands usually in the direction to the vascularized part of the rabbit retina - the optic disc and the medullary ray - and also against the posterior lens capsule.

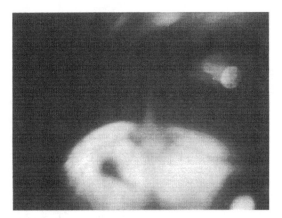

Figure 2. 1 week after implantation the strands started to pull the retina off and caused traction detachment which increased in size within the next 2 to 3 weeks.

Radioautography showed that proliferative activities started between the third and fifth day following intravitreal fibroblast injection, and reached peak activity during the second week (Figure 3).

The purpose of this report is to describe the results of several experiments which have evaluated the effects of extracapsular cataract extractions, and the use of Dexamethasonalcohol, 5-Fluorouracil in 1 and 5 mg dosages, and Cyclosporine A on the development of intravitreal cellular proliferation and traction detachments following intravitreal injections of 250,000 homologue fibroblasts.

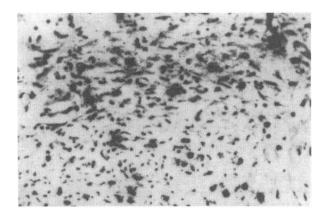

Figure 3. Radioautography showed the peak of proliferation in the second week.

EXTRACAPSULAR CATARACT EXTRACTION

Twelve rabbits had extracapsular cataract extractions with the posterior lens capsules remaining intact in 1/2 of the eyes, and having small central capsulotomies in the remaining eyes. Four weeks later, postoperative inflammation had cleared, and 250,000 fibroblasts were injected into the vitreous cavities. After four weeks the incidence of traction retinal detachments was identical occurring in 85% of both the eyes having intact posterior lens capsules, and those having central posterior lens capsulotomies.

An additional 10 rabbits had pars plana lensectomies combined with vitrectomies one week following preparation of an artificial ora serrata with peripheral retinal transcleral cryopexy. Four weeks following pars plana lensectomy-vitrectomy, the postoperative inflammation had cleared, and 250,000 fibroblasts were injected into the vitreous cavities. Within one week of the intravitreal fibroblast injection, 90% of the eyes had intravitreal cellular proliferation with retinal detachments complicated with PVR, with many also developing iris neovascularization (Figure 4).

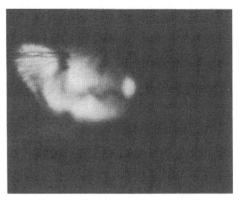

Figure 4. In the lensectomized and vitrectomized rabbit eyes the development of traction detachment was much quicker than in the unoperated eyes.

DEXAMETHASONALCOHOL

Twenty rabbit eyes received a single intravitreal injection of 1 mg of Dexamethasonalcohol in 0,1 ml NaCl simultaneously with the injection of 250,000 fibroblasts. Sixteen rabbit eyes served as controls and received 0.1 ml NaCl injection instead of the Dexamethasonalcohol. Four weeks later, traction retinal detachments occurred in only 6% of the eyes receiving Dexamethasonalcohol, but in 55% of the control eyes which had only received the NaCl injection (P < 0.01, χ^2 test) (Figure 5).

A G E N T	Dose	PVR-rate	
Control	0	85 ± 10 %	
Dexamethasone	1 mg intravitreal	12 %	(1981)
5 - Fluoruracil	1 mg intravitreal	30%	(1982)
	5 mg	85%	
Cyclosporine A	12.5 mg/kg oral	60%	(1983)

Figure 5. Number of traction detachments and PVR with various drugs after 4 to 12 weeks of observation.

Eight weeks following the injection, there was a gradual regression of the vitreous cavity membranes with the vitreous strands appearing thinner and elongated, producing a clinical impression that the active proliferative process had been completed.

Twelve weeks following fibroblast injection, there was no additional cellular proliferation, and histologic examinations failed to show any retinal damage outside the areas involved (13).

5-FLUOROURACIL

5-Fluorouracil is a cytostatic agent which interferes with DNA synthesis, and both 1 and 5 mg doses were evaluated. Both eyes of 10 rabbits received a 1 mg intravitreal injection of 5-Fluorouracil at the time 250,000 fibroblasts were injected into the vitreous cavity, and both eyes of 10 rabbits received 5 mg of 5-Fluorouracil at the time a similar injection of fibroblasts was made. Sixteen rabbit eyes were used as controls with 0.1 ml NaCl being injected into the vitreous cavity simultaneously with the intravitreal injection of 250,000 fibroblasts. Four weeks later, the incidence of traction detachments was significantly reduced to only 30% (6/20) of the eyes receiving 1 mg intravitreal 5-Fluorouracil compared with 75% (12/16) of the control eyes (P = 0.5, χ^2 test) (Figure 5).

The eyes that received 5 mg of intravitreal 5-Fluorouracil deteriorated rapidly. During the first day following injection, the retinal vessels were markedly narrowed with frequent occlusions associated with marked retinal edema and intraretinal flame-shaped hemorrhages presenting a clinical picture of venous thrombosis. Pigmented cells rapidly accumulated around the fibroblasts clouds with rapid cellular proliferation producing thick vitreous membranes and extensive and highly elevated traction retinal detachments. Further deterioration occurred with the development of huge retinal holes producing a combination of traction and rhegmatogenous retinal detachments in 85% (17/20) of the eyes. Light and electron microscopic examinations found degranulation and migration of pigment epithelial cells, incipient degradation of axons and myelin sheaths, migration of glial cells, and prominent edema of the inner retinal layers with extensive retinal damage (14).

CYCLOSPORINE A

The function of Cyclosporine A is not completely understood, but has its main effect on inhibition of the t-leucocytes, and acts on macrophages in chronic inflammatory conditions. It is primarily used in preventing organ rejection following kidney transplantation, to prevent corneal graft reactions, and occasionally in chronic cases of uveitis and sympathetic ophthalmia. We decided to test Cyclosporine A because of the possible effect on a potential autoimmune factor in eyes which develop PVR following perforating injuries (15,16).

When Cyclosporine A is injected intravitreally, its oily solution causes a severe foreign body reaction with total retinal detachment. Thus, 10 rabbits were given 12.5 mg Cyclosporine A per kg body weight orally daily starting two days before and continuing five weeks following an intravitreal injection of 250,000 fibroblasts. Blood levels were obtained at regular intervals to avoid toxicity and to maintain effective blood levels. Six weeks following injection of the fibroblasts, 61% of the treated rabbits had developed traction retinal detachments. A similar group of untreated control rabbits had a 90% incidence of retinal detachment. Histologic examinations failed to demonstrate any retinal or vascular toxicity in the treated rabbits (Figure 5).

DISCUSSION

Our results in producing traction detachments in a large number of rabbit eyes (75-95%) with the injection of 250,000 homologue fibroblasts into the vitreous cavity are similar to others previously published (9, 17, 18). This animal model provides an excellent means for evaluating the process of intravitreal cellular proliferation and secondary traction retinal detachments, and the potential therapeutic value of various drugs.

Tano (17) demonstrated that an intravitreal injection of 1 mg Dexamethasonalcohol significantly reduced the incidence of traction detachments in this animal model. Our results were essentially identical to Tano's, but the follow-up period was extended to 12 weeks during which there was no reactivation of the proliferating process. Blumenkranz (10) was able to reduce the incidence of traction detachments from 73%

to 31% with an intravitreal injection of 1 mg of 5-Fluorouracil. Our experiments found very similar results with a reduction from 75% to 30% with the use of this medication. However, when the dosage was increased to 5 mg of 5-Fluorouracil there was rapid and severe retinal damage with vascular occlusions, extensive intravitreal cellular proliferation forming dense vitreal membranes producing extensive traction detachments and subsequent large retinal holes.

The possible autoimmune origin of PVR proposed by Bonnet and Remy (15) is very intriging, and was tested in our experiment using oral Cyclosporine A with a dosage of 12.5 mg per kg body weight. This resulted in a decrease in the incidence of traction detachments from 90% in the untreated control animals to 61% of those receiving the Cyclosporine A. While this was a strong indication that the use of Cyclosporine A was beneficial, the difference did not reach statistical significance. Further experience with this drug will be necessary to determine its true value in preventing and/or treating PVR.

The rate and extent of PVR development, and the effects of various drugs in experimental animals and following pars plana lensectomy and vitrectomy may be significantly different than in the human eye which has not had pars plana lensectomy and vitrectomy. The clearance rate with which these drugs leave the eye may be considerably more rapid following pars plana lensectomy and vitrectomy, and may necessitate repeated applications to maintain therapeutic levels. The frequent use of intraocular tamponades such as silicone oil and gases significantly increase the concentration of the drugs compared to that obtained when the drugs are injected into a vitreous or fluid filled eye. These increased drug concentrations may result in retinal damage even when relatively low doses are used. Further evaluations are needed to test the efficacy and tolerability of these drugs in human eyes.

At this time, we believe that the multiple therapeutic qualities of Cortisone may offer the best form of treating the multifocal origins of PVR. Our animal experiments also suggest that the use of subconjunctival 5-Fluorouracil in human eyes would be safer in avoiding the retinal complications of intravitreal injections which exceed 1 mg doses.

CONCLUSIONS

Proliferative vitreoretinopathy (PVR) and secondary traction retinal detachments were produced in 75 to 95% of rabbit eyes within two to four weeks of injection of 250,000 homologue fibroblasts. The incidence of intravitreal cellular proliferation and traction retinal detachment was not influenced by extracapsular cataract extractions, but the rate with which these complications developed occurred much more quickly with eyes having pars plana lensectomy with vitrectomy.

A single intravitreal injection of 1 mg Dexamethasonalcohol at the time of intravitreal fibroblast injection significantly reduces the incidence of traction retinal detachments, and the intravitreal proliferative process did not reoccur during a three month follow-up observation. Retinal damage did not occur with this medication at this dosage.

The incidence of traction retinal detachments was significantly reduced from 75% to 30% with the injection of 1 mg of 5-Fluorouracil at the time of fibroblast injection.

However, when 5 mg of 5-Fluorouracil were injected there was extensive vascular and retinal damage combined with marked intravitreal cellular proliferation which produced extensive vitreal membranes and combined traction and rhegmatogenous detachments. Histologically, there was severe disruption of the retinal axons with loss of microtubular structure and mitochondria combined with generalized intra and extracellular edema. Similar but much less extensive changes were observed in those eyes receiving 1 mg of 5-Fluorouracil.

Oral Cyclosporine A appeared to reduce the instance of traction detachments from 90% of the untreated control eyes to 60% of these receiving Cyclosporine A during a four week follow-up period. Retinal changes were not observed in the animals receiving oral Cyclosporine A.

REFERENCES

1. Freilich DB, Lee DF, Freeman HM (1966): Experimental retinal detachment. Arch Ophthal; 76:393.
2. Landholm WM, Watzke RC (1965): Experimental retinal detachment with a sulphated polysaccharide. Invest Ophthal; 4:42.
3. Foulds WS (1963): Experimental retinal detachments. Trans Ophthal Soc UK: 83:153.
4. Machemer R, Norton EWD (1976): Experimental retinal detachment in the owl monkey. 1. Methods of production and clinical picture. Amer J Ophthalmol 66:3-388.
5. Kloti R (1967): Experimental occlusion of retinal and ciliary vessels in the owl monkeys. 1. Technique and clinical observation of selective embolism of the central retinal artery system. Exp Eye Res. 6:393.
6. Algvere P (1976): Retinal detachment and pathology following experimental embolization of choroid and retinal circulation. Av Graefes Arch Klin Exp Ophthal 201:123.
7. Muller-Jensen K, Mandelcorn MS (1975): Membrane formation by autotransplanted retinal pigment epithelium (RPE). Mod Probl Ophthal Vol 15:22, Basel: S Karger.
8. Machemer R, Laqua R (1975): Pigment epithelium proliferation in retinal detachment (massive periretinal proliferation). Amer J Ophthalmol 80:1.
9. Algvere P, Kock E (1976): Experimental fibroplasia in the rabbit vitreous. Retinal detachment induced by autologous fibroblasts. Av Grafes Arch Klin Exp Ophthal 99:115.
10. Blumenkranz M, Ophir A, Claflin AJ, Hajek A (1982): Fluorouracil for the treatment of massive periretinal proliferation. Am J Ophthalmol 94:458.
11. Fastenberg D, Diddie K, Sorgente N, Ryan S (1982): A comparison of different cellular in an experimental model of massive periretinal proliferation. Am J Ophthalmol 93:559.
12. Sugita G, Tano Y, Machemer R (1980): Intravitreal autotransplantation of fibroblasts. Amer J Ophthalmol 89:121.
13. Binder S (1981): Gibt es eine medikamentose Alternative in der Behandlung der massiven periretinalen Proliferation? Klin Mb, Augenheik 179:483.
14. Kulnig W, Binder S, Riss B, Skorpik C (1984): Inhibition of experimental intraocular proliferation with intravitreous 5-Fluorouracil. Ophthalmologica, Basel 88:248.
15. Bonnet M, Remy C (1982): Auto-immunity against the retina and massive vitreoretinal retraction. Presented during the XIII meeting of the Jules Gonin Club, Cordoba, March 29.
16. Remy C (1981): Recherche de Pautoimmunité contre la retine dans les decollements retinieus idiopathiques. Etude de 50 cas J Fr Ophthalmol Vol 4, 3:213.
17. Tano Y, Sugita G, Atrams G, Machemer R (1980): Inhibition of intraocular proliferations with intravitreal corticosteroids. Am J Ophthalmol 89:131.
18. Tano Y, Chandler E, Machemer R (1980): Treatment of intraocular proliferation with intravitreal injection of Triamcinolol acetonide. Amer J Ophthalmol 90:810.

Basic and advanced vitreous surgery
G.W. Blankenship, M. Stirpe, M. Gonvers, S. Binder (eds.)
Fidia Research Series, vol. II,
Liviana Press, Padova © 1986

OCULAR EFFECTS AND CLEARANCE OF INTRAVITREAL 5-FLUOROURACIL

George W. Blankenship, M. D., Beth R. Friedland, M. D. and Mark S. Blumenkranz, M. D.

The Bascom Palmer Eye Institute
University of Miami School of Medicine, Miami, Florida

Proliferative vitreoretinopathy (PVR) (1) continues to be a major cause of recurrent retinal detachments following scleral buckling procedures. Improved pars plana vitrectomy techniques (2) combined with intravitreal tamponades (3, 4) now permit successful reattachment of many of these cases. Recent studies have found that 5-Fluorouracil (5-FU) markedly reduces the proliferative activity of the fibroblasts and retinal pigment epithelial cells which result in recurrent retinal detachment.

During the past year, eyes with substantial inflammation following pars plana vitrectomy have been given 10 mg of intravitreal 5-FU with subsequent air/fluid exchanges. An analysis of these cases indicates that the eyes will tolerate this level of 5-FU, and that good therapeutic levels are maintained for 48 hours.

MATERIALS AND METHODS

During 1983, 20 eyes received 10 mg of intravitreal 5-FU within a few days of pars plana vitrectomy to try and minimize postvitrectomy intraocular inflammation. Ten of the eyes had air-vitreous cavity fluid exchanges 24 hours following the 5-FU injection, and the remaining 10 eyes had a similar exchange 48 hours following the injection. The vitreous cavity fluid specimens were analyzed for levels of 5-FU by a method previously described. Briefly, the drug was extracted from intraocular fluid specimens in N-propanol 1 diethyl ether, transferred to neutral diphasic phosphate buffer and levels determined by measurement of peak height at 7 minutes at 254 nm on a reverse phase C-18 HPLC column (8). Six months following vitrectomy and 5-FU injection, follow-up information was available on 15 of the 20 cases, with the remaining 5 cases being lost to follow-up.

Information regarding the best corrected visual functions, and ophthalmic findings with slit lamp microscopy, gonioscopy, fundus contact lenses, indirect ophthalmoscopy, and bright flash electroretinography was recorded at the preoperative and the 6 month follow-up examinations. Data regarding the operative procedures, complications, and findings were also recorded. All of the information was computerized.

RESULTS

The most frequent indication for pars plana vitrectomy for the 15 cases with 6 month follow-up was diabetic traction macular detachment for 7 cases, non-clearing diabetic vitreous hemorrhage for 3 cases, 2 cases had giant retinal tears with rolled over retinal detachments, and 1 case each had a diabetic vitreous hemorrhage and neovascular glaucoma, a combined diabetic traction and rhegmatogenous retinal detachment, and a retinal tear with combined vitreous hemorrhage and retinal detachment.

The preoperative and 6 month postoperative visual acuities are shown in Table 1 with 2 of the cases having essentially normal vision 6 months after vitrectomy and 5-FU injection, and an additional 5 having 6/60 or better vision. Of the 3 eyes with no light perception at the 6 month examination, 2 had neovascular glaucoma with irreparable retinal detachments, and the remaining case had become phthisical with irreparable retinal detachment.

There was a very wide range of 5-FU concentrations in the vitreous cavity fluid specimens obtained 24 and 48 hours after injecting 10 mg of 5-FU as shown in Table 2.

Fourteen of the eyes were phakic following vitrectomy and 5-FU injection, and the remaining 6 eyes were aphakic. Table 3 shows the average and range of vitreous 5-FU concentrations for both the phakic and aphakic eyes at 24 and 48 hours following

Table 1. *Intravitreal 5 FU visual acuities*

	Preop	6 mths
6/6 - 6/12		2
6/15 - 6/60	1	5
6/90 - 1/60	8	4
H.M. - L.P.	6	1
N.L.P.		3

Table 2. *5 FU intravitreal concentrations following 10mg intravitreal injection*

	Average	Range
24 hours	31μg	90 - 1.0
48 hours	2μg	4 - 0.1

5-FU injection. Surprisingly, the aphakic eyes had a higher average concentration 24 hours after injection, but 48 hours after injection the levels were slightly higher in the phakic eyes with wide ranges of levels in all groups. This disparity between the phakic and aphakic eyes may be partially explained as follows.

Many of the vitreous cavities were partially filled with gas bubbles at the time of 5-FU injections, and the average concentrations are shown in Table 4 with the part of the vitreous cavity being filled with gas. As expected the highest concentrations were in eyes with the largest intraocular gas bubbles.

Both of the 2 eyes with 6 months 6/6 to 6/12 visual acuity were aphakic without vitreous cavity gas bubbles at the time of 5-FU injection. Twenty-four hours following injection, the vitreous fluid 5-FU concentrations were 60 micrograms, and 54 micrograms.

Anatomically 11 of the 15 eyes with 6 month follow-up maintained clear corneas and anterior chambers with 4 of the 12 diabetic cases developing extensive iris neovascularization associated with retinal detachments. Eleven of the 15 eyes with 6 months follow-up had retained lenses of which 4 were clear, 3 had moderate lens opacities, but 4 had developed dense cataracts in association with other more serious problems such as irreparable retinal detachments.

Anterior segment opacities obscured 2 of the vitreous cavities 6 months following vitrectomy and 5-FU injection, but 11 of the 15 had clear vitreous cavities, and the remaining 2 had opaque vitreous cavities.

Of the 11 retinas that could be visualized at the 6 months examination, 10 were completely attached and 1 had a persistent inferior retinal detachment with macular

Table 3.   *5 FU intravitreal concentrations*

	Average	Range
Phakic		
24 hours (6 eyes)	27μg	90 - 1.0
48 hours (8 eyes)	2μg	4 - 0.1
Aphakic		
24 hours (4 eyes)	42μg	54 - 31.0
48 hours (2 eyes)	1μg	2 - 0.1

Table 4.   *5 FU intravitreal concentrations*

Gas	24 hrs	48hrs
None	5μg	1μg
<1/3	2μg	4μg
1/3-2/3	2μg	2μg
>2/3	31μg	2μg

involvement; however, in all probability the 4 remaining cases with obscured retinas had total retinal detachments.

Of the 11 retinas that could be visualized and were attached, 5 appeared to have normal maculas, 5 had atrophic macular changes, and 1 had cystoid macular edema.

Electroretinograms were obtained before vitrectomy, before 5-FU injection, 1 month after injection, and 6 months after 5-FU injection in most of the cases. Cases with postoperative retinal detachments, or extensive retinal treatment such as photocoagulation or cryotherapy were excluded. The 5 remaining cases had essentially identical bright flash electroretinograms 1 and 6 months following injection compared to those obtained prior to the vitrectomy procedure.

DISCUSSION

Recent laboratory findings evaluating 5-FU with fibroblast cell cultures (5) showed notable inhibition of proliferation in concentrations of less than 1 mcg per liter of 5-FU. More recent experiments with animal models (6) found that intravitreal injections of 5-FU markedly reduced the rate of traction retinal detachments following injection of intravitreal fibroblasts. These laboratory findings indicating that 5-FU may reduce the incidence of PVR are supported by the report of a 60% 6 months anatomical success rate utilizing intravitreal and subconjunctival 5-FU in conjunction with pars plana vitrectomy techniques (8).

Retinal toxicity studies of 5-FU found that a single intravitreal injection of 2.5 mg in the nonvitrectomized rabbit did not result in reproducible electroretinographic findings of permanent damage. When 5 mg of 5-FU were injected into the vitreous cavity there was a transient reduction of ERG B-wave amplitude which returned to normal at 2 weeks, but there appeared to be retinal thinning with subtle pigment epithelial derangement. Electron microscopy of the rabbit retina found no evidence of anatomical damage with the eyes receiving 1 mg of 5-FU, but unmistakable evidence of acute toxicity at levels of 5 mg of 5-FU (8). However, the average volume of the rabbit vitreous cavity is only 1.4 ml whereas the corresponding human compartment is more than twice this volume.

There were no visual or obvious retinal complications directly attributable to the use of 5-FU in the previously reported clinical trial (8). In that study a combination of subconjunctival 10 mg 5-FU and intravitreal 1 mg 5-FU were used and frequently repeated during the first few weeks following pars plana vitrectomy without visual or obvious retinal complications directly attributable to the drug. There may have been some delayed corneal epithelial healing and subsequent subcorneal epithelial scarring associated with the subconjunctivally administered 5-FU. Previous experimental studies have confirmed that 5-FU is rapidly cleared from the vitreous cavity of rabbits. The half life is 7.7 hours in normal phakic eyes, and 3.2 hours in aphakic vitrectomized eyes following a 1 mg intravitreal injection. This corresponds to levels of 7.8 micrograms/ml and 0.21 micrograms/ml for phakic and aphakic eyes respectively at 24 hours, and 2.3 micrograms/ml and 0.05 micrograms/ml at 48 hours (9).

In this study, a single injection of 10mg of 5-FU into the vitreous cavity following vitrectomy resulted in therapeutic levels of lmcg of 5-FU for at least 48 hours in this series of patients. The optimal time duration of therapeutic levels of 5-FU needed to maximally suppress proliferative activity is not known, nor is it known whether a single large intravitreal injection of 5-FU is advantageous to multiple smaller injections.

None of the cases in this study had evidence of detrimental effects of the 10mg of intravitreal 5-FU at the 6 month follow-up examination. The initial mild corneal edema was transient, clearing within 2 weeks of the injection without permanent damage. The disappointing visual and anatomical results which occurred in some cases were related to the underlying disease process rather than to the use of intravitreal 5-FU.

Future prospective and randomized studies will hopefully confirm the beneficial effects of 5-FU, and indicate the optimal strength, route, and frequency of injections.

REFERENCES

1. The Retina Society Terminology Committee (1983): The classification of retinal detachment with proliferative vitreoretinopathy. Opthalmology, 90:121-125.
2. Ratner CM, Michels RG, Auer C, Rice TA (1983): Pars plana vitrectomy for complicated retinal detachments. Opthalmology, 90-1323-1327.
3. Noton EWD (1973): Intraocular gas in the management of selected retinal detachments. Trans Am Acad Opthalmol Otolaryngol, 77:Op-85-98.
4. Grey RHB, Leaver PK (1979): Silicone oil in the treatment of massive preretinal retraction: 1. Results in 105 Eyes. BrJ Opthalmology, 63-555-60.
5. Friedland B, Blumenkranz MS, Jarus G, Pressman (1984): A new chromatographic technique for the determination of intraocular Fluorouracil (5-FU) - Submitted for publication.
6. Blumenkranz MS, Claflin A, Hajek AS (1984): Selection of therapeutic agent for intraocular proliferative disease cell culture evaluation. Arch Opthalmol, 102:598-604.
7. Blumenkranz MS, Ophir A, Claflin AJ, Hajek A (1982): Fluorouracil for the treatment of massive periretinal proliferation. Am J Opthalmol, 94:458-467.
8. Blumerkranz M, Hernandez E, Ophir A, Norton EWD (1984): 5-Fluorouracil: New applications in complicated retinal detachment for an established antimetabolite. Ophthalmology, 91:122-129.
9. Jarus G, Blumerkranz M, Hernandez E, Sussi N (1984): Clearance of intravitreal Fluorouracil: normal and aphakic vitrectomized eyes. In press, Opthalmology.